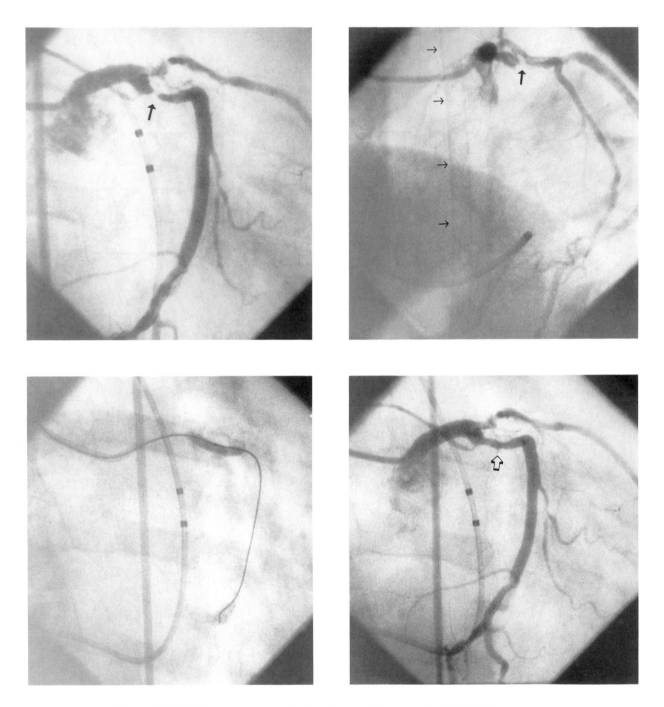

Top: *(Left) Left coronary artery, RAO projection. Severe proximal LCX lesion (arrow). (Right) Left coronary artery, LAO projection. Severe LCX lesion (large arrow). Note CPS venous canulla (small arrows).* **Bottom:** *(Left) Left coronary artery, RAO projection. Balloon inflation. (Right) Left coronary artery, RAO projection. Postangioplasty (arrow).*

CORONARY ANGIOPLASTY
— SECOND EDITION —

DAVID A. CLARK, M.D.

Physician Specialist
Division of Cardiology
Stanford University
School of Medicine
Stanford, California

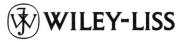

WILEY-LISS

A JOHN WILEY & SONS, INC., PUBLICATION
New York • Chichester • Brisbane • Toronto • Singapore

Address all Inquiries to the Publisher
Wiley-Liss, Inc., 41 East 11th Street, New York, NY 10003

Copyright © 1991 Wiley-Liss, Inc.

Printed in United States of America

While the authors, editors, and publisher believe that drug selection and dosage and the specifications and usage of equipment and devices, as set forth in this book, are in accord with current recommendations and practice at the time of publication, they accept no legal responsibility for any errors or omissions, and make no warranty, express or implied, with respect to material contained herein. In view of ongoing research, equipment modifications, changes in governmental regulations and the constant flow of information relating to drug therapy, drug reactions and the use of equipment and devices, the reader is urged to review and evaluate the information provided in the package insert or instructions for each drug, piece of equipment or device for, among other things, any changes in the instructions or indications of dosage or usage and for added warnings and precautions.

Library of Congress Cataloging-in-Publication Data

Clark, David A. (David Allen), 1939–
    Coronary angioplasty / David A. Clark. — 2nd ed.
      p.   cm.
    Includes bibliographical references.
    Includes index.
    ISBN 0-471-56074-X
    1. Transluminal angioplasty.   2. Coronary heart disease—Surgery.
I. Title.
    [DNLM: 1. Angioplasty, Transluminal. 2. Coronary Disease—
therapy. WG 300 C592c]
RD598.6.C57 1991
617.4'12—dc20
DNLM/DLC
for Library of Congress   90-13100
                                                    CIP

Cover: *(Left panel) Left coronary artery, preangioplasty. (Right panel) Left coronary artery, postsangioplasty.*

To CVC, NWC, Terice, Susan, and Lindsay
and
to the memory of Monroe

CONTENTS

PREFACE

The second edition of *Coronary Angioplasty* is designed to deal primarily with the practical aspects of coronary angioplasty as it exists today. There are several other excellent books available (see Bibliography) that document the history of angioplasty and the development of the technique. They also contain detailed discussions of the theories of the mechanism and pathology involved in the angioplasty process. Since the publication of the first edition of *Coronary Angioplasty,* the field has exploded from a publication standpoint, and selected references are presented in the Bibliography to provide more detailed reading for those interested. The goal of this book is again to present a practical and concise volume that will emphasize the rationale for the selection (or nonselection) of patients for angioplasty as well as the strategic approach necessary in specific anatomic situations to perform a safe and successful procedure.

To achieve this goal, the liberal use of case presentations will be employed to illustrate points of strategy and equipment selection. The addition of a teaching video tape with this second edition greatly enhances the selected case presentations, and the audio comments presented on the video tape should clarify points of technique that were difficult to demonstrate with the still photographs used in the first edition. It is hoped that this book will serve not only as a useful guide for the strategy of angioplasty for the experienced angiographer who is just beginning to learn angioplasty, but also as a reference book for experienced practitioners of angioplasty when confronted with certain strategic decisions in specific complex cases.

In the performance of a technical procedure such as angioplasty, there is no substitute for hands-on, repetitive experience in the development and maintenance of skill. The number of procedures that need to be done to become a competent practioner of angioplasty varies with the skill and expertise that the operator has developed as an angiographer. Certainly, the continued performance of a minimum of one case per week is needed to maintain technical expertise and keep abreast of the technical advances in this elegant, demanding, and rapidly developing field.

It is difficult to put into words the "touch" or finger calisthenics that are needed in performing percutaneous transluminal coronary artery angioplasty. Although attempts are made throughout this book to do just that, it should be recognized that words, pictures, and video tapes do not substitute for the actual tactile performance of maneuvers with angioplasty equipment in the laboratory.

Several chapters in this book serve as background and expand on the basic material presented. The first chapter detailing the history of angiography and angioplasty by Dr. Frank Hildner, the editor of *Catheterization and Cardiovascular Diagnosis,* is a thoughtful, witty, and unique presentation of the events that led to and made possible the field of angioplasty. This chapter expands on the marvelous lectures that Dr. Hildner has given on this subject and may also serve as a reference chapter for cardiologists to use as introductory material when presenting lectures to colleagues on the subject of angioplasty. The brilliance of Dotter, Gruentzig, Judkins, and Sones—and their enormous contributions to the field of angioplasty—should be enjoyed and understood by all angiographers. The chapter dealing with angioplasty equipment presents important groundwork for the rest of the book. It is recognized that not only will some of the comments in this chapter become outdated in years to come, but also the plethora of brands of equipment available has markedly increased since the first edition. In this book, therefore, the emphasis on equipment will be on type and style rather than on specific brand names. Comments and suggestions made in Chapter 2 (Coronary Angioplasty Equipment) are repeated elsewhere in the book, particularly in the section on selection of equipment in Chapter 4 (PTCA Strategy), but this repetition should serve only to stress the importance of equipment selection in terms of the successful and safe performance of PTCA. It is obvious that the technology and equipment of angioplasty is constantly and quickly changing. Comments in this book represent information pertaining to the most current catheter, balloon, and wire systems available.

A separate (and necessarily quite theoretical) chapter on recurrence has been included since this continues to be the "Achilles' heel" of angioplasty and is the most specific negative aspect of the procedure. In fact, when one considers that the type of "injury" produced in an artery by balloon inflation is the perfect way to produce an atherosclerotic lesion in experimental animals, the wonder of angioplasty is *not* that 25–30% of cases recur, but that 70–75% of patients do not experience recurrence. Over the past several years, the literature has been filled with articles dealing with the possible etiology, pathology, and immunology of recurrence, and a detailed reference list is included in the Bibliography of this book. The problems of recurrence and its treatment are dealt with in other chapters of the book, but I felt that a specific chapter emphasizing the practical aspects of treatment of recurrence was appropriate.

Drs. Geoffrey Hartzler and Joel Kahn have contributed an outstanding chapter detailing their experience with direct coronary angioplasty in the setting of an acute or evolving myocardial infarction. This subject is currently one of the most exciting and debated areas of angioplasty, and they have presented their successful strategy in dealing with a large series of patients.

Comments emphasizing patient-care aspects of PTCA have been prepared by Ms. Nonie Jenkins and Linda Kotrba-Ottoboni. This chapter presents recommendations about pre- and postangioplasty care of patients and should provide insight into the pre- and postprocedural problems and solutions that should make angioplasty an overall satisfactory experience for patients, their families, and their physicians.

The case presentations in Appendix I serve as a monograph within the book. The second edition is enhanced by the addition of a teaching video tape whose case numbers correspond to the case numbers in the book. Each case has been selected to illustrate particular strategic or technical aspects of angioplasty, and in that spirit, the clinical statements are very succinct. The "meat" of this section is in the discussion of the equipment selected and the strategy utilized in the approach to the case. The angiographic illustrations in the book for each case demonstrate the anatomy described and also give the reader some sense of motion and participation in the procedure. This allows the book to be used as a separate entity without having the capability of video replay immediately available. Specific cases are cited by number

throughout the book to illustrate various points made in the text, but perusal of Appendix I as an entity should also prove instructive to the reader.

The Bibliography and Suggested Readings section at the end of the book serves two purposes: First, references annotated in the text by number can be identified in this section by specific chapter and subject heading and the number that corresponds to it in the text. Second, since each chapter encompasses a particular topic, the articles referenced in the text as well as other suggested reading material are grouped by topic so that the reader can locate additional articles or texts dealing with a given subject.

As I did in the preface to the first edition, I would like to acknowledge two gentlemen with whom I had personal relationships that strongly directed my interest to the field of angiography and angioplasty. F. Mason Sones, Jr., the father of coronary angiography, was a wonderful physician, and my long relationship with him confirmed that his efforts were directed toward one goal, namely, the pursuit of excellence in angiography for the benefit of the patient. Dr. Melvin Judkins, while initially often seemingly at odds with Dr. Sones, in later years joined with Dr. Sones to pursue their goal to elevate the art of angiography to the highest possible level for the benefit of the patient. In that spirit, they co-founded The Society for Cardiac Angiography, now called The Society for Cardiac Angiography and Interventions. I strongly believe that this society is the most significant professional society to which angiographers and interventional cardiologists can belong. Now 14 years old, the society is composed of over 700 dedicated physicians who essentially are those physicians primarily performing quality angiography in the world and whose sense of dedication and pursuit of excellence has led them to join the society. I firmly believe that The Society for Cardiac Angiography and Interventions is a most significant contributor to excellence in the field, and I would encourage physicians in this specialty to strongly consider participation in the society's work.

Dr. Andreas Gruentzig is regarded as the true pioneer in the field of coronary angioplasty. Attendance at his early courses in Zurich was an exhilarating experience and one that had a profound influence on the life of anyone who journeyed to Switzerland to observe his dramatic work. Dr. Gruentzig often said that "angioplasty will change your life," and it is perhaps only after one becomes fully engrossed and involved with PTCA that the full impact of these words is understood. One of the most remarkable aspects of angioplasty is that Dr. Gruentzig shared, gave away, if you will, the technique by his demonstration courses and his teaching of others.

The deaths of Judkins, Sones, Gruentzig, as well as pioneer Charles Dotter in the year 1985 continue to provide bittersweet memories. Their conviction that patient care is a virtue that stands above all others should be the initial and lasting beacon to guide the practitioner of angioplasty.

The compilation of a teaching video tape for this second edition of *Coronary Angioplasty* is the natural use of a medium that lends itself well to teaching such procedures. Demonstration courses have provided the educational basis and exciting inspiration for practitioners beginning and continuing angioplasty since the late 1970s. The elegant courses, on video tape, produced by Dr. Geoffrey Hartzler and his colleagues at the Mid-America Heart Institute have been outstanding not only for their quality of teaching, but also for the quality of the video reproductions. It was at one of these meetings that I met David Liskin, who is the productional genius behind the video taping of Dr. Hartzler's courses. I greatly appreciate his collaboration with me on the video tape used with this book and would like to acknowledge his most significant contributions. I would also like to express my gratitude to Mr. Liskin and his organization for their help in leading me through the unique experience of transferring 35 mm cineangiograms to ¾ inch video tapes and the subsequent narration and editing that resulted in the final product. In particular, Mary Pluth and James Miller have been most helpful, encouraging, and patient with me during the video production process.

I would also like to recognize several individuals who assisted me tremendously in the preparation of this book: Mrs. Robyn Hillis, my long-time and faithful associate, for her technical skills as well as for her encouragement during this process of revising the book; the staff of Wiley-Liss, for their faith in producing a second edition and for their encouragement and help during this venture; and the cath lab crew and nursing staff at Stanford, Salinas, and Good Samaritan Hospital, without whom, as every angiographer knows, none of this would be possible. Last, but certainly not least, I want to thank my lovely wife Terice, my beautiful daughters Susan and Lindsay, and my old pal Duke for their encouragement and support during my period of authorship.

I would like to acknowledge the contributions to the materials, data, statistics, and illustrations made by the San Francisco Heart Institute and the San Francisco-Peninsula Cardiovascular Medical Group, Inc., during my tenure as director of Cardiovascular Intervention with them. I would also like to acknowledge the contributions and comradery of my colleagues at Stanford, particularly Drs. Tim Fischell, Michael Stadius, Ed Alderman, John Schroeder, and Norman Shumway, whose collegial help and encouragement embellish the pleasure of my practice of interventional cardiology.

David A. Clark, M.D.

ACKNOWLEDGMENTS

I wish to thank the following authors whose contributions appear in this book:

Tim A. Fischell, M.D.
Assistant Professor of Medicine
Stanford University School of Medicine
Stanford, California

Geoffrey O. Hartzler, M.D.
Consulting Cardiologist
St. Luke's Hospital
Mid-America Heart Institute
Kansas City, Missouri

Frank J. Hildner, M.D.
Editor-in-Chief
Catheterization and Cardiovascular Diagnosis
Professor of Medicine
University of Miami School of Medicine
Coral Gables, Florida

Nonie Jenkins, R.N., B.S.N.
Patient Care Coordinator
Cardiac Catheterization Laboratory
Stanford University Hospital
Stanford, California

Joel K. Kahn, M.D.
Cardiovascular Interventionalist
Michigan Heart and Vascular Institute
Ann Arbor, Michigan

Linda Kotrba-Ottoboni, R.N., M.S., C.C.R.N.
Nursing Education Coordinator
Coronary Care Cardiac Surveillance
Stanford University Hospital
Stanford, California

Michael L. Stadius, M.D.
Assistant Professor of Medicine
Stanford University School of Medicine
Stanford, California

David A. Clark, M.D.

1. A History of Cardiac Catheterization

AN OVERVIEW

In the history of medicine, few innovations have so profoundly influenced the future as has cardiac catheterization. In association with angiocardiography it has permitted investigation into the anatomy and physiology of the entire circulatory system, thereby laying the foundation for medical and surgical therapy of all cardiovascular diseases. Through invasive techniques, the effects of drugs on cardiac performance were observed, normal and abnormal values for physiologic parameters were determined, variations in anatomy were revealed, and effects of other organ function were related to the cardiovascular system. Without correlation of these invasive techniques, the results of noninvasive procedures including electrocardiography, exercise physiology, echocardiography, Doppler procedures, nuclear studies, bedside monitoring, and even physical examination could not have been developed to their current degree of excellence.

Although all of these incredible accomplishments have occurred in about 60 years, progress was slow and sporadic. After Forssman catheterized his own heart in 1929, prejudice against this type of invasion of the heart and fear of untoward consequences virtually halted all developments until the early 1940s. At this time, prompted by studies of basic cardiovascular physiology, Cournand and his co-workers began a systematic investigation into pulmonary and circulatory function using the techniques of right heart catheterization. Advances and facility with this technique came rapidly, but it was not until 1949 that Zimmerman successfully investigated catheterization of the left heart by a retrograde approach that proved reliable and relatively safe. Now that the entire heart was accessible to the exploring catheter, achievements and knowledge mounted rapidly.

Perhaps the time had come for these techniques to be discovered, but not all resulted from persistent plodding scientific research. The occurrence of fortuitous and even chance events played more than a minor role. Had not Forssman cultivated a social relationship with nurse Gerda, who volunteered to have her heart catheterized, he would not have gained access to the surgical equipment he needed, for she was custodian of the key. World War II occurred at an opportune time. Although Cournand had decided to embark on his physiologic exploration much earlier, by the time the 1940s arrived, he found a more immediate and practical reason for these investigations, namely, circulatory shock from wartime events. But the war effort also yielded technologic advances that permitted further development of invasive cardiology. Polymer chemistry produced plastics, which quickly supplanted the old rubber or nylon catheters. Metallurgy contributed alloys more suitable for human use. But all these marvelous accomplishments were relatively insignificant compared to the contribution derived from the science of electronics. Mechanical recording devices were replaced by strain gauges. X-ray tubes and generator systems became more powerful and easily controllable. But the single most important development, which set the stage for exponential future growth of invasive cardiology, was the cathode ray tube, which later was expanded into television. Up to this time, the physician would have had to accommodate his eyes to a green fluorescent screen by wearing red goggles for 15–20 min before performing fluoroscopy. Indeed, the faintly glowing image in a darkened room frequently failed to reveal even the position of the catheter. Radiation received by medical personnel was excessive, causing Zimmerman to remark to his students, "Don't use the x-ray as a light bulb." However, in the 1950s, with image amplification, catheters and cardiac structures became much more distinct. Further improvement permitted cineradiography replacing the single plate film or serial film changer images, which until this time had been called angiography. The late 1950s and early 1960s witnessed unprecedented exploitation of these new technologies. Seldinger contributed a percutaneous method for insertion of wires and catheters. New approaches to the left heart and coronary arteries were limited only by one's imagination; technology could now produce almost any type of instrument needed. Consequently, knowledge of physiology and anatomy of previously obscure diseases such as idiopathic hypertrophic subaortic stenosis, prolapse of the mitral valve, and cardiomyopathies was achieved. But at this time the issue of safety during catheterization became paramount. Contrast agents useful in peripheral angiography were found to be unsuitable for intracardiac use. Certain invasive techniques such as suprasternal, transbronchial, and paravertebral left atrial puncture were abandoned in favor of the transseptal approach. The percutaneous subxiphoid and transthoracic approaches to the left ventricle were abandoned in favor of other techniques with fewer complications. Most prominent among the problems of the time was ventricular arrhythmia. Development of ventricular tachycardia and especially ventricular fibrillation generally resulted in death of the patient even after administration of procaine intravenously and open-chest cardiac massage. The introduction of the AC defibrillator by Zoll in 1961 revolutionized catheterization practice, even though more reliable DC defibrillators soon replaced the AC units. Closed-chest compression of the heart replaced open-chest techniques in 1960. Without these achievements, the practice of invasive cardiology may not have reached a point where any physician would eagerly attempt to pass a wire and inflatable balloon into a sclerotic, mostly occluded, plaque-encrusted coronary vessel to relieve angina or limit the extension of an evolving myocardial infarction.

THE BEGINNING

Werner Forssman's classic experiment in which he catheterized his own right heart was a microcosm of intrigue, deception, and controversy as well as solid scientific determination. In his autobiography (1) he relates his dissatisfaction with the standard diagnostic methods of the 1920s. He states that percussion, auscultation, X-ray, and electrocardiography yielded results seriously different from autopsy findings. Furthermore, any dreams of heart surgery that he and the others held could never be realized unless access to the venous system was established to define essentials of physiology, metabolism, and pathology. His determination was fueled by knowledge of prior work done by nineteenth century physiologists. Claude Bernard (2), in the 1840s, named the procedure he performed on animals "cardiac catheterization." While investigating whether oxidative metabolism occurs in all body tissues or in the lung alone, he passed a long thermometer into a horse's left and right ventricles via carotid artery and jugular vein cutdown. Through subsequent years, he continued his basic investigations utilizing animal catheterization. His detailed descriptions of the method for left and right ventricular entry in the living dog are remarkable. Somewhat later, in 1861, two French physiologists, A. Chaveau and E.J. Marey, set out to investigate the pronouncements of William Harvey (3) that ventricular contraction began with systole. Chaveau had an interest in the timing of cardiac events and heart sounds. Marey had already recorded pressure wave forms from the heart

utilizing his sphygmograph. Together, using recording devices described by others and modified for their own purposes, they inserted two long tubes into the heart of an unanesthetized horse and described the pressure curves obtained. They should be credited with the first systematic investigation of intracardiac pressures through the use of catheters (4). It is likely that a picture of this experiment in the horse haunted Forssman when he conceived his own experiment.

Convinced of the plausibility and safety of human venous heart catheterization, Forssman determined to proceed despite the proscriptions given by his confidant and chief. He captured the attention of Gerda Ditzen first with an exchange of books and later with his ideas for heart investigation. After a short time had passed and their relationship was faring well, he asked her to provide him with venesection equipment from the stock under her control. When questioned whether he intended to perform his experiment against orders, Forssman reassured her that she needn't be aware of any of the details, and besides it would be quite safe. Her reply was that she should be his subject! To this he quickly agreed, explaining that she would be the first person to have this done while still fully intending to do it on himself. Once the equipment was assembled, Gerda was asked to recline and was firmly strapped to the table unable to move. Out of her sight, he then completed the cutdown and inserted the rubber ureteral catheter a short distance into the vein. Upon realizing what had happened, Gerda became furious and accused him of deception. Nevertheless, she continued to assist him, and by the time the pair had walked down some steps to X-ray, a short distance away, the nurse attendant was ready with the fluoroscope. He assumed a position behind the fluoroscopic screen, and while watching the dim picture in a mirror held in front, he proceeded to advance the catheter further into the vein and ultimately into the cardiac silhouette. Although he states that the tip entered the right ventricle, because he had measured the length, the radiographic plate he had made to document the event clearly reveals the tip centered in the right atrium. A short time later the same day, Forssman was summoned to the chief's office and was berated for a violation of trust and confidence. Schneider informed him that he had undoubtedly made a remarkable discovery, which should be published immediately. He advised the young physician to tell no one so as to prevent theft of the idea and results. Forssman was also informed that such work was not suitable at that small clinic in Eberswalde and that he would have to seek training elsewhere. But before he left, the procedure (without the benefit of fluoroscopy) was used to treat a patient dying of a septic abortion. The intracardiac administration of medications proved to be acceptable, although we do not know how worthwhile. Before leaving that place, Forssman met with a visitor, Dr. Wilhelm His, discoverer of the "His bundle." Forssman's future plans to record electrical activity from various points in the heart were discouraged by His as probably being unproductive.

Shortly after his arrival in a new training program located at the Charite in Berlin on November 5, 1929, Forssman's paper was published to much acclaim and disdain (5). The popular press praised the work as masterful, but his associates and chief viewed it as a trick appropriate for a circus. Soon thereafter, he learned that he was, indeed, not the first man to catheterize a human heart. Three prominent German physicians had been engaged in vascular catheterization for years. In 1912, Bleichoder, Ungar, and Loeb had published three short articles entitled "Intra-arterial Therapy" about their work in humans (6). They had passed catheters through the femoral artery to the aortic bifurcation for administration of "Collargol" in cases of puerperal sepsis. In fact, Ungar had actually performed two procedures on Bleichoder, passing a catheter from the forearm to the armpit and another from the groin to the inferior vena cava. One of these efforts caused Bleichoder severe chest pain, which they attributed to the heart. Consequently, to avoid scientific criticism, this was never mentioned in writing. Moreover, no publication of their efforts occurred, nor were any X-rays taken. The outcry by Ungar that his priority in catheterization had been usurped and that his work had been plagerized was answered cleverly in a way devised by the editor of *Klinische Wochenschrift,* the journal in which Forssman's paper had appeared. In an appendix to his paper, Forssman would acknowledge all previous work, and in so doing would obviate any need for further debate (7). The episode was not to end without another blow. Dr. Sauerbruch, chief of the Surgical Clinic, called Forssman to his office for an explanation of the matter, which did not, after all, mention the clinic and which attempted to steal the eminence of a senior physician. Any explanations were to no avail, and Forssman was once again out of a job. Although he continued to investigate catheterization techniques, including angiocardiography in dogs and himself (8), Forssman could not break through the resistance and prejudice that met his efforts. The story, however, was not completed until 1956, when, because of their pioneering efforts in cardiac catheterization, Forssman, Cournand, and Richards were awarded the Nobel Prize (9).

RIGHT HEART CATHETERIZATION

Guided right heart catheterization was immediately recognized as a valuable clinical tool, but exploitation was slow. Klein, at the German University in Prague (10), utilized the method to perform Fick cardiac output measurements. Others recognized the method's usefulness in the performance of pulmonary angiography to define congenital anomalies (11). It was in 1932 that Richards and Cournand first agreed to investigate systematically cardiopulmonary function, but only in 1936 did they consider right heart catheterization to be crucial to their task. It was not until 1941, when Cournand and Ranges (12) published accounts of their first experiences in man, that the acceptability of the method for scientific purposes and patient tolerance was finally confirmed. The right ventricle was entered in 1942 and the pulmonary artery in 1944 (13). There followed a series of experiments that laid the foundation for all future invasive cardiovascular research. Pressure recordings and blood gas sampling were now possible simultaneously from the right atrium, right ventricle, and pulmonary artery. Analyses of different types of circulatory shock and their treatment were made and the results reported to the Committee on Medical Research of the Office of Emergency Management. Cardiac failure resulting from hypertension, rheumatic heart disease, and cor pulmonale was studied. Others expanded the use of venous catheterization to renal (14) and hepatic (15) veins. Warren and colleagues (16) and Noble and colleagues (17), respectively, presented the first reports on diagnosis of atrial and ventricular septal defects. McMichael and Sharpey-Schafer (18), despite criticism from their British colleagues, persevered in their exploration of cardiovascular pathology and ultimately studied intravenous digoxin for the first time. It was then, during the period of 1940–1945 (19), that right heart catheterization assumed its place in modern medicine. Through it, new concepts of basic physiology were established that quickly led to improved clinical diagnosis and new methods of therapy.

LEFT HEART CATHETERIZATION

From a contemporary point of view, initial efforts to enter and study the left heart were crude and unsophisticated. The intensity of interest in this pursuit is adequately demonstrated by the large number of methods ultimately used, including transthoracic parasternal puncture, subxiphoid puncture, apical puncture, suprasternal left atrial puncture, paravertebral left atrial puncture, transseptal atrial puncture, and retrograde left ventricular catheterization. Each of these played a role in the development of this technology and deserves some attention.

Perhaps the first person to catheterize—or at least attempt to catheterize—the left heart was Johann Dieffenbach in 1831 (19). This effort involved an attempt to bleed a patient with cholera. At no time did he obtain any blood at all even from the brachial artery he initially attempted to enter. It is therefore doubtful that the left ventricle was ever entered.

Parasternal Left Ventricular Puncture

In 1933, Reboul and Racine (20) used an intercostal anterior parasternal route to the right and left ventricles of dogs for the injection of contrast. Apparently, the first human use of the method occurred in 1936, when Nuvoli attempted to visualize an aortic aneurysm (21). The patient expired from what he describes as overdistension of the ventricle.

Subxiphoid Puncture

A popular approach to the left ventricle was from the subxiphoid area across the right ventricle and through the interventricular septum. Ponsdomenech and Nunez (22), in 1951, performed 45 subxiphoid and direct left ventricular punctures for contrast visualization with 70% Diodrast. They reported no major complications. In 1954, Smith et al. (23) reported 60 human cases in which right and left ventricles were opacified with Diodrast and viewed fluoroscopically and radiographically. An intercostal approach used for the first 15 cases was abandoned in favor of the subxiphoid route after the laceration of a coronary artery. This technique flourished for some time and included reports by Cregg et al. (24) and ultimately Lehman et al. in 1957 (25), who used the phrase "left (or right) cardiac ventriculography." These investigators introduced the concept of quantitation of mitral regurgitation (on a 1 to 4+ scale) derived from left atrial opacification.

Apical Puncture

Although retrograde left ventricular catheterization was already in use, systematic apical left ventricular puncture was pursued in 1956 by Brock et al. (26) in 23 patients. Technology for crossing stenotic aortic valves in a retrograde fashion had not yet been settled. Thus, left ventricular puncture proved useful for mea-

suring transvalvular gradients. In 1957, Fleming and Gibson (27) reported 115 additional cases, and in 1958, Yu et al. (28) added 30 more. In 1959, Ross (29) used this method to cross the aortic valve in 75 cases. The instrumentation introduced by Brock et al. was consistently modified and improved. Ultimately, ventriculography became and remains a standard feature of this technique. In selected cases, particularly in patients who are postoperative with prosthetic valves and in patients with peripheral vascular diseases, apical left ventricular puncture remains a useful adjunct to invasive study.

Suprasternal Puncture

Access to the left atrium is highly desirable in patients with mitral stenosis as well as certain other diseases. When congenital and rheumatic heart diseases occupied the majority of laboratory practice, far greater attention was given to the left atrium than is current practice in the United States. In 1954, Radner (30) described an extension of his practice of suprasternal aortic puncture. When the aorta was small, the puncture needle could be passed more deeply and enter the left atrium selectively. When the aorta was moderate in size or when more physiologic data were desired, measurements from the left atrium, pulmonary artery, and aorta could be obtained in sequence simply by withdrawing the puncture needle (30). Hansen et al. (31) documented their experience with 500 punctures in 1955. In 1959, Lemmon et al. (32) used this technique for coronary arteriography.

Transbronchial Left Atrial Puncture

The technique of posterior left atrial puncture via a rigid bronchoscope was introduced by Facquet et al. in 1952 (33). Allison and Linden in 1953 (34) and Morrow et al. in the United States (1957) (35) continued the method. As was frequently the case, this technique was combined with others such as left ventricular puncture and right heart catheterization to achieve complete left and right heart pressure and angiographic investigation (36).

Transthoracic Paravertebral Left Atrial Puncture

In 1953, Bjork et al. (37) introduced direct posterior paravertebral left atrial puncture as an alternative to other techniques for measurement of left atrial pressures. Fischer and McCaffrey in 1956 (38) modified the original method by utilizing a prone position instead of the lateral decubitus and adding fluoroscopic control. Wood et al. in 1956 (39) modified the equipment to allow simultaneous recording of left ventricular and left atrial pressures. Blakemore et al. (40) inserted two tubes for pressure monitoring. Later, Litwak et al (41), in order to investigate exercise physiology, performed the left atrial puncture. After removing the needles, they left soft polyethylene tubes in the atrium, turned the patient into the supine position, and completed the study with separate right heart catheterization and left ventricular puncture if needed (41). With the introduction of successful transseptal left atrial catheterization, external atrial puncture was largely abandoned.

Transseptal Left Atrial Puncture

Since the interatrial septum is approached at a 45° angle from the inferior vena cava, straight catheter passage into the left atrium occurs frequently if the fossa ovalis has not become sealed. This favorable geometric arrangement and the fact that the fossa ovalis can be crossed in 30% of adults without puncture suggested this route for entry into the left heart. The concept of transseptal left atrial puncture was introduced by Ross in 1959 (42). Because it is entirely intraatrial, potential problems inherent in any of the external techniques such as hemopericardium and laceration were largely eliminated. Initially, the procedure was performed by saphenous vein cutdown and insertion of a #11F blunt catheter sheath to the right atrium. A long 16-gauge needle was then passed to the tip on the catheter, and both were positioned against the septum. After puncturing the septum, the left atrial pressure could be recorded immediately. If left ventricular pressures were desired, a thin polyethylene tube (PE-50) was passed through the needle in most cases (75–90%) reaching the ventricle. Subsequent passage through the aortic valve was described but seldom practiced. To correct the obvious potential problems of polyethylene tube knotting or shearing and the local consequences of venous cutdown, major modifications were made. Cope in 1959 (43) introduced a percutaneous method of entry followed by multiple exchange of needles and catheters. The technique described by Brockenbrough and Braunwald in 1960 (44), however, except for minor modifications remains unchanged today. In this modification, a preformed catheter is passed percutaneously into the right atrium over a standard guide wire. A long needle with a 17-gauge shaft and 20-gauge tip is then ad-

vanced through the catheter and positioned against the septum. Once puncture has been completed and documented by left atrial pressure contours, the catheter is advanced into the left atrium and the needle withdrawn. Ordinarily, the catheter can still be advanced into the ventricle for pressure measurement and angiography. Attempts at septal puncture from the external jugular vein were described by Bevegard et al. (45). Although successful, the technique was not pursued.

After a decade of decline of use because of a diminished incidence of rheumatic valvular disease in the United States, transseptal catheterization may soon return as a therapeutic tool. In children, atrial balloon septostomy has been practiced successfully for years after being introduced by Rashkind and Miller in 1966 (46). Blade septostomy, introduced by Park et al. in 1975 (47) extended the usefulness of this concept. Recently, modification in the transseptal equipment and concept by Mullins (48) allowed a pigtail catheter to be introduced in the atrium and ventricle for more successful angiography. Balloon mitral valvuloplasty has already been described (49) and may become the next major use for transseptal left atrial puncture.

Retrograde Left Heart Catheterization

Documentation of attempted retrograde arterial catheterization dates back to 1831 (19). Successful aortic catheterization and administration of drugs were accomplished by Bleichoder, Ungar, and Loeb in 1930 (6). From that time through the 1940s, many other groups reported entering the aorta, measuring pressures, and performing arteriography (50–52). By 1950, the anatomy of all branches of the aorta and especially the coronary arteries was well known and was under further study. Retrograde entry of the left ventricle had also been performed in desultory fashion. But Zimmerman in 1949 (53) reported the results of a systematic approach to left ventricular catheterization.

The ease and safety of crossing the aortic valve, which he later achieved, was not evident in Zimmerman's original paper (54). He expresses concern about moving the catheter against a pressurized flow and through the valve only during "that short ejection interval (0.22 sec) during which the aortic valves are open." He quotes Wiggers' (55) concern that eddy currents cause some leaflet approximation and partial valve closure even during systole and speculates that this may be the reason the procedure was unsuccessful in five normal subjects. At this time, successful entry into the left ventricle was achieved in 11 patients with syphilitic aortic insufficiency. But, in the one patient with rheumatic aortic insufficiency, attempted entry was associated with ventricular fibrillation. Despite administration of intracardiac procaine and adrenaline and open-chest massage, survival did not occur.

For his initial report, Zimmerman used the ulnar artery 8–9 cm distal to the medial epicondyle. After infiltration with procaine, isolation of the vessel was accomplished and bleeding controlled with umbilical tapes. A 6F catheter of Cournand's design was inserted over a Bing wire. The catheter was well lubricated with sterile olive oil and filled with a 1% solution of heparin in saline. Vasospasm was a major concern such that reinsertion of a catheter once withdrawn was usually unsuccessful. Likewise in this initial trial, Zimmerman also relates that 20% of attempts at traversing the subclavian-aortic junction were unsuccessful. After completion of the procedure, the ulnar artery was repaired and the patient was given 75 mg of heparin intramuscularly every 6 hr for 3 days.

Also in 1950, Limon Lason and Bouchard (56) reported safe and successful entry into the left ventricles of 17 subjects using a catheter with a "J" tip configuration. Strangely, in view of the problems encountered by others in crossing the aortic valve, this method was not pursued. During this period, transaxillary retrograde arterial catheterization was reported by Pierce (57) but complications prevented further development. Shortly thereafter, in 1953, Seldinger (58) introduced his method for percutaneous entry into arterial vessels. Despite this event, reports regarding left heart investigation lagged until 1957, when Prioton et al. (59) modified Seldinger's technique by passing a polyethylene catheter over a long guide wire directed at the left ventricle. This development was followed by a host of reports indicating that left heart entry had come of age.

CATHETERS

The first major improvement in catheter design occurred in 1941, when Cournand and Ranges (12) employed a catheter with a radiopaque coating. Double lumen modifications were introduced later for right heart procedures, but the same basic catheter was used by Zimmerman in 1949 and others through 1960. Polyethylene, a new synthetic plastic for catheters, was introduced by Ingraham et al. in 1947 (60). It quickly became popular and was used by Pierce in 1951 (57) and Seldinger in 1953 (58). Its major advantages were a large internal lumen compared to wall thickness and great flexibility, but its major disadvan-

tage, a lack of radiopacity, prompted many investigators to modify it for better visualization. These efforts included use of a metal tip, insertion on a wire core, and filling it with contrast medium. In 1956, Odman (61) introduced radiopaque polyethylene color coded for size. Soon thereafter, Dacron and Teflon became available.

It is not possible to detail all the investigators responsible for modifications of catheter styles and configurations. End-hole-style Cournand catheters were found to be unsatisfactory for ventricular angiography because of their recoil, which produced arrhythmias, but the addition of side holes facilitated angiography and blood sampling. Odman suggested individual modification of a catheter tip for special purposes. Olin in 1958 (62) introduced a loop-end catheter with multiple side holes for ventriculography in animals. Littman et al. (63) demonstrated its easy passage across normal aortic valves. Bellman et al. in 1960 (64) and Williams et al. in 1960 (65) used it successfully for coronary arteriography. Also in 1960, Dotter (66) reported use of a spring guide wire, a technique he had encountered abroad. Since these were not yet available in the United States, he purchased coiled wire used for stringing musical instruments and found this a suitable alternative. Later, Dotter and Gensini (67) described selective visceral angiography with straight-tip modifications. Stimulated by the knowledge that organ visualization was feasible and safe, and prompted by the availability of new materials and technology, development of catheters was only a matter of time.

The contributions made by Sones in 1958 (68) and Judkins in 1968 (69) for coronary arteriography were monumental. The need for bedside monitoring led Swan, Ganz, Forrester et al. (70) to develop the flow-directed balloon catheter in 1970. The feasibility of peripheral angioplasty resulted in the development of the coronary angioplasty catheter by Gruentzig and Hopff in 1974 (71).

CATHETERIZATION TECHNOLOGY

Angiocardiography

The contemporary practice of cardiac catheterization relies on angiocardiography more heavily than at any other time in the past. The requirements of coronary angioplasty stress the limits not only of catheters and dilation hardware but also of the apparatus through which heart structures and especially the coronary vessels are visualized. It is sobering to reflect on the fact that none of this was available until the late

1950s and early 1960s. References to cardiac angiography or coronary arteriography until the late 1940s usually meant a single radiographic plate resulting from injection of massive amounts of contrast into a limited vascular space. A revolution in radiography occurred with the introduction of serial film changers in 1949. A cassette-loaded device was developed by Sanchez-Perez and Carter (72). Roll film was utilized in changers described by Dotter, Steinberg, and Temple (73), Scott and Moore (74), and Gidlund (75). Evolution of true motion cinematography, however, awaited the development of a radiographic source that could produce enough light to permit film exposure at rates of 15–60 frames per second. The answer was the image intensifier, which was developed largely through the efforts of Sturm and Morgan in 1949 (76) and Moon in 1950 (77). Technologic advances were slow and did not keep pace with desired applications. Initial viewing was possible only with mechanical optical magnifying devices. The coupling of cameras to the intensifier frequently prevented simultaneous viewing. The persistent efforts of Janker in 1954 (78) and Sones in 1958 (79) advanced cineangiography substantially. Now not only was it possible to better visualize intracardiac structures as they moved through systole and diastole but this could be accomplished with a fraction of the contrast volume and substantially less X-ray exposure for both patient and operator.

Coronary Arteriography

The first person to attempt visualization of the coronary arteries in a living patient was probably Peter Rousthoi (80), closely followed by Reboul and Racine in 1933 (20). The outcome of their work is in doubt, and certainly no clear demonstration of coronary vessels was accomplished. In 1945, Radner (81) successfully demonstrated the coronary arteries in a living patient and published the results. This was followed by a similar report in 1948 by Manses-Hoyos and Gomez del Campo (82). Jonsson (83), using the same technique of ascending aortic contrast flush chiefly by retrograde catheterization, succeeded in clearly demonstrating all branches of the coronary tree. DiGuglielmo and Guttadauro in 1952 (84) reported a series of 153 coronary opacifications also by a flush technique. By this time it was clear that use of large amounts of contrast was not satisfactory. Not only did use of massive quantities interfere with proximal coronary visualization because of overlap but it frequently caused side effects of neurologic and cardiovascular importance. The chance occurrence

of a period of asystole in a dog following contrast injection prompted Arnulf to utilize acetylcholine for production of transient asystole in man. Dotter and Frische (85) introduced a balloon occlusive device, which was inflated above the coronary arteries to limit outflow of contrast for a very short interval. Bellman et al. in 1960 (64) devised a spiral-tipped catheter with side holes that would direct a jet of contrast at the coronary orifices while also flooding the aorta. In clinical use, the results were disappointing.

None of the techniques in use in 1958 was ideal for consistently excellent coronary arteriograpy. At this time, Sones was seriously engaged in investigating selective cineangiocardiography of all types. Coronary arteries were opacified by contrast, frequently 20–25 ml, injected into a sinus of Valsalva through an NIH catheter with a power injector. The physical arrangement of his laboratory at that time required the patient and operator to occupy a position on a platform several feet off the floor while the observer was forced to view the procedure in a pit under the table—a matter of 8 feet from the operator. One day in 1958, during a usual procedure, the catheter migrated into the right coronary artery before injection. Before Sones could stop the power injection, the bolus of contrast was delivered virtually totally into the vessel. The patient experienced relatively little ill effect, but the incident convinced Sones that selective coronary cannulation for arteriography was possible. Between 1959 and 1962, the first 1,000 selective coronary arteriograms were performed by the cutdown method. Only two deaths and a 2% incidence of ventricular fibrillation proved the safety of the method. Selective coronary arteriography by the percutaneous route was soon proposed by Ricketts and Abrams (86), who introduced performed polyethylene catheters in 1962. Design of a more practical group of preformed catheters made of more durable, torqueable material by Judkins (69) completed the task.

Ancillary Procedures

From the beginning of cardiac catheterization, ventricular tachycardia and fibrillation were the most devastating and feared potential complications. Development of either of these arrhythmias before 1961 was likely to result in death of the patient. Once again, technology and the new knowledge of physiology gained from invasive procedures permitted development of external defibrillation. As early as 1936, Ferris et sal. (87), and somewhat later Wiggers (88), described the effects of electric current on the heart.

In 1961, reports by Zoll et al. of the use of AC defibrillation (89) across an intact chest wall revolutionized practice in the catheterization laboratory. The greater reliability and safety provided by DC defibrillation introduced by Lown et al. in 1962 (90) removed the fear of ventricular arrhythmias and permitted even more aggressive investigation of invasive techniques.

It is inappropriate to separate cardiopulmonary resuscitation into its various component parts in that one is of limited value without the others. In 1960, the demonstration that closed-chest cardiac compression was at least as effective as open-chest massage revolutionized resuscitative procedures. Kouwenhoven, Jude, and Knickerbocker reported their initial findings in 1960 (91). The results of the method in 118 patients appeared in 1961 (92). Within a 2 year period, external cardiac massage and defibrillation were added to laboratory practice, making catheterization far safer than ever before. Thirty years had passed since Forssman worried about what could happen to his heart when a catheter was introduced. Twenty years had passed since Cournand worried about his patients' welfare. Ten years had passed since entry into the left ventricle became commonplace. Three years had passed since coronary arteriography added a new and more immediate risk to laboratory practice. It was about time.

Coronary Angioplasty

The transluminal dilation of stenotic coronary arteries is just another in the long series of accomplishments punctuating the 60-year history of cardiac catheterization. As in the development of cardiac surgery, the first portions of the body to receive attention were in the periphery. Through the genius and foresight of Charles Dotter, attempted transluminal dilation of the leg arteries was begun in a variety of ways. The first report of a successful approach was published by Dotter and Judkins in 1964 (93). Through the use of coaxial sheaths, they demonstrated that perfusion could be restored by sequential dilation. This idea captured the attention of many investigators, but accomplishments were halting. In 1969, inspired by a presentation given by Dotter, Myler devised a mechanical dilation device to be used in coronary vessels, but he was unable to devise a method with which to deliver it to the coronary circulation. In 1970, Andreas Gruentzig moved to Zurich and began investigation of balloon angioplasty of leg vessels. Soon thereafter, he miniaturized the balloon with which he entered dog coronary arteries and cleared experimentally induced strictures. His first report in 1976, which dealt only with work in animals, was met with little acclaim and great skepticism (94). It was at this conference in Miami in November of 1976 that Myler and Gruentzig first met. This relationship was to bear fruit in May of 1977. To pursue the development of coronary angioplasty, Myler invited Gruentzig to San Francisco. After careful planning, it was decided to attempt balloon dilation of a single lesion in a patient undergoing multiple-vessel bypass. Thus, during the operation, a short balloon-tipped catheter was passed retrograde through an arteriotomy made in a left anterior coronary artery. Dilation was performed, and outflow monitoring failed to reveal any debris or other untoward effect. Shortly thereafter, the patient was studied by arteriography, and the lesion requiring bypass that was the target of angioplasty was found to be minimally visible. The experiment had been successful. A total of 16 such experiments were carried out by this team in San Francisco and Zurich. Upon return to Switzerland, Gruentzig awaited the perfect patient for a trial of PTCA. The opportunity arrived, and dilation of a discrete lesion of the left anterior descending vessel was successful. Gruentzig reported his results encompassing four patients in Miami in November of 1977. It is interesting to note that the published abstract did not contain mention of the clinical work in humans (95). This time his presentation was greeted with excitement and enthusiasm. A rush to learn the procedure and its exponential use in many institutions, which had already begun, prompted the leaders of the field to convene a workshop under the auspices of the NHLBI, in Bethesda during June of 1979. In the finest tradition of medicine, the participants agreed to limit the centers performing the procedure to those with clearly defined protocols approved by their institutional boards. Even the commercial provider of most of the equipment would abide by this and all the other guidelines. The participants then agreed to pool their results in a unified systematic fashion, from which statistical and other data could be derived for the benefit of all. The initial chapter of the history of coronary angioplasty had been concluded.

2. Coronary Angioplasty Equipment

Coronary angioplasty equipment—guiding catheters, dilatation catheters, guide wires, inflation devices, and other ancillary pieces of equipment—have evolved from very primitive models in the early 1980s to extremely sophisticated devices in the early 1990s. It is largely because of this technologic advancement that the field of angioplasty has been extended to more complex disease and has also been made less difficult for the practitioner and safer for the patient.

In reviewing the chapter dealing with coronary angioplasty equipment in the first edition of this book, it was very clear that most of the diagrams were woefully out of date and that some of the commentary was no longer pertinent because much of the equipment used in 1987 had become obsolete 3 years later. With that in mind, this chapter will be redesigned to describe, in general, the equipment and types of equipment available with less emphasis on the brand names and minute specifics of the devices.

In the early days of angioplasty, it was clear that two or three companies were dominant in the field of producing equipment, and through the 1980s, several other companies emerged as significant factors in providing equipment for angioplasty. Most of the companies have excellent representatives and clinical specialists who are willing to provide the practitioner with features and details of their equipment. Since it is unreasonable to expect that every hospital laboratory stock all of the equipment currently available, it is important that each institution settle on an adequate variety of equipment to allow appropriate choices during angioplasty and to be certain that the physician does not enter a procedure without the material back-up support needed to meet and conquer the challenge of the case.

In some instances in this chapter, I will comment on some equipment that I have found particularly useful in certain situations, but it should be recognized that in the majority of cases, several companies have nearly identical guiding catheters, dilatation catheter systems, and guide wires available with similar characteristics.

GUIDING CATHETERS

The selection of the proper guiding catheter is one of the most important steps in successful coronary angioplasty. It is vital to recognize the differences between diagnostic and guiding catheters. The curves of guiding catheters in the Judkins style differ slightly from the standard diagnostic curves, and the tip lengths also vary. Usually, the difference between guiding and diagnostic catheters is slight and not important, but in some cases, the generally shorter tip length of guiding catheters may not quite reach the left coronary ostium, for example, and another style catheter may be necessary to achieve coaxial intubation. Most guiding catheters now have a soft material at the tip, and the potential for proximal coronary artery trauma that was present with the early models of guiding catheters is no longer a severe limitation. Guiding catheters, in general, are somewhat thinner walled than are diagnostic catheters, and the torquing capabilities of the guiding catheter may be somewhat less than that of a diagnostic catheter. Most guiding catheters have three layers. An outer layer provides memory and stiffness, a middle layer consisting of a wire braid gives support and allows for torque control, and an inner layer of Teflon or some coated material provides lubricity for the passage of the dilatation catheter system (Fig. 2–1).

There are many different types and sizes of guiding catheters available. Reports in the literature have indicated the use of small diagnostic catheters as guides with balloon-over-wire systems, and certainly a large variation of guiding catheter sizes and styles can be used when unusual circumstances prevail. In general, however, the femoral guiding system is 8 French with both 8.3 French and 9 French catheters available, and the brachial guiding catheter systems are usually 8.3 French with 8 French systems also available. To choose the optimum catheter, it is important to review the diagnostic studies for several key features: 1) the coaxial engagement of the diagnostic catheter; 2) the anatomy of the proximal vessel; 3) the anatomy of the aorta; 4) the anatomy of the lesion; and 5) the anatomy of the distal target vessel.

The guiding catheter performs two primary functions: 1) forming a conduit to transport the balloon catheter into the diseased vessel, and 2) providing a

Schematics and drawings provided by USCI, C.R. Bard, Inc.; ACS, Division of Eli Lilly Co.; Scimed Life Systems, Inc.; and Baxter Healthcare Corporation, Edwards LIS Division.

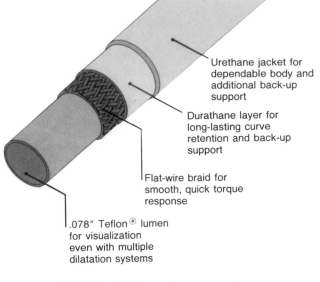

Urethane jacket for dependable body and additional back-up support

Durathane layer for long-lasting curve retention and back-up support

Flat-wire braid for smooth, quick torque response

.078″ Teflon® lumen for visualization even with multiple dilatation systems

Fig. 2–1. Guiding catheter construction.

platform launching pad for advancing the balloon catheter system through the stenotic lesion. To fulfill these requirements, the guiding catheter must have a sufficiently large lumen and low-friction inner surface to allow for easy transport and passage of the balloon catheter. The guiding catheter must also have the strength and rigidity in the shaft for stable positioning in the coronary ostium. The softened tip of the guiding catheter is important to provide safety once the coronary ostium is engaged. Secure proximal positioning enables the catheter to serve as back-up support for advancing the balloon catheter across the lesion. However, this needed stiffness in the shaft must be combined with sufficient overall flexibility for good torque control and maneuverability.

Although adequate cine angiograms of the coronary arteries are possible without true coaxial engagement, particularly if side hole catheters are used, the chances for success are greatly reduced, and the potential for complications is increased when proper coaxial alignment is not achieved by the guiding catheter in PTCA. In the case of a vein graft or unusual coronary anatomy, for example, it is often advisable to begin the angioplasty procedure with a diagnostic angiogram, particularly if the original angiogram was performed at another facility, and it is not known exactly which diagnostic catheter was used or how easily it seated. This approach is more economical than is the insertion of several guiding catheters to determine coaxial conformance. It also provides the immediately necessary current angiograms prior to the angioplasty procedure and the availability of digital subtraction or videodisc images necessary during angioplasty.

Whether the femoral or brachial approach is used is determined by the training and experience of the operator, by the anatomic pattern of the diseased vessel, and, to a lesser extent, by the pathologic appearance of the vessel. Both approaches are equally viable alternatives in most cases, assuming that the operator is equally proficient in performing diagnostic angiograms by both approaches. The brachial approach may be preferred in the relatively small subset of cases, with eccentric anatomic variations in the native vessels or obstructive disease in the distal aorta or iliofemoral vessels. The choice for approach in the majority of cases, however, depends more on operator training, experience, and skill than on anatomic criteria.

While the guiding catheter must provide sufficient selective engagement of the catheter tip to provide a stable platform for the advancement of the dilatation catheter system, engagement that is too deep or too firm may cause decreased flow in the vessel and ischemia of the affected myocardium. This is generally identified by damping of the pressure tracing obtained from the tip of the catheter and by poor flow when injections of contrast are made. Damped pressure resulting from a wedged guiding catheter reflects compromise of coronary artery flow with decreased myocardial perfusion, which can result in ischemic pain, electrocardiographic changes, and myocardial injury, if prolonged. In addition, catheter wedging results in the loss of the proximal pressure monitor and subsequent inability to obtain a reliable transstenotic gradient if pressure gradients are utilized. However, the ability to transiently seat a guiding catheter deeply markedly enhances the possibilities of successful passage of the balloon catheter across a very tight and/or hard or long lesions. Therefore, a common guiding catheter dilemma is that super-subselective intubation of the proximal coronary artery by the guiding catheter may greatly increase the chance of crossing difficult lesions but risks decreased coronary flow and significant myocardial ischemia. Careful attention must be paid throughout the procedure to the position of the guiding catheter tip, including withdrawal of the guide from the coronary ostium at appropriate times during the procedure to allow flow to continue. This will tend to minimize the potential problems of catheter wedging and enhance the safety of the procedure. The timing of these strategic manipulations is discussed elsewhere in this book.

To further alleviate the problem of catheter wedging and decreased coronary flow, guiding catheters with side holes are available (Fig. 2–2). This situation most frequently occurs in the right coronary artery. Although side-hole catheters allow for more coronary

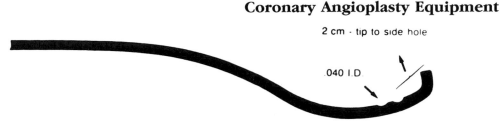

Fig. 2-2. USCI perfusion port guiding catheter.

flow and allow the guide tip to be seated in a more stable position, there is decreased ability to inject contrast selectively through the guiding catheter into the target artery because of the reflux of dye through the side holes into the sinus of Valsalva. This loss of good contrast injection and subsequent good visualization of the vessel impairs one's ability to localize precisely the lesion-balloon relationship and to define postangioplasty angiographic results before the wire is removed. If the dilatation catheter system is advanced beyond the side holes, often little or no contrast can be injected in an antegrade fashion. Therefore, after balloon inflations, to assess results, the balloon catheter must be withdrawn so that the entire dilatation catheter is proximal to the side holes, thereby usually allowing adequate antegrade contrast injections to be made.

The choice of size in femoral guiding catheters is usually 8 or 9 French. The 9 French catheters may provide increased torque control, better contrast delivery, and more reliable pressure recording, but the less stiff 8 French guiding catheters allow for safer subselective engagement, decreasing the potential for proximal coronary artery intimal trauma, and, because of the smaller arterial puncture, less likelihood of puncture-site complications. Most commonly available 8 French guiding catheters have adequate torqueability and injection capabilities and are used in preference to the 9 French catheter systems. Guiding catheters with a variety of tapered sizes making even smaller tips possible are available and perform in an exemplary manner. Large lumen catheters provide better contrast injection capabilities but have somewhat decreased torquing capability and are a bit more difficult to form into a power position because of increased stiffness and a less flexible tip.

Anatomic Considerations in Catheter Selection

Both the anatomy and pathology of the vessels to be dilated are taken into account in guiding catheter selection. Anatomic variations in the origin of the coronary arteries are of primary importance in the selection of the guiding catheter, and the location and

severity of lesions within the vessels are of secondary importance (Fig. 2-3). Characteristics that must be taken into consideration in selecting guiding catheters include the internal diameter of the shaft and tip, the softness of the tip, the amount of support provided by the guiding catheter, torque control, the ability to provide adequate contrast injections with the dilatation catheter system in place, the radiopacity of the catheter and the tip, and the ability to measure proximal pressures if needed. The catheter companies all have information available regarding their products, but evaluation among all of the excellent products currently available usually must be done by individual use and comparison (Appendix II–F).

Left Anterior Descending Coronary Artery Lesions

If the left anterior descending coronary artery arises in the classical anterior and superior direction, the standard Judkins-type catheter is the most commonly selected. Although this catheter conforms well to the classic configuration, in some cases the guide wire will tend to be directed toward another branch (circumflex or ramus intermedius) instead of the LAD. This is particularly true in patients with a short left main trunk. To overcome this technical difficulty, the guiding catheter is rotated in a counterclockwise motion (Fig. 2-4). A shorter tipped guiding catheter can also be used, and these are available from several companies. The counterclockwise rotation of the catheter is performed with the balloon catheter and guide wire well back in the guiding catheter. Through this manipulation, the heel of the secondary curve is repositioned in a posterior direction in the aortic route, thereby redirecting the tip of the guiding catheter in a superior position toward the LAD.

This maneuver can be accomplished, provided that the secondary curve of the Judkins-type catheter is short enough to allow the catheter to be advanced downward into the aortic root so that the segment between the primary and secondary curve lies transversely in the aorta. If the secondary curve is too long,

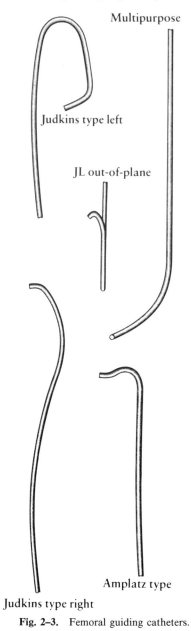

Fig. 2–3. Femoral guiding catheters.

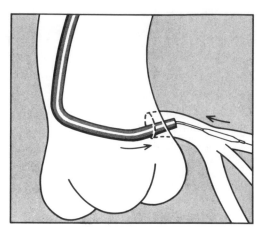

Fig. 2–4.   Left coronary guide catheter.

branch. Alternatively, an Amplatz-type catheter may be used. This catheter tip is often directed inferiorly so that the guide wire will pass selectively into the circumflex system (Fig. 2–5).

Right Coronary Artery Lesions

When the proximal right coronary artery originates in a transverse or downward direction, the right Judkins-type catheter is commonly used (Fig. 2–6). When the orientation of the vessel is superior, however, the Judkins-type catheter may not provide adequate back-up support to advance the dilatation catheter system. In such cases, the use of an internal mammary guide has proven useful and either an Amplatz-type catheter or multipurpose catheter with a 45–90° distal curve may be used (Fig. 2–7). The Arani 75° or 90° long or short catheter tip (depending on vessel orientation

that segment will lie axially in the aorta and cause the guiding catheter tip to point inferiorly toward the circumflex branch.

Circumflex Coronary Artery Lesions

A Judkins-type catheter with a longer secondary curve may be used to direct the dilatation catheter system selectively toward the circumflex artery because the tip of the guiding catheter will tend to point inferiorly to transport the balloon into the circumflex

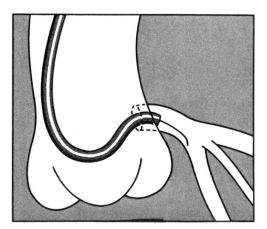

Fig. 2–5.   Amplatz guide catheter, circumflex.

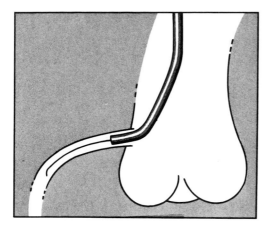

Fig. 2–6. Right coronary guide catheter.

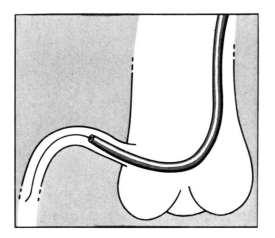

Fig. 2 7. Multitip guide catheter to right coronary artery.

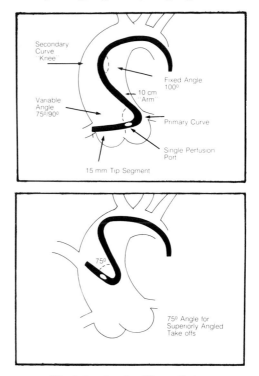

Fig. 2–8. Arani guiding catheter.

from the aorta) is an excellent alternative catheter choice to achieve better back-up when solid seating in the right coronary ostium is difficult (Fig. 2–8).

Even though a Judkins-type catheter may conform well to the origin anatomy of the right coronary artery, it may not supply the necessary support to advance the balloon catheter across a severely stenotic or hard (particularly distal) lesion. In such cases, attempts to advance the balloon catheter will cause the guide tip to "back-out" of the orifice when forward pressure is exerted on the dilatation catheter system. If this occurs, the operator may be able to advance the Judkins-style catheter into a power position by a push-pull technique that results in the tip of the catheter being seated more deeply in the right coronary ostium and the elbow of the catheter backing up against the opposite wall of the aorta. This maneuver must be done with care and should be done only by experienced operators. An alternative solution is to use an Amplatz, Arani, or multipurpose-type guiding

catheter that can be advanced safely over the balloon catheter and farther into the ostium to provide support to advance the balloon catheter system. The back-up pressure on the opposite aortic wall is one of the prime factors in gaining enhanced platform support.

Vein Graft Lesions

Selection of the guiding catheter for a saphenous vein bypass graft cannulation may be challenging, particularly when the graft originates from the aorta from the anterior position. Because of the short distance between the aortic arch and the origin of such grafts, the Judkins right coronary catheter may not provide adequate support for advancement of the balloon catheter system (even though the position of the catheter for angiography may be entirely satisfactory). The guiding catheter must span the aorta, braced on the opposite wall, thereby attaining a stable position for advancement of the balloon catheter system.

A single curved catheter such as the multipurpose or El Gamal modified multipurpose catheter with a 90° or greater distal curve may achieve this purpose.

Amplatz-style catheters may also provide adequate cannulation and back-up in vein graft lesions.

Internal Mammary Bypass Graft Lesions

If lesions exist in the internal mammary artery, which has been used for a bypass graft, or if the internal mammary must be traversed to reach a lesion distal in the (usually) LAD system, there are a variety of tips of catheters designed for the variation in origin configurations of the internal mammary artery (Fig. 2–9). Great care must be taken in the positioning and use of these catheters during the procedure, since the origin of the internal mammary is a very friable area. In most cases, the femoral approach will provide adequate back-up for either right and left internal mammary guiding catheter positions. If, however, more stable positions are needed, the femoral guides may be positioned via a brachial approach utilizing the right brachial artery for the right internal mammary and the left brachial artery for the left internal mammary artery. This approach may provide excellent guiding catheter support.

Brachial Guiding Catheter Design

The most commonly used brachial guiding catheter has a 3 inch medium curved flexible guiding tip that, with proper manipulation, can be molded to conform to anatomic problems created by the diseased vessel (Fig. 2–10). In smaller aortas, a 2 inch medium tip may prove beneficial, and for larger aortas, larger curves are also available. Brachial guides with Amplatz-style tips can also be used to more subselectively engage the circumflex coronary artery in particular and to provide better back-up for either left or right coronary intubations. The molding of the brachial guiding catheter is easily done by experienced practitioners who have utilized the brachial approach and does provide some advantage over most femoral guiding catheter systems that are preformed and cannot usually be molded within the aorta into any other shape than their original configuration. This provides an advantage in selectively and appropriately cannulating coronary ostia if some variation in origin exists.

Brachial Approach to Right Coronary Artery, Left Anterior Descending Coronary Artery, and Circumflex Coronary Artery Lesions

In cases where it is necessary to advance the guiding catheter deeply into the target coronary artery to achieve back-up support, this maneuver can generally be accomplished more safely with the brachial guiding catheter because of its soft, flexible, nonformed tip and lack of preformed secondary curves. In the presence of severely stenotic lesions, and in the absence of proximal disease, the brachial approach allows deep subselective penetration into the proximal artery to provide solid support to advance the guide wire across the stenosis and subsequent support and stability for advancing the dilatation catheter system across the lesion. This maneuver is quite safely accomplished by experienced brachial practitioners and is the counterpart of "Amplatzing" or achieving a power position with femoral guiding catheters to provide support for crossing severely stenotic lesions. With the brachial approach, multiple-vessel angioplasty can be performed rapidly with the same guiding catheter in some patients. The same guiding catheter and dilatation catheter systems can often be used in several arteries if balloon sizing is similar. Subselective intubation of the left anterior descending and circumflex branches of the left main coronary artery is often possible with the brachial guiding catheter system.

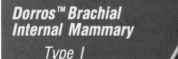

Dorros™ Brachial Internal Mammary

Type I
Type II
Type III

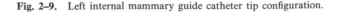

Fig. 2–9. Left internal mammary guide catheter tip configuration.

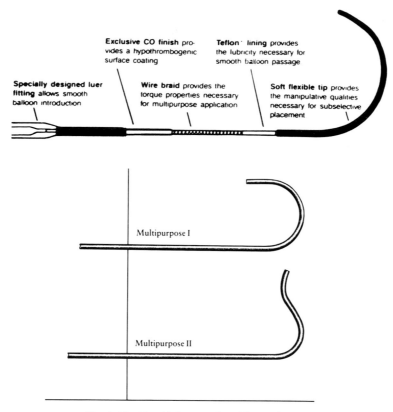

Exclusive CO finish pro- vides a hypothrombogenic surface coating

Teflon lining provides the lubricity necessary for smooth balloon passage

Specially designed luer fitting allows smooth balloon introduction

Wire braid provides the torque properties necessary for multipurpose application

Soft flexible tip provides the manipulative qualities necessary for subselective placement

Multipurpose I

Multipurpose II

Fig. 2–10.   Brachial-approach guiding catheters.

Brachial Approach to Vein Graft Lesions

The position of the aortic anastomosis and the anatomy of the aorta can be used to predict whether the brachial approach will offer advantages or disadvantages over the femoral approach in each individual case. As with native vessels, 90% of the catheterizations can be done with equal ease from either approach. A "bent tip" or "Amplatz-style" brachial guiding catheter may be advantageous in vein grafts for cannulation and support. The high or anterior orientation of the origin of a vein graft may necessitate the use of larger curved brachial guiding catheters to reach and coaxially enter the vein graft with the appropriate support needed for the advancement of wire and dilatation catheter systems.

DILATATION CATHETER SYSTEMS

One of the most important considerations in the mechanics of PTCA is the dilating force applied directly to the arterial wall. The force acting against the arterial wall varies with the balloon pressure, the area

of stenosis, the balloon diameter and length, and the degree of stenosis.

Selecting a balloon size is usually straightforward, but must not be done in a casual manner. "Eye-balling" of lesions to select size of catheters is often woefully inaccurate. Caliper measurements, either with mechanical calipers or a caliper computer system, should be routinely performed and, if possible, at least three views, two of which are orthogonal, measured and averaged to assess not only the preprocedural stenosis but also the size of the adjacent "normal" artery. It is obvious that in diffusely diseased vessels, the artery proximal and distal to an area of severe stenosis is probably somewhat diseased as well, but the appropriate sizing of the balloon catheter is usually accomplished using the widths of these segments. The goal should be to dilate the severely diseased portion of the artery to equal the caliber of the adjacent "nondiseased" segment. However, there are some exceptions to this rule. If restenosis has occurred, the possibility of slight oversizing of the balloon should be considered. This should be minimal, and it should be recognized that more than *slight* oversizing of the balloon catheter may cause not only intimal tearing but also medial disruption in the artery. Similarly, a slight oversizing when dealing with graft stenoses has been shown to correlate positively with increased initial success and decreased chance of recurrence. The size of the artery or graft may be determined by comparison with a diagnostic or guide catheter seen on the angiogram. This corrects for the magnification factor of the variety of imaging systems used. In comparing vessel size to size of angiographic catheters, 3 French equals 0.039 inch, which equals 1 mm; 7 French equals 2.3 mm; 8 French equal 2.67 mm; and 9 French equals 3 mm. A 6 French catheter system that is commonly used in diagnostic procedures today equals 2.0 mm. Using these comparative figures, measurement of the vessel in three different angiographic views and averaging the three measurements (with a mechanical or computer caliper system) will give the most accurate possible measurement of vessel size.

When selecting dilatation catheters, it is important to know exactly how the balloon will respond at higher pressures. Some balloons maintain their size and shape, whereas others expand beyond the predicted size at higher pressures. Some balloons have been shown to conform to curves and angles in the vessels better than others, and these balloon characteristics should be taken into consideration when selecting a balloon for each individual lesion. Most catheter companies have a variety of balloons available that have combinations of these characteristics, and the operator should be familiar with the characteristics of the balloon catheters available in his/her institution. One must also continually update his/her knowledge regarding the variety of available dilatation catheter systems. In general, polyethylene balloons will not become larger at higher pressures, but balloons made of polyvinyl chloride will become slightly larger at higher pressures in a predictable fashion. Balloon inflation charts are available from various companies, and one of these are presented in Appendix II–E to indicate the expected balloon size at various pressures for this latter type of balloon. For example, the Sci-Med balloons achieve their advertised size at 8 atm, whereas pressures below that produce smaller balloon diameter and pressures above that expand the balloon in a rather predictable fashion. This knowledge can be used to "build" the desired balloon size in various circumstances. The current availability of quarter-size balloons also allows for more accurate balloon-size choice. Undersizing of the balloon may be considered when the target lesion is on a bend or when the patient is elderly or has diffuse disease. Angled balloons are available, and some balloon catheter systems (particularly the ACX

balloon from ACS and the Skinny balloon from Sci-Med) conform nicely to curves and bends in the artery even at high inflation pressures. The prototype patient who would require undersizing of the balloon would be an elderly female with a lesion on a bend of the right coronary artery. This type of situation is particularly prone to dissection, and often "drilling" an adequate lumen in the vessel will relieve symptoms and achieve a good result.

As mentioned above, polyvinyl chloride and other balloon catheter material can be increased in size by inflating at high atmosphere pressures. In doing so, a 3 mm balloon may be increased to approximately 3.3 mm, or a 2.5 mm balloon may be increased to 2.7 or 2.8 mm, and this may provide a useful alternative to exchanging for other balloon sizes (see balloon inflation chart in Appendix II–E). The choice of the balloon size is of paramount importance in both the success of the procedure and safety of the procedure to the patient. If a smaller than ideal balloon is chosen, the result may be inadequate dilatation with significant residual narrowing and increased risk of restenosis. Failure to select the proper balloon size carefully may also lengthen the procedure if exchanging for a larger-size balloon is necessary, and this inadequate preprocedural preparation may not only prove more costly to the patient, but also expose the patient to more radiation and heavier contrast amounts. On the other hand, an oversized balloon may result in dissection, uncontrolled intimal injury, and also the need to exchange for a smaller balloon initially if the oversized balloon cannot cross a tight lesion. Meticulous attention to the selection of the proper balloon size prior to the procedure should be the trademark of an expert practitioner of angioplasty.

The stiffness of the shaft of the dilatation catheter system provides the support necessary to cross very tight stenoses. Some balloon catheter systems have very flexible shafts in order to conform with vessels, and these do not have the "pushability" necessary to cross tight lesions, particularly in distal vessels. On the other hand, balloon catheter systems with good "pushability" may not have the maneuverability to traverse tortuous vessels, particularly if tight curves are present. Preprocedural evaluation of the artery proximal and distal to the lesion, as well as the lesion itself, is important in choosing the proper dilatation catheter system that will result in the best chance for success of the procedure. The consistency of the tip of the dilatation catheter is also important. The softer the tip, the easier it usually is to get through a lesion. A tapered tip may be advantageous in successfully traversing severe stenoses. The characteristics of the individual balloon catheter material and tip configurations are available from the catheter company representatives.

The "balloon-on-wire" systems are sometimes very advantageous in crossing severely stenotic lesions. Any operator with reasonable experience has had the problem of being able to get a wire across a lesion but not having the proper back-up support to push the higher profile of the dilatation catheter through the lesion. The balloon-on-wire systems tend to minimize this difficulty, and if, indeed, the lesion can be wired, the balloon is then in position to be inflated. Hartzler-type catheters (Fig. 2–11) and the ACE catheter from Sci-Med (Fig. 2–12) are particularly good examples of this type of catheter system. They are, in general, less steerable but more pushable and trackable than are the over-the-wire systems.

Rapid-exchange catheter systems, such as the RX dilatation catheter or the Piccolino system from Schneider-Shiley, offer the advantage of utilizing a standard-length guide wire and being able to rapidly exchange the balloon catheter system for different sizes. This has particular implication in the crossing of very severely stenotic lesions with a small balloon diameter and then upsizing to the appropriate balloon size for the vessel. These catheters are quite flexible and maneuverable and have good pushability. Some balloons have the unique ability to conform to the shape of the vessel even at high-pressure inflations. These catheters should be selected if the lesion is on a curve in the artery such that a less compliant balloon might straighten the curved segment during inflation and cause shearing forces on the vessel wall, thereby inviting dissection.

GUIDE WIRES

The safety and success of an angioplasty procedure often lies with the choice of an appropriate wire. Selection of the wire must consider the size and the need for the following qualities: steerability, flexibility,

formability, trackability, and pushability. I prefer to use 0.014 inch wires, and the "workhorse" wire at present is the 0.014 Hi-Torque Floppy II from ACS. The flexible wire from USCI is also quite good, and both of these wires afford good steerability with very flexible tips and a high degree of safety. The 0.016 inch and 0.018 inch wires are also made with very safe tips, and many practitioners prefer these larger-size wires since they are a bit more steerable. As mentioned elsewhere in this book, the 0.014 intermediate wire from ACS is a "magic" wire in terms of crossing total occlusions, and often if a total occlusion is present, this is the wire that is used as first choice. Most of these wires afford excellent steerability, and the ability to custom-form the shape of the tip of the wire is facilitated as is the ability to track along a tortuous vessel. The coefficient of friction of the wire is greatly enhanced by the application of Microglide or other slippery substances, which is probably most important in the passage of the dilatation catheter system over the wire and not the initial wiring of the artery itself. All these wires also provide superior support to enhance the trackability and pushability of the dilatation catheter system over the wire.

In wires with tapered inner cores (mandril) that end a variety of lengths before the tip of the wire, the tip of the wire is very safe but may tend to buckle. Advancement of the dilatation catheter system over the mandril junction can stiffen the tip of the wire, and although this maneuver provides better pushability, it does decrease the safety of the procedure. One must be careful in this concert between dilatation catheter and wire to avoid using the tip of the wire as a spear. If the dilatation catheter is advanced too far toward the tip of the wire, advancing the wire results in pushing a very sharp and stiff object within the artery, and this may result in arterial perforation. A newer generation of USCI guide wires is available in fully silicon-coated configuration, and this wire has been proven to be very steerable, and the ability to advance various dilatation catheter systems over it has been excellent. A 0.018 high-torque floppy wire manufactured by ACS has an excellent one-to-one torque response as well as a safe, formable tip, and is favored by many practitioners (Appendix II–G).

Extendible wire systems have proven to be a great advantage during angioplasty. The ability to increase the length of the wire allows removal of an entire dilatation catheter system with the wire still across the lesion. This provides the safety of not having to re-cross an area that has already been dilated. The use of an extendible wire or an exchange wire can also provide better postangioplasty evaluation of results.

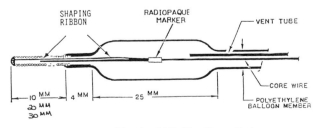

Fig. 2–11. Hartzler LPS dilatation catheter.

1.5 ACE™ Catheter

Atraumatic, radiopaque, 20 mm spring tip has shaping characteristics to make custom curves and traverse tortuous anatomies

Design of core wire to distal tip provides 1:1 torque

Dual bonding system for tip stability

Smooth taper from tip to balloon for crossing of tight stenoses

Heat set memory of the POC balloon maintains its low profile, even after multiple inflations. It has minimal postpurge winging

Proximal marker band for precise placement

Uni-body core wire provides steerability for negotiating tight bends

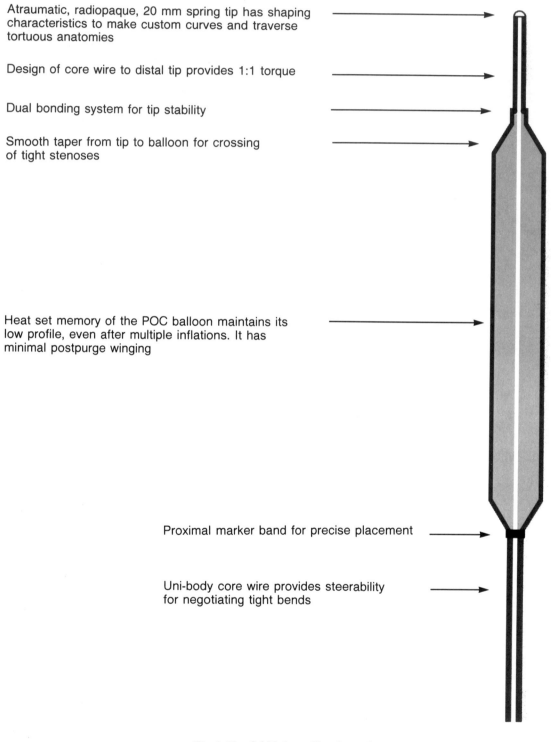

Fig. 2–12. Sci-Med ace dilatation catheter.

Injecting through the guiding catheter with the balloon catheter withdrawn just slightly from the tip of the guide is sometimes difficult, depending on the profile of the balloon catheter and the winging of the previously inflated balloon, but withdrawing the dilatation catheter system entirely from the guide over an extended or exchange wire provides only the impediment of the wire diameter to dye injection, and the contrast flow is excellent. If the imaging system present does not allow for adequate visualization with minimal contrast injection, this maneuver can be used to provide nearly normal injection of contrast through the guiding catheter for result assessment. Examples of this type of system are shown in Figure 2–13.

The "feel" of the guide wire is something that must be gained by experience and cannot be learned by reading or by observation. Advancement of the guide wire within the dilatation catheter should always be free, and *any* resistance to motion is excessive and may indicate a faulty wire or lumen in the dilatation catheter. This movement should be thoroughly checked prior to insertion of the dilatation catheter and wire into the guiding catheter system. In general, with over-the-wire systems, the guide wire is moved independently and first into the target vessel and across the lesion with the distal vessel then being wired for support. Moving the guide wire independently of the dilatation catheter provides valuable tactile information. Bends or kinks in the wire shaft will destroy torque, and whippy intracoronary wire movements resulting from kinked wires are a negative factor in both safety and steerability. Wire movements should be measured in millimeters, not centimeters, and any impedance to advancement of the wire in the target vessel probably indicates that it is either beneath a plaque or in a small side branch. In these situations, the wire should be slightly withdrawn, the tip moved into a different orientation, and then advancement tried again. Buckling of the wire tip with advancement pressure generally indicates a problem, but is sometimes acceptable for tight lesions and/or total occlusions. If mandril-buckling impedes wire progress, as noted above, advancement of the dilatation catheter in a careful manner over the mandril can solve this problem. Advancement of the dilatation catheter to an area just proximal to the lesion and subsequently changing a buckling wire for a "stiffer" wire, such as the 0.014 intermediate wire from ACS, provides a combination of safety of proximal wiring through a tortuous diseased vessel as well as enhanced ability to cross a severely stenotic lesion.

If an abrupt closure has occurred and the patient is returned to the laboratory, or in the case of dissection and impending closure in the laboratory during the procedure, a soft, very flexible-tipped wire is the safest for crossing or recrossing the previously dilated segment. In the use of wire systems with mandrils, the floppy tip of the wire should be advanced 2–3 cm beyond the lesion so that the mandril is distal and the segment of wire across the lesion provides stability and ease of advancement of the dilatation catheter system over it.

Some basic parameters should be checked before the dilatation catheter system complete with wire is advanced into the guiding catheter for use. It must be made certain that the torquing device is tightly adherent to the wire. This can be checked by turning the torque device and watching the tip of the wire. A 1:1 ratio should be present. When extendible wires are used, the torque device should not be back on the hypo tubing lumen since the appropriate tightness of the torque device could pinch the lumen and the extension option would then be lost.

When adding shape to the wire tip, one should not tug on the distal tip weld. This may snap the tip weld from the tapered safety-forming wire and could cause dangerous unraveling or breaking of the wire distally in the vessel. Torqueability may also be lost. The tip of the wire can be reshaped either by using one's fingernail or by using an instrument, such as a needle, to shape the wire. If the wire becomes caught in a vessel and starts to unravel, this is identifiable since the tip of the wire stays in place and there is an apparent discontinuity between the proximal and distal wire. The safety wire is usually still in place but is not readily radiopaque. The administration of intracoronary nitroglycerin may relax the vessel (particularly a small septal or side branch in which the tip of the wire may be caught), and then gentle tugging on the wire may cause it to come back. Advancing the dilatation catheter up to the unraveled wire tip while pulling the wire back can facilitate easier removal of the dislodged tip from then ensnaring coronary vessel. Torquing of the wire in vivo more than three or four times in the same direction can also cause the distal soldered tip in some wires to snap loose.

In vivo forming of the tip of the wire is sometimes helpful. By selecting a small vessel and engaging the wire tip in it, the tip can be made to buckle, thereby producing a more acute angle in the tip of the wire. By pulling back and turning the wire toward the target vessel, this tip can be made to "flip" across a curve in the vessel. This maneuver is not recommended if one uses a stiff wire. For the "hooking wire" technique, a softer wire should be used. With this technique, one can hook the wire tip in a small vessel distally, thereby anchoring the wire to facilitate balloon advancement. For example, in the right coronary

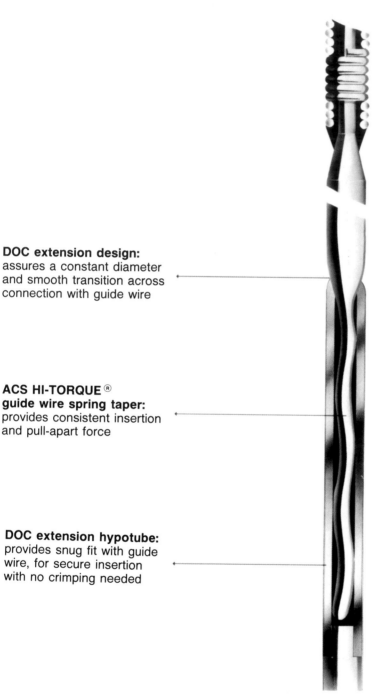

**DOC™
Guide Wire
Extension**

DETACHABLE: Design
provides a rapid,
reliable method for
extending any 175 cm
ACS HI-TORQUE®
guide wire to 320 cm
exchange length.
Extension also permits
detaching, to revert
to original 175 cm
guide wire length.

DOC extension design:
assures a constant diameter
and smooth transition across
connection with guide wire

**ACS HI-TORQUE®
guide wire spring taper:**
provides consistent insertion
and pull-apart force

DOC extension hypotube:
provides snug fit with guide
wire, for secure insertion
with no crimping needed

Fig. 2–13.   DOC guide wire extension.

artery, the atrioventricular nodal artery, posterior descending artery, posterolateral branches of the right coronary artery, or inferior septal branches may be used. In the circumflex, the second or third obtuse marginal branches may be used, and in the left anterior descending coronary artery, the distal LAD around the apex or septal branches in the LAD may be used for this technique. During these maneuvers, great care must be taken to observe the EKG for arrhythmias and the patient for anginal symptoms.

In dealing with diffusely diseased arteries or, in particular, diffusely diseased vein grafts, advancement of the wire is sometimes difficult because the tip of the wire may become lodged beneath the irregular surface of the vessel. Preforming of the tip of the wire into a "U" configuration allows the wire to pass through a sufficiently large vessel with the leading "U" bouncing off the irregularities rather than a straight tip digging under them. This is similar to the use of a "J" wire to advance diagnostic and guiding catheters through diseased aortic segments. An example of this technique is seen in Case 16 in Appendix I and on the video tape accompanying this book.

One of the principal keys to successful angioplasty is controlled wire manipulation and successful intraluminal wiring of the vessel. Haphazard or "roto-rooter" style of advancement of a wire is dangerous, and in any wire manipulation, excellent visibility of the tip of the wire as well as the availability of proximal contrast injections are necessary to successfully complete the procedure. Today's high-resolution images and excellent videodisc and digital subtraction systems can generally provide this information. Good preliminary angiograms are necessary to identify the view necessary to separate the lesion from overlapping anatomy or vessels, and angulated and inventive views are often helpful.

INFLATION DEVICES

A variety of mechanical devices to inflate and deflate the balloon are available. All of these have accompanying pressure gauges. Some have digital readouts that not only show the atmospheres of inflation pressure, but also the time of inflation and the number of inflations performed. Some degree of pressure measurement is necessary to give the angiographer a method of quantifying the amount of pressure applied to the balloon. Although it is sometimes common practice in peripheral angioplasty to inflate balloons without accompanying pressure-measuring devices, this is not appropriate in coronary angioplasty. With the availability of high-pressure balloons,

an inadvertent amount of very high pressures could be used in an unintended setting. The amount of pressure necessary to get the advertised size of the balloon catheter is available from the various manufacturers, and this is another reason for always using pressure manometers with the procedure.

The mechanical inflation devices are also capable of applying greater pressure to the balloon than can be achieved by hand inflation alone. The fatigue factor of hand inflations also plays a factor, and in most of the mechanical systems, a "lock" is present in order to hold a steady pressure for a long period of time.

OTHER DEVICES

The manifold and injection syringe assembly must be both stable and comfortable and capable of allowing the operator to firmly and safely inject contrast throughout the procedure to identify the wire route and monitor progress during angioplasty. Most of the manifolds and injection syringes are now made of plastic-type materials, and the marriage between the manifold and injection syringe must be stable and not conducive to the forming or trapping of air bubbles. Whether a two-, three-, or four-port manifold is used is entirely the operator's choice and usually reflects that which the operator is comfortable with during diagnostic angiography.

I find a 6 inch extension tubing between the Y-adaptor and the manifold to be helpful in allowing the manifold to be out of the field of manipulation during the wire and dilatation catheter movement phase of PTCA.

The immediate presence of a baseline EKG strip visualized on the monitor (or taped to it) throughout the procedure allows the operator to have an instant comparison with the real-time EKG tracing, rather than relying on one's memory of the configuration.

It is strongly advised that the operator and technicians protect themselves to the fullest with lead glasses, thyroid shields, and room shields against the prolonged X-ray exposure inherent to the procedure of PTCA.

FUTURE TECHNOLOGY

Balloon catheter research and development have exploded in recent years. Many companies now are competing to produce the ideal balloon catheter, the ideal wire, and ideal ancillary equipment. I do not believe that any one company has the franchise on all of these systems, and each operator should be aware of the variety of instruments available and keep well versed on advancements in technology. Refinements will undoubtedly center on decreasing the balloon shaft diameter, increasing the strength of the balloon, and decreasing the balloon resistance to passage over the wire. Multidirectional wire-tip guide wires may also become available in the near future.

Other devices, such as atherectomy catheters, lasers, and stents, are described in Chapter 13 (New Technologies for the Treatment of Obstructive Arterial Disease). Additional comments regarding equipment are made in Appendix II–E—G and also in the audio portion of the video tape accompanying the book.

HARDWARE ASSEMBLY

In the first edition of this book, detailed instructions regarding the preparation of a few catheter systems were presented. This is no longer appropriate since a large number of dilatation catheter systems are available and this information is readily available from the manufacturer. After the proper guiding catheter, balloon, and wire have been selected, the balloon must be properly prepared. Various balloon catheter systems prep in different manners, and the operator and his/her staff should be fully conversant with the proper way to inflate and test the balloons.

In some balloon catheter systems, it is possible to prep the balloon with the balloon tip shield still in place over the balloon itself. This minimizes winging and allows one to have the smallest possible diameter of the balloon available to cross severe stenoses.

The solution used to fill the balloon should be contrast medium diluted with normal saline. The mixture of contrast, be it Renografin, Hypaque, or Amipaque, should be a 50/50 ratio for balloons 2.0–3.0 mm in size and a 40/60 ratio in larger balloons so that the inflation and deflation time is not compromised because of thicker contrast medium.

The insertion of the guide wire into the dilatation catheter can be accomplished either in a forward manner or by back loading the dilatation catheter. Forward loading has the advantage of advancing the softest portion of the wire through the inner lumen of the balloon catheter system, whereas in back loading

(which always is the case with extendible systems when balloons are changed during the procedure), the stiff end of the wire is inserted through the tip end of the dilatation catheter. This has some advantage in the initial preparation of the system in that the soft steerable end of the wire is then protected from any damage in passing through the balloon catheter system.

Once the balloon catheter system is prepared—the wire in the inner lumen, the balloon tested, and the inflation device connected—the entire system can be passed through the "Y" adaptor and then the "Y" adaptor connected to the pressure and contrast manifold. Whether a two, three, or four-port manifold is used is entirely the operator's preference, and in most cases it should be the same as that which the operator comfortably uses during diagnostic angiography. Care should be taken in advancing the dilatation catheter system through the "Y" connector that no bubbles of air are trapped and carried along with the system.

Once the dilatation catheter system has been passed through the guiding catheter and is in position in the artery, when balloon inflation occurs, it is sometimes necessary to loosen the "Y" connector so that the pressure can be transmitted to the balloon itself. When guiding catheter injections are made, the Touhey-Boorst connection must be tight so that there is no retrograde flow of contrast and that the dye is injected into the target artery.

When the dilatation catheter system is advanced through the target artery, at least 2 or 3 cm of wire should lead this in (in over-the-wire systems) so that the tip of the wire has its usual flexibility and is not made stiffer by the advancement of the dilatation catheter over the flexible tip. When the procedure is completed, removal of the wire and dilatation catheter should be deliberate, firm, and slow and should be done under direct vision on fluoroscopy. This assures that the tip of the wire is not caught and comes along with the maneuver and also that the guiding catheter tip does not dive deeply into the target artery because of the withdrawal of the dilatation catheter.

The proper selection of guiding catheter to coaxially intubate the target coronary artery, the careful sizing and selection of balloon catheter types, and the use of a safe flexible and steerable guide wire all work in concert to ensure a successful result of angioplasty and also to protect the safety of the patient.

3. Selection of Patients for PTCA

The initial clinical indications for selection of patients for angioplasty included only those patients with demonstrated reversible myocardial ischemia, who were absolutely or relatively refractory to medical therapy such that the patients were considered to be candidates for bypass graft surgery. From an anatomic standpoint, an acceptable lesion had to be a proximal, discrete, concentric, noncalcified stenosis that was both approachable and crossable with the equipment available. It was estimated in the late 1970s and early 1980s that 3–5% of patients who were candidates for bypass graft surgery could be treated by balloon angioplasty.

The indications for percutaneous transluminal coronary artery angioplasty markedly widened in the 1980s for several basic reasons. In 1980, the material and process used to manufacture guiding catheters was changed, making them more manipulable and at the same time safer for use. These developmental changes in guiding catheters allowed for better torque control and, at the same time, enhanced the ease of passage of balloon catheter systems through them as well as the ability to inject contrast material through the guide for better visualization even with the balloon catheter in place. These changes made the entire procedure more efficient and safe for the majority of appropriately selected patients. A more striking change occurred in the balloon catheter system with the development and introduction of the steerable mechanism in 1983. This steerable catheter system made it much more likely that, in experienced hands, a lesion could be reached and crossed safely. The development of the guiding and balloon catheter systems is well documented by Jang et al. (see Bibliography).

Throughout the 1980s, continued progress was made by various catheter companies toward the production of safer and better guiding catheters and countless variations of balloon dilatation catheter systems to deal with specific problems. This progress has further widened the anatomic indications for angioplasty. Many balloon catheters are now available that enhance "trackability" to accommodate very tortuous vessels. At the same time, these catheters have a high degree of "pushability" to allow severe lesions to be crossed, once reached. High-pressure balloons now extend the procedure to patients with calcified, or "harder," old lesions.

Advances in techniques have also expanded the horizons of angioplasty. The development and frequent use of the "kissing balloon" technique for bifurcation lesions has made safe angioplasty available to patients with that anatomic configuration. Initially performed with two guiding catheters and two balloon and wire systems from either the bifemoral or brachial-femoral approach, it is now common to use one guiding catheter with two guide wires with one exchangeable balloon to protect and sequentially dilate bifurcation lesions. This development has not only broadened the application of the "kissing balloon" or "kissing wire" technique to practitioners not familiar with the brachial approach, but also has made it faster and safer.

The development of techniques to cross total occlusions in patients with recently totally occluded arteries has expanded the indications to this subset of patients as well. Better back-up from guiding catheters and several new wire configurations has enhanced the ability to cross total occlusions (see Chapter 2, Coronary Angioplasty Equipment).

The current clinical indications for angioplasty remain much the same as originally described. The patient should have a severe stenosis in one or more major coronary arteries with a significant amount of myocardium at risk and with demonstrated reversible ischemia in the distribution of the stenotic vessel. These patients should be refractory either absolutely or relatively to medical treatment and should be considered candidates for bypass graft surgery by the individual practitioner's own criteria for that selection process. Exceptions to these situations exist and should be recognized particularly in patients who are elderly or who have concomitant serious diseases of other organ systems.

Because of the aforementioned developments in guiding and balloon catheter systems as well as techniques, the anatomic indications for angioplasty have been greatly expanded. Prior to 1983, it was estimated that 95% of cases performed were patients with single-vessel disease and only 5% fell into the "complex" category. Since the advent of the steerable balloon catheter system in 1983, the percentage of "complex" cases has markedly increased, and now approximately 60% of patients treated by experienced practitioners fall into the "complex" category with less than 40%

having straightforward, single-vessel disease. Table 3–1 outlines the relative incidence of subsets within the category of complex angioplasty. Patients in this complex group include those with left main coronary disease, bifurcation lesions treatable by the kissing balloon technique, recent total occlusion in major epicardial coronary arteries, stenotic lesions in vein bypass grafts or internal mammary bypass grafts, multiple-vessel disease in which all lesions are amenable to angioplasty treatment, and tandem or multiple lesions in one artery or long segmental stenoses in a single coronary artery.

Anatomic contraindications to angioplasty are important to recognize. It should be understood that the evaluation of the suitability of anatomic configurations for PTCA is an evolutionary situation dependent on changes and advances in both technology and technique. For example, calcified lesions were initially thought to be a contraindication for PTCA because the "hardness" of such lesions predictably would not respond to the amount of pressure that could be exerted by the early balloon catheter systems. The development of higher-pressure balloons has virtually ended this concern, and we have had "hard" lesions that have been successfully dilated by the application of pressures in excess of 20 atm. Tortuous arteries that could not be successfully negotiated by the early dilatation catheter systems can now be successfully and safely wired with delicate steerable systems in the hands of experienced operators. Once such a vessel has been "wired," one now has an excellent chance to cross the lesion successfully with the dilatation catheter because of both technological advances in guiding catheter configurations (e.g., Arani) to provide back-up force and the "trackability" of the more advanced dilatation catheters to allow the balloon to reach and successfully cross the lesion in a tortuous vessel. If long segmental disease and/or tandem lesions are present, a situation previously thought to be a relatively strong contraindications to PTCA, this type of lesion is now approachable because of the delicate maneuverability of the guide wire across such stenoses and the

favorable experience that has been gained by attempting such lesions. Long (3–4 cm) balloons are also available to provide complete rather than multiple sequential inflations to mold an area of long stenosis. Figure 3–1 demonstrates one such case. Lesions in saphenous vein grafts, an increasingly common disease as more and more post-CABG patients reach the 5–10 year postoperative interval, can now be safely treated in a large number of cases, but the older vein grafts still represent a relative contraindication to PTCA (see below).

Severely stenotic lesions that might previously have been considered a contraindication to angioplasty can now be attempted because of the technologic development of lower dilatation catheter profiles and better guiding catheter back-up systems (see Chapter 2, Coronary Angioplasty Equipment). Nearly all companies now produce an extremely low profile catheter system that can often solve the problem of crossing a severely stenotic lesion and result in successful dilatation in cases in which the older equipment was simply too high profile to allow the dilatation catheter system to cross the stenosis. The tapered tips of newer balloon catheter systems are very helpful in the successful engagement and crossing of these difficult lesions. Low-profile, trackable, and pushable balloon catheters such as the ACX system from ACS and the new "shadow" from Sci-Med as well as multiple balloon-on-wire systems are the latest versions of the new generation of "problem-solving" catheters.

Eccentric lesions, which might have been viewed with dismay and concern 10 years ago, are now approachable and crossable because of the steerability and extreme flexibility available in dilatation catheter systems. The wires allow for micromanipulation of the guide wire to assure crossage in the true lumen of an eccentric lesion. It should be strongly emphasized that the increased success rates in all of these areas are greatly dependent on the remarkable advances that have been made in imaging systems over the past 10 years as well. Better visualization by videodisc systems and magnification of areas of stenosis by digital subtraction techniques (Fig. 3–2) also allow the experienced operator to see the exact nature of the eccentricity and thereby maneuver the guide wire safely across the stenosis.

With advances in imaging techniques, guiding catheters, and dilatation catheter systems, the time may be approaching when there will be no absolute anatomic contraindications to an angioplasty attempt on the basis of the location or configuration of a lesion. There are, however, several anatomic problems that should be recognized as, if not absolute,

TABLE 3–1. Complex Angioplasty

	Percent
Multiple vessel	39
Tandem and long segmental stenoses	22
Total occlusion	16
Bifurcation lesions	6
Grafts (SVG/IMA)	12
Left main stem	5

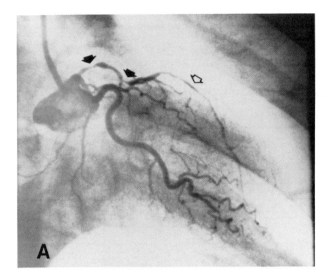

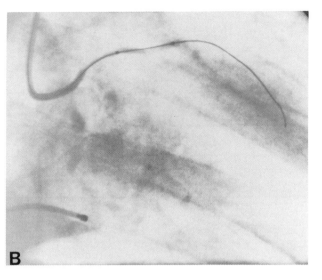

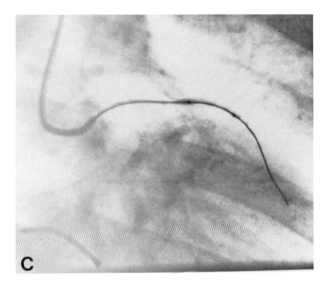

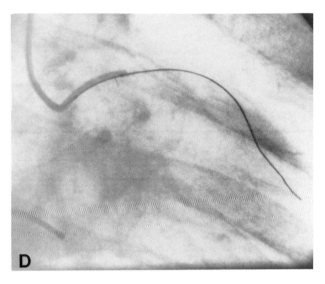

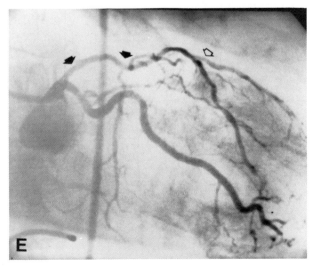

Fig. 3–1.   A: Left coronary artery. RAO projection. Arrows indicate long segment of severe disease in LAD. **B:** Left coronary artery. RAO projection. Initial balloon inflation at site of most severe stenosis to allow passage through the rest of the long diseased segment. **C:** Left coronary artery. RAO projection. Balloon inflation in distal portion of long segmental disease. **D:** Left coronary artery. RAO projection. Balloon inflated in proximal portion of long segmental disease. Inflations seen in B–D overlapped entire area of long segmental stenosis. **E:** Left coronary artery. RAO projection. Post-PTCA angiogram shows excellent improvement in lumen of LAD with increased distal flow (arrows).

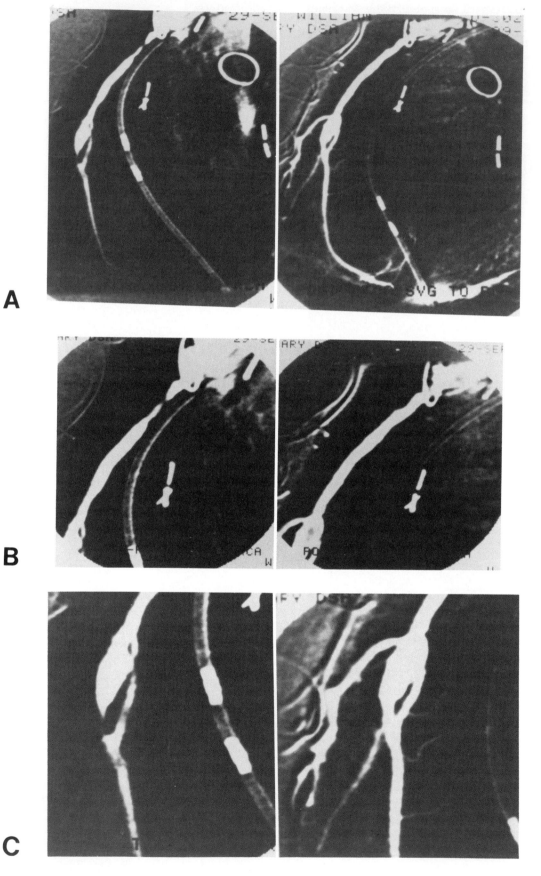

certainly strong relative contraindications to the procedure.

Unprotected left main coronary disease, which will be discussed at length elsewhere, remains a strong relative contraindication to angioplasty. If there is no "protection" of the left main trunk, either by previous bypass surgery or by excellent collateral filling of either the left anterior descending or circumflex branches of the left main trunk, then, in most cases, left main coronary disease stenosis should be treated by surgery. The position of a lesion in the left main trunk, in an unprotected setting, obviously affects nearly two-thirds of the myocardium in most individuals. With the concept of supported angioplasty, utilizing the cardiopulmonary bypass support system, prolonged balloon inflations in the left main coronary or a left main "equivalent" lesion do not cause great concern when this technique is employed; however, a dissection, spasm, or abrupt closure of a dilated segment in that position obviously could have catastrophic consequences and mitigates against safe presentation of the patient for emergency bypass surgery. In addition to this, the development of restenosis in the left main trunk theoretically could present with sudden closure and fatal infarction because of the large amount of myocardium distal to the potential recurrence site.

Origin stenosis of the right coronary artery is also a relative contraindication to angioplasty. Lesions in this particular anatomic position are often a combination of lesions of the coronary artery and the aorta, and successful dilatation is certainly a lower percentage procedure than are dilatations of lesions truly in the coronary artery. However, with higher-pressure balloons and longer molding dilatations available, orificial disease can be approached by angioplasty in selected cases (Fig. 3–3).

Although ectasia of coronary arteries is not by itself a contraindication to angioplasty attempt of severely stenotic sclerotic segments in such vessels, particularly if the ectasia is just proximal or distal to the area of stenosis to be dilated, it does represent a relative contraindication to angioplasty (Fig. 3–4). These aneurysmal segments potentially contain thrombotic or friable material that can be dislodged by the guide wire manipulation necessary in that area or by balloon inflations and cause distal emboli resulting in infarction or the need for emergency bypass surgery. In addition, there appears to be an increased risk of significant dissection of localized lesions with adjacent aneurysmal dilation in this type of artery (Appendix I—Case 21).

Old total occlusions of coronary arteries represent a strong relative contraindication to angioplasty when viewed in the context of likelihood of success. As will be discussed in more detail in Chapter 6 (Complex PTCA II: Total Occlusions), if a total occlusion has been present for more than 4 months, the chance of success drops dramatically to less than 20%. In such cases, the organization of the area of total occlusion is such that the ability to traverse the solid occlusion with the safe guide wires utilized simply is prohibited. The use of the hot-tip laser may in the future enhance the ability to cross older total occlusions (see Chapter 13, New Technologies for the Treatment of Obstructive Arterial Disease). Several new guide wires, such as the 0.014 intermediate wire from ACS, have been demonstrated to have dramatically higher success rates in crossing total occlusions and should be kept in the laboratories' armamentarium available for cases of total occlusions. The early encouraging experience with thermal laser angioplasty in peripheral vessels suggested that such old total obstructions in coronary vessels could be successfully dilated using the thermal laser probe to cross the area of occlusion initially and provide a small lumen through which a standard coronary guide wire and dilatation balloon catheter system could be passed with subsequent successful balloon angioplasty carried out. In fact, the deliverability of such laser catheter systems to the area of total occlusion has frustrated the success of this technique.

Old, diffusely diseased saphenous vein bypass grafts are strong relative contraindications to angioplasty. One must view a graft over 5 years old as being lined with friable material amenable to dislodgment and distal embolization by the guide wire or dilatation catheter system. Figure 3–5 demonstrates problems encountered in such situations and demonstrates why stenotic lesions involving older vein grafts should be viewed as strong relative contraindication to angioplasty. As experience with PTCA continues, and as improvements in technology and technique progress, anatomic indications and contraindications to angioplasty will evolve and be clarified.

A general rule that should be followed in viewing angiograms to assess whether the patient is a candidate for angioplasty is as follows: Review of the diagnostic angiogram should result in determining whether the patient is a candidate for medical therapy or bypass graft surgery. It should be viewed in the context that PTCA does not exist as a therapeutic alternative. If, by the practitioners own criteria, the

Fig. 3–2. **A:** Digital subtraction angiogram of SVG to RCA demonstrating proximal and distal stenoses pre- and post-PTCA. **B:** Digital subtraction enlargement of proximal stenosis pre- and post-PTCA. **C:** Digital subtraction enlargement of distal stenosis pre- and post-PTCA.

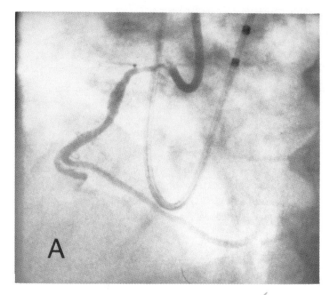

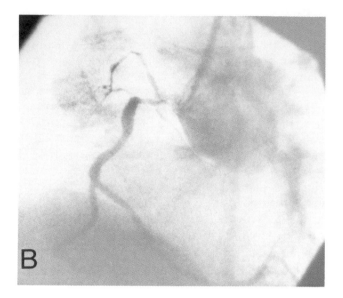

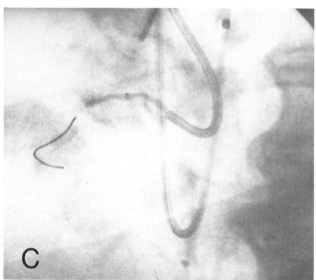

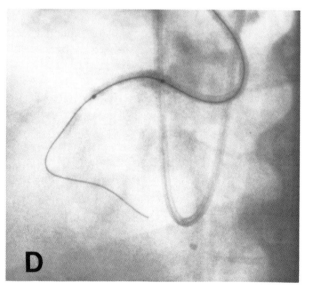

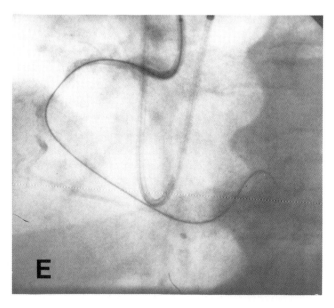

Fig. 3–3. A: Right coronary artery, LAO projection, severe ostial stenosis. **B:** Right coronary artery, left lateral projection, severe ostial stenosis. **C:** Right coronary artery, LAO projection, Hartzler dilatation catheter across ostial stenosis with balloon inflated (2 mm). **D:** Right coronary artery, LAO projection, 3 mm balloon inflated across ostium after entry gained by 2 mm Hartzler balloon. **E:** Right coronary artery, LAO projection, post-PTCA double injection through guide and dilatation catheter showing excellent proximal lumen and good distal flow. Note wire left in artery as stent for post-PTCA angiogram to avoid trauma to dilated ostium.

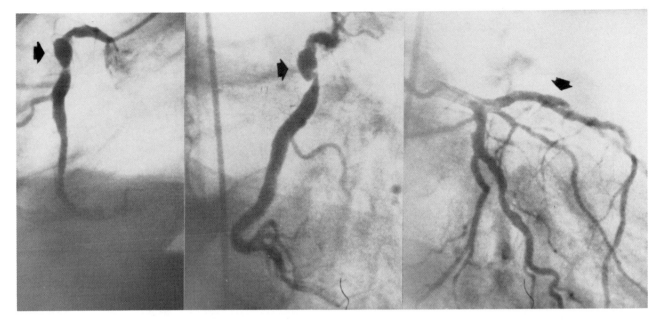

Fig. 3–4. The left and center panels demonstrate LAO and RAO views of the right coronary artery with proximal aneursymal dilatation not favorable for PTCA attempt. The right panel shows a similar area in the patient's left anterior descending artery.

patient would not be considered for bypass graft surgery, but would be treated medically, then that patient is generally not considered to be a good candidate for angioplasty. If, however, the patient is thought to be a good candidate for bypass graft surgery, then the angiogram should be rereviewed with an eye toward whether all arteries to be bypassed could be as effectively treated with angioplasty. In general, the goal of angioplasty should be to achieve as complete revascularization as can be achieved by bypass graft surgery, although some exceptions to that goal exist and will be discussed below.

In viewing the angiograms and deciding whether the patient is a candidate for angioplasty, the safety of the patient should be the foremost factor in the equation. If the angiographer believes that all the significant coronary lesions can be approached by angioplasty and a revascularization result achieved that would equal the result achieved by bypass graft surgery, then one must decide if the patient can be safely treated with angioplasty. One must keep in mind that between 3 and 5% of patients undergoing an angioplasty attempt at experienced centers will require emergency bypass graft surgery. The question should then be asked, In a worst-case scenario, were the patient to require emergency bypass graft surgery, could that be accomplished in a safe manner for the patient? One example of this situation in which a patient may be more safely treated by elective bypass graft surgery than by a PTCA attempt would be a patient with severely compromised left ventricular

function resulting from previous myocardial infarctions and a severe lesion in the major artery supplying the remaining amount of the patient's viable functioning myocardium. Were this vessel to close abruptly during the angioplasty procedure, one could predict that the patient would then have no significant amount of functioning myocardium, and, certainly, this patient could be more safely treated by calm, elective bypass graft surgery than by being transported to emergency bypass graft surgery under cardiopulmonary resuscitative efforts. Even though the lesion may appear ideal for angioplasty, the ability to transport the patient safely to the surgical suite for bypass graft surgery, should arterial closure occur, must dictate whether the patient should undergo an angioplasty attempt. The use of supported angioplasty (CPS) using the cardiopulmonary support system has extended the procedure of angioplasty to many such patients, but it should be cautioned that each case must be viewed individually and the procedure recommended should be that procedure that is the safest for the patient. In many cases, the use of supported angioplasty in such a setting could be argued to be safer than even calm, elective bypass graft surgery since the inherent surgical risk in such patients is also increased. Figure 3–6 represents a high-risk situation that, although anatomically suitable for PTCA, is better treated by elective bypass graft surgery.

It is suggested that the physician reviewing an angiogram to assess a patient for angioplasty should be ischemia-oriented rather than lesion-oriented. This is

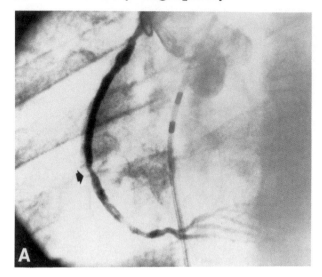

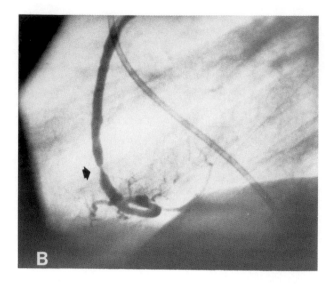

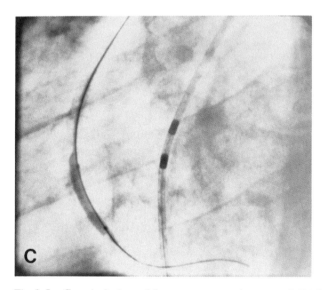

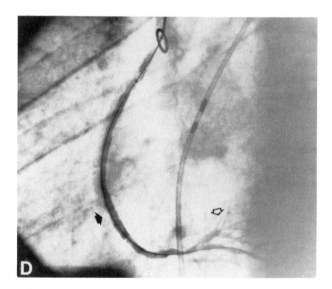

Fig. 3–5. Case A. A: Aortoright coronary artery bypass graft. LAO projection. Lesion in graft body 80% (arrow) with extensive distal distribution dependent on graft. **B:** Aortoright coronary artery bypass graft. Left lateral projection. Stenosis indicated by arrow. **C:** Aortoright coronary artery bypass graft. LAO projection. Balloon fully in- flated and distal native vessel wired. **D:** Aortoright coronary artery bypass graft. LAO projection, post-PTCA. Area of stenosis fully dilated (solid arrow). Note decreased flow in distal native vessels (open arrow) compared with A.

particularly true in case of multiple-vessel disease. The primary goal of angioplasty should be to achieve complete revascularization of ischemic myocardium. In almost all cases of multiple-vessel disease, one or more lesions appear anatomically ideal for angio- plasty. Except in special circumstances, patients in whom complete revascularization by PTCA cannot be anticipated should be referred for bypass graft sur- gery.

Incomplete revascularization by PTCA is accept- able in certain special circumstances, which include patients who are poor surgical candidates because of concurrent noncardiac diseases such as severe pulmo- nary disease, cancer, liver disease, or hematologic dis- orders. The referral of a patient who is a poor surgical risk often comes to the practitioner of angioplasty from the cardiac surgeon. If such a case is presented, the dilemma exists that the very fact that makes the patient a high surgical risk makes him a poor angio- plasty candidate as well. If a patient is deemed to be a poor elective surgical risk by the cardiac surgeon, then that risk must necessarily increase if angioplasty fails and the patient has to go to emergency bypass graft surgery. On the other hand, there is no question that in some cases patients who are poor surgical candidates can benefit from avoidance of that high-

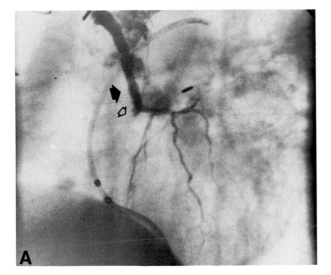

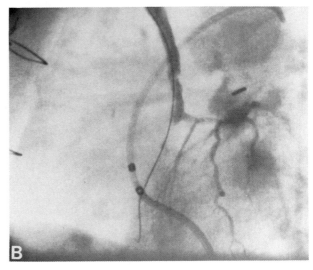

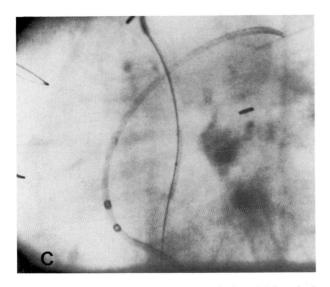

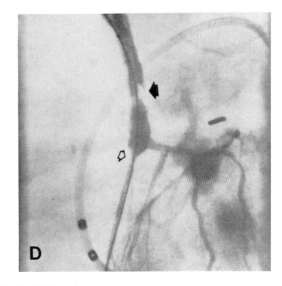

Fig. 3–5.   Case B. A: Aorto-LAD bypass graft. Steep LAO projection. The vessel is totally occluded at the distal anastomosis to the LAD (open arrow) with no antegrade flow into distal LAD. Note the area of interest in the graft (solid arrow). **B:** Aorto-LAD bypass graft. Steep LAO projection. This injection demonstrates wire across the area of total obstruction into native LAD. **C:** Aorto-LAD bypass graft. Steep LAO projection. Balloon inflated at distal anastomotic site. **D:** Aorto-LAD bypass graft. LAO projection. This double injection demonstrates patency of the distal anastomotic site (open arrow) with good flow into native LAD and also obvious filling defect (solid arrow) in body of graft.

See following page for continuation of figures.

risk surgery by angioplasty. In such cases, the risk of the angioplasty procedure including the potential for emergency bypass graft surgery must be weighed against the risk of the major surgical procedure itself. It is imperative that the patient and the patient's family be fully informed of the risks and benefits of both procedures and included in the decision.

Incomplete revascularization may also be acceptable in older patients with multiple-vessel disease, but in whom one target stenosis can be identified as the symptom-producing lesion. Because of the increased surgical risk in older patients, if the clinical syndrome can be "de-fused" by dilatation of the most severe lesion, perhaps other 70 or 80% lesions that are not producing ischemia and angina can be left alone and successful dilatation of the most severe lesion will allow the elderly patient to resume activity and achieve an acceptable quality of life without undergoing the trauma of open-chest bypass surgery.

Comment should also be made regarding an approach to patients with multiple-vessel disease who are either very unstable or in the early stages of an

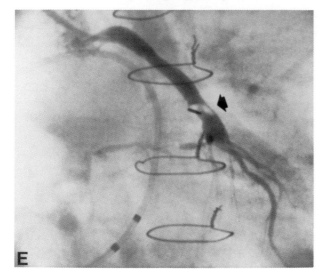

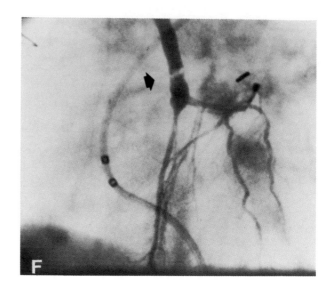

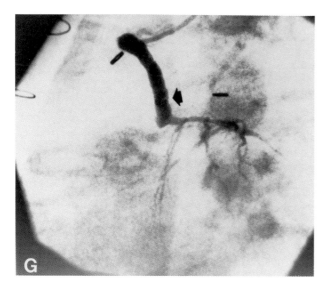

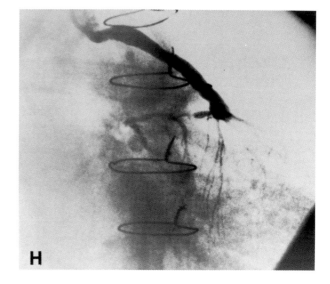

Fig. 3–5. Case B. E: Aorto-LAD bypass graft. RAO projection. Filling defect in graft post-PTCA (arrow). **F:** Aorto-LAD bypass graft. Steep LAO projection. Filling defect in graft (arrow). **G:** Aorto-LAD bypass graft. Steep LAO projection. Four months after PTCA. Arrow shows healing of filling defect in graft. Note recurrent total obstruction of LAD anastomotic site. **H:** Aorto-LAD bypass graft. RAO projection. Compare with E.

acute myocardial infarction. In these patients, it is important that only the target vessel producing the unstable clinical syndrome or causing the myocardial infarction should be treated at the first angioplasty procedure. These cases should then be staged with the patient brought back to the laboratory at a later date to have the other vessels dilated. This concept is important in that, if one segment of myocardium is in trouble from either ischemia or early infarction, and another segment at a distant site becomes jeopardized by the abrupt closure of a dilated vessel during angio-

plasty, then the risk to the patient is dramatically increased concomitant with the increased amount of myocardium jeopardized. The other advantage of a staged procedure in this set of circumstances is that the early results of the angioplasty of the first lesion can be assessed angiographically, and if excellent antegrade flow through the dilated vessel persists, then the other vessels can be approached in a safe manner. The safety factor provided by collaterals from recanalized arteries to other jeopardized vessels cannot be overemphasized. Therefore, in acute situations, only

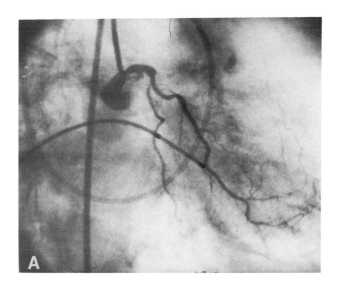

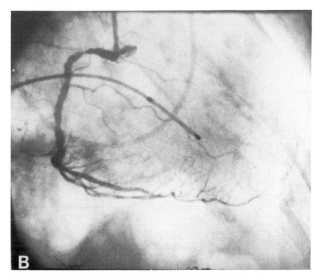

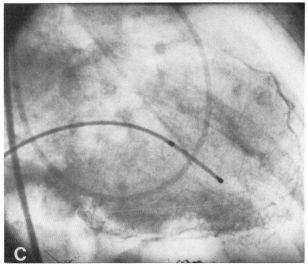

Fig. 3–6. **A:** Left coronary artery. RAO projection. Total occlusion of LAD (age unknown). **B:** Right coronary artery. RAO projection. Severe proximal RCA lesion with early septal collaterals to LAD. **C:** Right coronary artery. RAO projection. Late phase of B showing more complete collateral filling of LAD system via collaterals through septum.

the target vessel should be approached during the first procedure and the patient should be returned for a second stage to have other vessels dilated.

More specific comments regarding selection for angioplasty in patients with complex disease will be made in later chapters. Each patient must be assessed individually and the decision as to whether the case is appropriate for PTCA made with the safety of the patient considered first, and other factors, including technical appropriateness, viewed in that context.

4. PTCA Strategy

SELECTION OF EQUIPMENT

The selection of equipment for any lesion for angioplasty is determined by the appearance of the lesion, the position of the lesion in the artery, the size of the artery, and the configuration (i.e., tortuosity) of the artery both proximal and distal to the lesion or lesions to be dilated. Many catheter companies now have guides, balloons, and wires of similar configuration and excellence available. The differences between catheter companies, such as was seen in the early days of angioplasty between the ACS systems and the USCI systems, have now melded toward the midzone of equipment, and all are very similar. For example, for a straightforward lesion, there is little to choose between the ACX balloon catheter (ACS), the "skinny" system (Sci-Med), or the new "slinky" balloon from Baxter. The selection of equipment becomes more important when lesion aberrations are present. It is then important to know the advantages and disadvantages of various catheters, wires, and guides in order to successfully accomplish cases that are not straightforward. The main consideration is that all the basic components of angioplasty equipment—the guiding catheter, the dilatation catheter, and the guide wire—must function in harmony to provide the proper support, maneuverability, and trackability to accomplish angioplasty. The brand name used is not important, but operator familiarity with the system to be used is a very important factor.

In most cases of angioplasty, a right heart catheter with pacing capabilities is desirable. Many operators have discontinued the use of this insurance factor, but I still believe that it provides an important safety net that is not very time-consuming to introduce. The placement of a right heart catheter with pacing capabilities prior to the angioplasty gives the physician immediate access to pacing if needed during the procedure, and if a catheter with a central lumen is used, the ability to measure pulmonary pressures as well as the availability of a large central line is also present throughout the procedure. Balloon-tipped flow-directed catheters are easily maneuverable, and the balloon tip makes passage through the tricuspid valve and right ventricle into the pulmonary system significantly easier technically and also safer than with non-balloon-tipped catheters. Flow-directed pacing catheters pace more reliably if the tip is positioned in the right pulmonary artery than in the left.

SELECTION OF APPROACH

It is estimated that the femoral or brachial approach can be used with equal efficacy in approximately 90% of cases. In the other 10% of cases, an advantage may exist if either the femoral or brachial technique is chosen.

The first consideration in selection of the approach should be familiarity of the operator with the technique. Particularly with angiographers who are trained in the femoral (Judkins) technique, attempts to do angioplasty by the brachial approach may prove both frustrating and dangerous. It is somewhat easier for the physician trained in the brachial technique to adapt to the femoral approach for either angioplasty or diagnostic procedures. In general, the rule should be that the practitioner select the approach for angioplasty based on his/her expertise in the diagnostic angiographic field. If equal proficiency with both techniques is available, a preangioplasty assessment of the diagnostic angiograms can be used to determine which approach will provide better selective cannulation of the coronary ostium and ultimately better back-up for the launching of the balloon catheter system during angioplasty.

SELECTION OF GUIDING CATHETERS

Femoral Approach: Left Coronary Artery

If the diagnostic angiogram has been performed by the femoral approach, the seating of the angiographic catheter in the left coronary ostium will give the operator a hint as to the selection of a guiding catheter. It should be remembered that the tip of most Judkins-style guiding catheters is slightly shorter than is the tip of most diagnostic catheters. If a 5 or 6 French diagnostic system has been used, it is particularly important to note that they have slightly different curves and tip lengths than does the guide. If a Judkins 4-curve diagnostic catheter has been used with success, then the operator should start with a 4-curve

35

Judkins-style guiding catheter. If the tip of this catheter seats securely and coaxially, it is the guiding catheter of choice. If the tip goes somewhat below the left coronary orifice, particularly as seen in the LAO projection, a deep breath by the patient will often seat the guiding catheter tip in the left coronary ostium. If this fails, then a 3.5-curve guiding catheter may better selectively cannulate the left coronary ostium. This 3.5-length curve, however, sometimes is detrimental later in the procedure if a power position of the guide is necessary to achieve proper push to cross the lesion. The shorter curve in the 3.5 guide will provide less satisfactory back-up for this power position of the guiding catheter than will the 4-curve. If the patient has a very wide aorta, of course, a 5-curve might be selected for better cannulation.

If Judkins-style catheters do not provide adequate selective cannulation, then an Amplatz-style catheter may solve the problem. These catheters, however, are somewhat stiffer, and it is important that great care be taken in both entering and leaving the left coronary orifice to avoid trauma to the left main trunk. Obstruction of the left main trunk is somewhat more common with Amplatz-style catheters during the procedure. If obstruction occurs, demonstrated by either ventricularization of the pressure curve recorded from the guiding catheter tip or reduced flow of contrast during injections, the guiding catheter should be backed out of the left coronary orifice when not in continuous use. This technique is important with all guiding catheters in both coronary arteries and not just with the Amplatz catheter in the left coronary artery. In removing the Amplatz-style catheter from the left coronary ostium, simply pulling back of the catheter may actually advance the catheter tip into the left main trunk and abrasion or dissection of the inferior wall of the left main trunk may occur. Advancement of the entire catheter system will usually result in coaxial withdrawal of the tip from the ostium and is the recommended maneuver.

The Schoonmacher-style multipurpose guide catheters can be successfully used mainly by operators who are familiar with their use in diagnostic procedures. If the operator is not familiar with them, they feel somewhat stiff and are more difficult to manipulate safely.

A longer version of the brachial catheter is available for use from the femoral artery and very nicely cannulates the left coronary orifice in a manner similar to the angulation that the catheter takes when introduced from the brachial approach. If this catheter is used from the femoral approach, a 9 French long sheath must be used to accommodate the guide and facilitate movement of the catheter.

If damping occurs in the left main trunk with retardation of flow in the vessel, side-hole catheters are available in various styles and should be used to insure the ability to cannulate the vessel for the time necessary to carry out the procedure without undue ischemia. For further comments regarding side-hole catheters, see the discussion regarding the right coronary artery below.

There have been reports of 7 French diagnostic catheters being used as guides with balloon-on-wire dilatation systems, and there has even been a report of 5 French catheter being used as a guiding catheter (see Bibliography). These innovations from the usual 8 French system can obviously be successful, but at the present time, there is no advantage to using the smaller guides as equipment of choice.

Femoral Approach: Right Coronary Artery

The selection of a guiding catheter for the right coronary artery is again usually based on preliminary knowledge gained by the diagnostic study. If a Judkins 4-curve diagnostic catheter seated nicely, then the initial guiding catheter to try in the right coronary artery should be the 4-curve guide. It is again noted that the tip of the catheter is somewhat shorter than is the tip of the diagnostic catheters, and this may alter the approach and the capabilities of the system. The right coronary guiding catheter will not infrequently "damp" on entry into the right coronary orifice, and if this occurs, a side-hole guiding catheter should be utilized. If the 4-curve guide is not appropriate, then longer or shorter Judkins curves can be used depending on the orientation of the right coronary orifice.

One of the most frequently encountered problems with the guiding catheter system in the right coronary artery is the lack of back-up with the Judkins-style catheters when an attempt is made to cross a severely stenotic or distal lesion. As was mentioned above, this ability to cross the lesion must result from a concert among the guiding catheter, balloon catheter, and guide wire, but the lack of guiding catheter back-up will often preclude a successful result. If lack of back-up occurs with the Judkins-style system, then an Arani- or Amplatz-type of curve can be tried. Often, an Amplatz left guiding catheter will provide better back-up for the right coronary artery than will the Amplatz right catheter in a normal-sized aorta. The goal is to provide coaxial intubation and gain back-up support from the opposite aortic wall, and the right curve Amplatz catheters are somewhat short to achieve this. The brachial-style catheter or multipurpose catheter can be used, but these are somewhat more difficult to manipulate. The Arani-style catheter is excellent in providing back-up and currently exists in several tip angulations and lengths that must be selected based on the orientation of the origin of the right coronary artery and the size of the aorta. This catheter provides for a buttress effect with back-up against the aorta on both the left and right sides and will often provide the stable intubation necessary for crossing a lesion. Most styles of this catheter have side holes. El Gamal guide catheters are often useful in dealing with "back-up" problems and will often solve that problem by bracing against the opposite wall of the aorta.

The presence of side holes in the guiding catheter is both positive and negative. It is positive from the standpoint of allowing flow through the system, and this can easily be demonstrated not only by the lack of damping of the pressure tracing achieved from the tip of the catheter, but also by small injections of contrast, which clear rapidly through the artery. This assures that there is flow through the artery and that prolonged ischemia does not occur during intubation. Once the balloon catheter has been passed into the coronary artery and has gone beyond the side holes and the guiding catheter, the pressure measured at the tip of the balloon catheter will often reflect a damped contour since the side holes are now effectively closed by the shaft of the balloon catheter. This not only effects a reliable pressure gradient measurement if that technique is utilized, but also inhibits antegrade injection from the tip of the guide catheter since much of the injected contrast will now exit the guide through the side holes. Therefore, to measure a reliable gradient with a side-hole system, either an "intrinsic" gradient measured proximal to the lesion with the balloon catheter in the artery (and across the side holes of the guide) must be subtracted from the gradient once the lesion is crossed or the lesion must be crossed and then the guiding catheter withdrawn from the coronary ostium so that the effect of damping does not occur. This latter maneuver is preferable in that it also assures flow through the artery during the procedure. Great care must be taken when withdrawing the guide catheter since it will often "fling" once it leaves the coronary ostium and has the capability of withdrawing the entire system from the coronary artery.

The approach to the right coronary artery with the longer version of the brachial guiding catheter is often more difficult from the leg. It frequently assumes the shape of a reverse loop with the tip of the guide entering the right coronary ostium with a loop in the area of the left cusp. The usual clockwise maneuvers to achieve intubation of the right coronary artery using the brachial approach are often not successful when the longer brachial-style guide is used from the leg.

Brachial Approach

The brachial introduction of the guiding catheter is similar to the introduction of a diagnostic catheter. The entire system, including the smaller Teflon introducing catheter to provide a traumatic introduction into the brachial artery should be advanced over a guide wire and positioned in the ascending aorta in the usual manner. The curved tip of the standard brachial guiding catheter makes selective cannulation of both the left and right coronary arteries somewhat easier than with the standard brachial diagnostic catheters. Torquing of the brachial guide should be done very carefully since this catheter is somewhat thinner walled than the standard diagnostic catheter, and twisting and kinking of the guide can occur. If a lot of torque transmission is necessary, performing this with the indwelling tracker catheter and wire in place will sometimes provide the stability needed. It should be noted that the standard brachial guide is 8.3 French, although 8 French sizes are available for smaller brachial arteries. The standard 3 inch medium curve is generally the catheter to start with, but if the aorta is small, a 2 inch curve can prove efficacious, and in some cases, a "bent tip" or Amplatz-style-tip brachial catheter is helpful in achieving selective cannulation of the target vessel.

In disease of the left coronary artery, one advantage of the brachial system is the ability to cannulate selectively either the left anterior descending or circumflex coronary arteries. This often provides excellent back-up power to cross lesions. In the right coronary artery, the catheter can often be advanced far down the vessel to achieve excellent back-up force. This must obviously be done with care and presents a potential danger in diffusely diseased arteries.

Care must be taken in the manipulation of the brachial guiding catheter system so that excessive torque is not used. The thinner wall of the guiding catheter can kink, particularly in the brachiocephalic area, if excessive torque is applied. This can be recognized by damping of the pressure or difficulty in passing the dilatation catheter system through the guide (see above).

The selection of the left or right arm approach is predicted from the anatomy. The right brachial approach is most frequently used, as it is in diagnostic procedures. In some cases, an approach from the left arm to cannulate the right coronary artery selectively often provides excellent back-up to cross lesions in that vessel. The main drawback to the left brachial approach is frequently the configuration of the room in which the operator works.

Another use of the guiding catheter, of course, is to perform the postangioplasty angiograms. This can generally be done safely, but it should be remembered that the tips of the femoral catheters are often a bit stiffer and longer than those of diagnostic catheters.

Great care should be taken during the postangioplasty angiography if dilatations have been carried out in the proximal segments of the right coronary artery or if a short left main trunk is present and proximal dilatations have been carried out and the proximal portions of either the left anterior descending or circumflex systems. Once balloon inflation has been carried out, the lining of the artery is obviously roughened, and the presence of the tip of a diagnostic or guiding catheter can result in dissection if great care is not taken. In some cases, it may be desirable to perform the postangioplasty angiograms with the wire still in the artery and across the lesion and with the balloon catheter withdrawn into the guiding catheter system or entirely out of the guide over an extended or exchange wire. With the current high-flow catheter technology, excellent-quality angiograms can often be obtained with the wire still in the vessel, and the use of the wire as a stent to preclude trauma by the guiding catheter is a valuable tool in postangioplasty angiograms. If digital subtraction angiography is available in the laboratory, this often will produce excellent-quality pictures in such situations when smaller amounts of contrast can be infused.

The selection of the guiding catheter can usually be predicted by the anatomy observed in the diagnostic angiogram performed prior to angioplasty. In selecting the guiding catheter and the route of entry, the prime consideration should be safe cannulation of the coronary orifice and anticipated excellent back-up to provide the power necessary to cross the lesion. The characteristics of the more commonly used guiding catheters are detailed in Chapter 2 (Coronary Angioplasty Equipment).

SELECTION OF DILATATION CATHETERS

The selection of the proper dilatation catheter to work in concert with the guiding catheter and guide wire is of utmost importance in achieving successful angioplasty. The characteristics of the various dilatation catheter systems most commonly used are described in Chapter 2 (Coronary Angioplasty Equipment). During review of the preangioplasty an-

giogram, one should keep in mind the need for trackability of the system as well as the need for stiffness of the dilatation catheter to cross the lesion (pushability). This is particularly important in lesions in the distal vessel segments.

The size of the balloon selected should be determined very precisely. Measurement of a relatively normal segment of artery just proximal and just distal to the lesion should be accurately made with calipers or a computer system; one should not trust the "eyeball" method to select balloon size. If the lesion is on a tortuous segment of artery, "downsizing" of the balloon slightly is advisable to reduce the chance serious intimal disruption. It has been reported by some groups that a slight oversizing of the balloon, particularly in the vein bypass grafts, may reduce the likelihood of recurrence. This oversizing should be undertaken very carefully, however, and should be of a minimal nature or one risks serious intimal and even medial disruption.

Several balloon materials have a characteristic whereby slight variances in the balloon size can be predicted based on the atmospheres of pressure used. It should be noted that these manufacturer's measurements are usually made in water and probably vary from the very precise figures provided by the catheter company when inflation is carried out in a rigid arterial system. For example, a 3 mm PVC balloon when inflated at 4 atm produces a balloon size of 2.70 mm. When the same balloon is inflated at 10 atm, the predicted balloon size is 3.28 mm. Polyethylene balloons do not have this characteristic and will assume a specific balloon size regardless of the atmospheric pressure. The current availability of quarter-size balloons (i.e., 3.25 mm) allows for more specific sizing of the balloon to approximate the adjacent nonstenotic artery. Therefore, the knowledge of specific balloon characteristics will help in accurate balloon selection.

The trackability of the balloon over the wire is particularly important in vessels in which considerable tortuosity is present proximal to the lesion. In early generations of equipment, the dilatation catheters manufactured by ACS always exhibited more favorable tracking characteristics than those of other companies. Currently, however, all companies have catheters with excellent trackability and a variety of coatings (e.g., Microglide) such that the choice of a dilatation catheter renowned for exhibiting excellent trackability is more dependent on the type of catheter produced by a variety of companies than by the company itself. The operator should be knowledgeable of the characteristics of a variety of catheters so that one that is exceptionally trackable can be chosen.

The price paid for trackability, however, is sometimes the softness of the shaft of the dilatation catheter. A common dilemma is the need for trackability proximal to the lesion and stiffness at the lesion in order to cross the stenosis. In difficult cases, compromise in balloon catheter selection is often necessary to achieve satisfactory angioplasty results. Initial downsizing of the balloon catheter system with the use of an exchange of extendible wire to reintroduce the proper-sized balloon after a tight stenosis is minimally dilated will often solve this dilemma. Very low profile systems such as the Hartzler fixed-wire dilatation catheters or a variety of balloon-on-wire systems will often provide a very trackable catheter that has the stiffness to cross the lesion once reached. One method that can be successfully used in crossing severe lesions distal to tortuosity is to advance the wire as far as possible through the tortuosity and then, when further wire advancement becomes difficult, to advance the dilatation catheter over the wire as far as possible, thus stiffening the wire and providing some back-up support to allow better tip control and maneuverability of the wire further down the artery. This can be done in sequence with small advancements of the wire followed by small advancements of the balloon catheter until the proper position in the artery is achieved.

In the early 1980s, many experienced physicians believed that the measurement of pressure gradients before and after balloon dilatations was a very important part of the procedure. The ability to measure simultaneous pressures from the tip of the guiding catheter and from the tip of the dilatation balloon catheter across a lesion gave several very valuable bits of information.

The measurement of a pressure gradient across a lesion gives the operator an initial indication of the severity of the stenosis and also an indication of the success of the procedure. Continual pressure measurements during the procedure demonstrate the progress (or lack thereof) being made with each balloon inflation. As an endpoint, the general goal was to achieve a pressure gradient reduction to 15 mmHg or less, demonstrating a good hemodynamic result. The persistence of a high-pressure gradient made one concerned about the presence of a dissection or flap, and if pressure gradients wax and wane during the procedure, one must be concerned about spasm in the area of stenosis.

A few pitfalls regarding the validity of pressure gradient measurements were understood and taken into consideration when assessing the meaning of pressure gradient measurements: 1) If significant collaterals are present, the pressure gradient will be less than expected because of the increased pressure dis-

tally through retrograde collaterals. Therefore, an angiographically significant stenosis may yield a surprisingly low-pressure gradient, and the presence or absence of collaterals should be considered when assessing the validity of that pressure gradient. 2) Once balloon inflations have been carried out, particularly at higher pressures, a falsely high-pressure gradient can be measured for several reasons. First, a "flagging" of the balloon occurs with inflation. With deflation, the balloon does not completely rewrap around the dilatation catheter and the presence of "wings" will produce a falsely high gradient. This can be overcome in most cases by withdrawing the balloon into the dilatation catheter to rewrap the balloon around the dilatation catheter shaft and then recrossing the lesion to obtain a more valid pressure gradient. 3) Inflations at very high pressures of 10 atm or more can collapse the lumen of the dilatation catheter through which pressures are measured, and this can produce erroneous pressure measurements. A brief injection of contrast through the lumen briefly reestablishes its continuity and transiently produces a more true pressure reading.

It has certainly become common practice to not measure pressure gradients in all cases. The improved imaging systems and in particular the improvements in the videodisc and digital subtraction replays gives one a very true sense of the angiographic results in the area dilated, and in most cases, measurements of pressure gradients are now considered to be time-consuming and do not add significantly much to the procedure.

One instance that I believe that initial pressure gradients are very useful is in the assessment of the hemodynamic significance of an angiographically borderline lesion. Although angiographic appearance of a lesion if accurately measured in three views or more and then averaged is very reliable, there are anatomically "borderline" lesions, and, certainly, the presence of superimposed spasm on significant lesions can occur. The initial pressure gradient across the lesion should be 20 mmHg or more to be considered hemodynamically significant. Again, the presence of collaterals must be put into the equation to assess the significance of pressure gradient measurements, and also the tortuosity of the vessel proximal and distal to the lesion can produce fictitious gradients. An example of an angiographically severe lesion that was proved not to be hemodynamically significant is demonstrated in Case 5 in Appendix I.

Once the lesion has been dilated and a pressure gradient measured, another gross assessment of hemodynamic significance of the residual stenosis can be made by injecting a small amount of contrast beyond the lesion and observing its washout characteristics. If hang-up of contrast or slow washout occurs, then the lesion is probably still significant in terms of coronary flow. If the contrast washes out rapidly in spite of the presence of the dilatation catheter across the area of stenosis, then the hemodynamic significance of the lesion should certainly be questioned. The winging of the balloon catheter should be taken into consideration in this maneuver.

Pressure gradient measurements can also be effectively used to assess the severity of a particular stenosis in multiple-vessel disease to decide if the patient is a candidate for angioplasty or bypass graft surgery. This is particularly true in suspected left main lesions. In many cases, the significance of a left main stenosis is questioned even after multiple angiographic views have been obtained. For example, if a questionable left main lesion is present angiographically in a patient with a severe lesion or lesions elsewhere that appear acceptable for PTCA, whether or not the patient is a candidate for for angioplasty depends on the hemodynamic significance of the left main lesion. In such as case, the approach would be first to measure a pressure gradient across the left main stenosis. If no significant stenosis is measured in either the proximal LAD or circumflex arteries, then it can be assumed with certainty that the left main lesion is not hemodynamically significant and dilatation of the discrete stenoses in either the right coronary artery or the distal circumflex or LAD vessels can be offered to the patient as a viable and safe alternative to bypass graft surgery. If, however, the pressure gradient measured across the left main trunk is significant (usually 20 mmHg or higher), then, because of the presence of that hemodynamically significant lesion in a position not advisable for PTCA, the patient should be referred for bypass surgery.

Thus, the current status of the importance of pressure gradient measurements is, in general, to assess the significance of lesions, particularly in the left main trunk, and, in some cases, to provide additional information regarding the success or nonsuccess of the angioplasty procedure. Certainly, most practitioners, including this author, do not routinely measure pressure gradients. With the current technology available, the availability of pressure gradients provides the operator with one more parameter to evaluate the severity of the initial lesion, to assess the progress of the procedure as it is taking place, and to assess the results of the procedure at the end.

Although several catheters are available that claim to provide good pressure gradient measurements, a particularly good system to use is the ACS Pinkerton balloon catheter system (which is designed to be used with a 0.018 wire), with an 0.014 wire in this system. This provides one with a very trackable and pushable balloon catheter, and, in my experience, the pressure gradient measurements have been exceptionally good and reliable.

Several catheters have been produced by many companies that fall into the category of "balloon-on-wire." Some of these have worked quite well, and others have not been exceptional in their performance characteristics. The currently existing "balloon-on-wire" systems provide a very trackable catheter with an extremely low profile that will often cross severe stenoses when conventional steerable over-the-wire systems will not. The main negative characteristics of this type of catheter system include the facts that the lesion must be recrossed if a larger balloon is needed, pressures cannot be measured, and distal contrast injections cannot be made. These these systems are also less maneuverable than are the over-the-wire steerable systems.

SELECTION OF GUIDE WIRE

Guide wire selection is crucial not only to the success of the procedure, but also most certainly to the safety of the procedure. The advent of the steerable guide wire has allowed the expansion of angioplasty to include tortuous vessels and distal lesions. This also presents the operator with more potential dangerous situations. The characteristics of the more commonly used guide wires are discussed in Chapter 2 (Coronary Angioplasty Equipment). Preangioplasty assessment of preliminary angiograms must include a judgment as to the specific type of wire that will give the highest chance of success and the lowest chance of complication as the initial guide wire of choice for each specific case. Currently available wire systems provide a variety of stiffness of tip and also a variety of sizes, the most commonly used being 0.014, 0.016, and 0.018. The "floppiness" of the tip of the wire varies, and this information is readily available from the descriptive material provided by the catheter companies. Most of the wires have very good torque characteristics, and their flexibility yields a high safety quotient.

More gentle steerable wires with very flexible tips can be helpful in extremely tortuous vessels to essentially float through the artery to reach the lesion. These wires, however, by design do not have significant stiffness characteristics once the lesion is reached, and the extreme flexibility may be counterproductive when trying to cross a tight lesion downstream. The very characteristic that may have been necessary to reach the lesion safely then potentially thwarts the success of the case. In this situation, the balloon and guide can be used in concert with the wire to overcome the floppiness of the tip. If the floppy wire has approached and reached the tight stenoses but will not cross it, advancing the balloon catheter over the proximal portion of the wire to "stiffen" the distal segment will sometimes provide the back-up necessary to cross a tight lesion. Another maneuver that can be used, particularly in tortuous vessels, is to advance the wire as far as possible down the vessel and then advance the balloon over the wire to take some of the tortuosity out of play and give better tip control and maneuverability of the wire system.

If one type of wire is needed to reach a lesion and another type to cross the lesion, this same technique can be used. The wire needed to reach the lesion can be positioned just proximal to the stenosis and the balloon advanced nearly to the end of that wire. The wire can then be removed and replaced with the type of wire needed to cross a tight or total stenosis (i.e., a 0.014 intermediate ACS wire to cross a total occlusion).

The mandril position in the various guide wires may pose problems in crossing lesions. Guide wires commonly tend to buckle at the mandril junction if the tip of the wire is engaged either in the lesion or in a side branch. Advancing the balloon catheter over the tip of the wire to the area of the mandril junction thereby stiffens this junction and allows the flexible tip to remain safe and eliminate the mandril-buckling problem. All these maneuvers should be done with caution, however, since advancing the balloon catheter a bit too far can produce a stiffer tip of the wire, thereby diminishing the safety of the flexible tip.

The size of the wire used is generally 0.014 inch. The 0.016 inch wires are a bit stiffer and more pushable, but that characteristic diminishes the safety of the wire. The 0.018 inch high-torque floppy wires are very safe but do have the disadvantage of a larger profile. Many people prefer the 0.018 wires, and this simply becomes a matter of personal preference and touch with experience.

Extendible and exchange wires can be safely used, particularly if a downsized balloon has been necessary to cross a very stenotic lesion. The extension wire systems available from various companies are excellent, and this provides the ability to leave a wire across the lesion while changing for a larger or smaller balloon size as the case demands.

Although some very experienced and talented practitioners routinely cross and recross areas of lesions that have been dilated in order to change balloon sizes, I personally feel much more comfortable leaving a wire across an area of previous dilatation and exchanging balloons over a lengthened or exchange wire. I believe that this decreases the chance of the tip of a wire digging into the roughened area of dilatation and thereby dissecting the vessel.

The coatings on wires vary greatly. Fully Teflon-coated wires or wires coated with silicon, Microglide, or other slippery substances are prevalent, and each company seems to have their own material. The appropriate coating on the wire certainly enhances the ability of the balloon catheter to track over the wire, and this is important particularly in tortuous vessels.

In selecting the guide wire, the goal should be to advance the wire throughout the distal vessel as far as possible for anchoring and safety in manipulations during the procedure as well as for support to advance the balloon catheter system. Therefore, the distal vessel must be assessed as well as the proximal vessel in terms of the selection of the guidewire. The tip of the guide wire as it is commercially available is often not adequately curved to manipulate rigorous tortuosities or to avoid side branches. Viewing the preangioplasty angiograms can give one the sense of how much additional curve is necessary on the tip of the wire to traverse the artery successfully. The tip can be reshaped either by gentle manipulation with the thumb and index finger or by rolling the tip on a rounded instrument such as a needle or introducer. Great care should be taken not to fracture the tip of the wire, and this should be assessed before the wire is placed in the balloon and guiding catheter system.

It should be emphasized that this entire section should be read incorporating the comments presented in the sections on selection of guiding catheters and dilatation catheters, since the successful crossing of a lesion is dependent on the harmonious relationship of guiding catheter for back-up support, the wire for initial cannulation and wire support, and the trackability, pushability, and profile of the balloon catheter system.

USE OF DIGITAL SUBTRACTION ANGIOGRAPHY DURING ANGIOPLASTY

The use of digital subtraction angiography during angioplasty is very helpful during the procedure. Care must be taken when considering pre- and postangioplasty assessments of lesion stenoses to not use the ability to add or subtract darkness from the area of concern to give erroneous information to the operator. There are major advantages, however, to having digital subtraction angiography available. A preangioplasty digital picture of the artery to be approached can be run on a continuous loop providing a repetitive motion study of the vessel. This has advantage over the static videodisc system views in showing the branches and configurations of the target vessel in motion. Many of the newer videodisc systems also provide this advantage and are quite good in terms of sharpness of image.

Magnification of the lesion by digital subtraction angiography is very helpful and displayed on a monitor in the laboratory, and the impressive magnification obtainable can often assist in the exact manipulation of the tip of the guide wire across the area of stenosis. This type of magnification is also available in some videodisc systems. Digital subtraction angiography is also helpful during the procedure to assess the results and the progress. When injections through the guide are made with the wire still across the lesion, often the videodisc image is not too clear because of the diminished amount of contrast delivered into the artery. The digital subtraction system can enhance this smaller amount of contrast, and the area of dilatation is better seen. Again, care must be taken not to produce a fictitious of the area of lesion by excessive or undersubtraction.

Digital flow studies are available using digital subtraction equipment. These provide color assessments of flow pre- and postangioplasty and are of some minor physiologic interest. They are time-consuming, however, and in terms of practical value on a routine basis are probably not the strong point of digital subtraction angiography. The clear benefit of digital subtraction angiography is the magnification of the lesion and the ability to assess an in-motion image during the procedure.

Another helpful advantage of digital subtraction angiography is demonstrated in cases of total occlusions. In cases of totally occluded vessels where retrograde or antegrade collateral opacification of the distal vessel beyond the area of total occlusion is seen, two digital images can be taken in an exactly angled view and then matched: the antegrade injection of the stump of the total occlusion and an injection into the vessel that supplies the collateral flow to allow visualization of the distal vessel. The early and late phases of these two injections can then be displayed on the screen simultaneously, and a reconstructed picture of the entire artery, including the length of the totally occluded segment and the route that the wire must take in the distal vessel, can be visually available during the procedure.

HIGH-RISK CASES

In certain patients who are deemed to be at high risk for angioplasty, particularly patients with compromised left ventricular function, the presence of an intraaortic balloon pump during the procedure is sometimes a valuable prophylactic safety measure. Preliminary assessment must again be geared toward the ultimate safety for the patient, and assuming the possible need for emergency bypass surgery, the ability to transport the patient safely to the surgical suite must be considered. In patients with compromised left ventricular function, the preliminary availability of an intraaortic balloon pump is often very valuable. This could take several forms. If marked left ventricular dysfunction is present, the intraaortic balloon pump can be inserted in place and functioning during the procedure. If moderate left ventricular dysfunction is present, access to the left groin with a sheath can be achieved ahead of time and the intraaortic balloon pump device present in the room during the angioplasty so that immediate insertion of the IABP can be carried out without any delay because of technical factors of access or availability of the balloon pump. This prophylactic measure should be kept in mind in assessing the ability to present safely a stable patient to the surgeons in case of any complications during the procedure.

PTCA WITH CARDIOPULMONARY SUPPORT

The concept of "supported" angioplasty is relatively new. This refers to angioplasty during which the patient has functioning or standby cardiopulmonary support with a heart-lung machine in place and either functioning or on standby.

Supported angioplasty is used for patients who are otherwise high-risk candidates for both angioplasty and for bypass surgery. This should be reserved for those patients who, after evaluation of the diagnostic angiogram, are believed to be at extremely high risk for elective bypass surgery and also at extremely high risk should any problems develop during the angioplasty attempt. Most commonly, these patients will have very severe left ventricular dysfunction usually secondary to previous multiple myocardial infarctions and who present with a lesion in a major coronary artery that essentially supplies the remaining functioning myocardium in the individual.

Using cardiopulmonary support during angioplasty allows for stability of the patient during balloon inflations and longer balloon inflations in order to mold lesions than would be possible without the CPS and also reduces the anxiety factor of both the patient and the physician performing angioplasty. Having a functioning heart-lung bypass device in place during angioplasty stabilizes the patient, and if arterial closure should occur either during the angioplasty or abruptly in the short period thereafter, the patient can be more quickly transported to the surgical suite in a stable condition and surgery accomplished much more quickly than if the heart-lung machine had to be put in place after the patient arrived in the operating room.

The disadvantages of utilizing cardipulmonary support during angioplasty are nearly all related to local phenomenon in the femoral area due to the positioning of the arterial and venous cannulae necessary for the cardiopulmonary support system to function. These cannulae are very large, and if positioned percutaneously, they cause a sizable rent in the artery and vein that is particularly difficult to close with external pressure, particularly in the rigid vessels of older patients. The prolonged compression of the groin necessary following percutaneous placement of these cannulae is quite uncomfortable for the patient, and there have been both vascular and neurologic problems reported. Recent communications with Shawl indicate that the use of activated clotting times during and after the procedure with the arterial and venous cannulae not being removed until the ACT approaches normal results in much shorter groin compression times and fewer complications.

The very large size of the hole in the femoral artery and vein, however, has encouraged me to favor the direct cutdown approach versus the percutaneous approach. Having a vascular or cardiac surgeon in the room performing a localized cutdown on the femoral artery and vein and then placing the cannulae under direct vision and after the procedure repairing the incisions in the cannulae under direct vision has been very satisfactory and prolongs the time in the laboratory only by about 45 min.

It is necessary to place the CPS system cannulae from the right femoral approach, since utilizing the left femoral vein causes some kinking of the femoral venous cannula and restricts the amount of flow in liters per minute that can be achieved with the CPS system. The general procedure that I have utilized has been to first gain access to the left femoral artery and vein with the angioplasty sheaths, and if a pacing catheter is to be used (and it is usually necessary in these circumstances), then this is positioned first. The use of a flow-directed pacing catheter with pulmonary pressure measurement capabilities is very advisable in all these cases. The pacing catheter should be posi-

tioned first since the multiholed venous sheath used for CPS is quite large and would make positioning of the flow-directed catheter more difficult after the venous CPS cannula is in place. With the long sheath in the left femoral artery, the surgeon then exposes the right femoral artery and vein and properly positions both the venous and arterial sheaths. These are then connected to the CPS machine, and under the surgeon's direction, the pump technician tests the equipment to make sure that a 4–5 liter flow can be achieved. Once this is done, then the usual angioplasty equipment is positioned and angioplasty is carried out.

During the procedure, the patient is under high heparin dose because of the use of the CPS equipment, and this usually is in the 20,000–25,000 unit range. If cardiopulmonary support is to be instituted prior to angioplasty, this should be done and then angioplasty carried out with the patient on a several liter flow of support. If a standby mechanism is desired, the surgeon and heart-lung technician should be in the room and ready to institute cardiopulmonary bypass in case any problems develop during the procedure.

Often, the angioplasties are quite rapid and straightforward since they frequently involve proximal lesions in major arteries. Following postangioplasty angiography, if the result looks quite good, the surgeon can remove the equipment and sew up the femoral access incisions. If there is some question as to the result of the angioplasty, then the arterial and venous cannulae can be left in place even overnight with continued heparinization.

This approach has widened the indications for angioplasty to patients viewed as salvage cases. These patients all are extremely fragile, but with cardiopulmonary support can be quite safely approached with angioplasty.

GENERAL STRATEGY DURING THE PROCEDURE OF ANGIOPLASTY

In preparation for PTCA, all patients are maintained on their usual medications up until the time of angioplasty, with the exception of Coumadin, which is stopped 2–3 days prior to the procedure. Twelve to twenty-four hours prior to the angioplasty attempt, the patient is started on a regimen of aspirin 325 mg daily, and dipyridamole 50–75 mg orally two or three times per day.

The immediate pre-PTCA regimen consists of a mild sedative and a calcium channel blocker (usually nifedipine 10 mg orally). Once arterial and venous access has been obtained and prior to the insertion of the angioplasty equipment, a bolus of 10,000 units of heparin is administered and supplemented as needed based on the duration of the procedure. In general, an additional 5,000 units of heparin is given each hour.

Once the lesion has been crossed with the wire and the distal vessel wired, the placement of the dilatation balloon at the site of stenosis should be carried out in an expeditious fashion. Following confirmation of the proper positioning of the balloon by guiding catheter injections, the first balloon inflation is carried out at an atmospheric pressure that results in full balloon inflation. Once full balloon inflation has been achieved (and the lesion is conceptually cracked), the balloon is then held inflated for approximately 1 min in order to mold the lesion at that pressure. Subsequent balloon inflations are then carried out for longer periods of time if possible and often at lower pressures in order to compact or remodel the area of stenosis and dilatation. If a slightly larger balloon is needed and a polyethylene-type catheter is in place, higher pressures can be used to minimally enlarge the size of the balloon diameter. The length of time that the balloon is inflated is dependent on the symptomatic tolerance of the patient and the tolerance of the operator while assessing electrocardiographic changes of ischemia. In general, I try to keep these molding inflations in the 45 sec to 1 min range, but occasionally 90 sec or 2 min is possible. Longer balloon inflations certainly produce significant ischemia unless a Stack-type of perfusion balloon is used. If the tacking back of a dissection flap is thought to be necessary and longer balloon inflations are needed, the use of such a flow providing catheter is recommended. If pressure gradient measurements are being performed, the "flagging" or "winging" of certain balloon catheter systems following inflation should be kept in mind after a few balloon inflations. If the residual pressure gradient is unacceptably high, then the balloon catheter should be withdrawn into the guiding catheter to accomplish "de-flagging" of the balloon. Once this has been done, the lesion can again be crossed and a more valid pressure gradient obtained.

When the balloon catheter is being withdrawn into the guiding catheter, either to de-flag the balloon or to provide a channel that is not obstructed by the balloon catheter profile, one must be careful that the guiding catheter does not inadvertently advance into the coronary orifice or the proximal portion of the target artery. If this is allowed to happen, intimal damage caused by the tip of the guiding catheter can occur, and this can either cause immediate dissection of the artery or provide a nidus for future atherosclerotic formation and "restenosis." This is usually preventable by a push-pull technique of pulling back on the guiding catheter as the balloon catheter is being withdrawn and the wire held forward. This technique develops with practice among colleagues working together during angioplasty. Once an apparent good result has been obtained as assessed by injections through the guiding catheter, a better visualization can be obtained if the wire is extended and the balloon withdrawn completely out of the guiding catheter with just the wire left in the guiding catheter and across the lesion. This provides nearly perfect angiographic injectability because of the very small profile of the wire.

The postangioplasty angiography should be used to assess the results of the procedure. In particular, the presence or absence of side branches arising from the area of dilatation should be observed since the loss of small side branches during the procedure, although not hemodynamically significant overall, can produce some transient postprocedural pain as well as a small rise in enzymes and perhaps minor EKG changes. The angiographic recognition of the loss of these branches can often provide a satisfying explanation to the operator following the procedure if persistent pain or EKG changes are present. The other sign to look for is the "hang-up" of contrast in the area of dilatation following dilatation following angioplasty. This would suggest that a significant intimal tear has occurred and is a predictive precursor to an abrupt reclosure later. Patients exhibiting this should be kept on heparin for a longer period of time, and in cases of severe retention of contrast but a patent lumen and good antegrade flow, the possibility of repeat angiographic assessment 24 or 48 hr following the procedure to assess the healing of the area should be considered.

Following the balloon inflations, I favor a short time interval (3–5 min) at the end of the procedure during which time the wire alone is left across the area of dilatation and then further injections through the guide carried out to ascertain that no abrupt reclosure or thrombus formation is occurring. Once these several minutes have passed, the balloon and guide wire can be removed slowly, firmly, and under fluoroscopic view and the postangioplasty angiograms performed usually using the guiding catheter if it assumes a safe position in the ostium of the coronary artery. If there is any question about the guide position or safety, a diagnostic catheter should be used if that seems to be a safer method of injection. If very proximal inflations are carried out, the use of the guide wire as a stent during postangioplasty angiography will often provide the safety factor to avoid intimal disruption of a dilated segment by the tip of the guiding catheter. In general, after the removal of the balloon and wire and before the final angiography is carried out, intracoronary nitroglycerin is administered in small doses after the removal of the equipment from the coronary artery. The use of intracoronary nitroglycerin during the procedure is also helpful in improving flow in distal vessels and diminishing the chance of spasm.

Full surgical standby is necessary in all cases of angioplasty. There are no predictors for the need for emergency bypass surgery that can be accurately utilized, and even in patients with total occlusions and good collaterals, the emergency surgery rate hovers between 2 and 3%. The safety factor in angioplasty is the ability to transport the patient quickly and safely to surgery, and this is necessary for the safety of all procedures.

The performance of PTCA in free-standing catheterization laboratories or in hospitals without surgical back-up should not occur. Even in cases where a very distal, symptomatic lesion is being dilated in a vessel small enough that the operator would think that even if the vessel closed he/she would not send the patient to surgery, the chance of dissecting the proximal artery with the wire or with the guiding catheter exists and lifesaving surgical back-up would be immediately needed. Some hospitals differentiate between various severities of surgical back-up necessary during cases. This certainly is a reasonable solution to logistic problems, but the fact remains that in all cases of angioplasty some degree of surgical back-up should be immediately available.

Our post-PTCA medical regimen is well described in Chapter 12 (Patient Care Aspects of PTCA). This usually consists of allowing the intraprocedural heparin to wear off and then removing the sheaths when the femoral approach is used. We have stopped using protamine routinely to reverse the heparin effect in order to avoid abrupt changes in clotting mechanisms and also to prevent the possibility of protamine allergic reactions. In patients with total occlusions who have undergone successful PTCA, we generally restart the heparin and continue this until full anticoagulation with warfarin is achieved. We may also continue heparin for 24 hr post-PTCA with or without the sheaths remaining in place (for ready access should abrupt reclosure occur) in patients who have a significant intimal tear demonstrated on demonstrated on post-PTCA angiogram or when a less than satisfactory result has been achieved.

It should be noted that I have seen several cases in which heparin was continued for a longer than usual period of time, and then upon the cessation of IV heparin (2–4 days postprocedure), abrupt reclosure has occurred approximately 4 hr later. These cases demonstrate the importance of continuing in-hospital observation of the patient for at least 8–12 hr after stopping heparin.

All patients are sent home on calcium blocker, if tolerated, for 6 months or until the 5–6 month post-PTCA treadmill is performed. Long-acting nitrates are used for shorter periods of time if tolerated. Most patients are sent home on aspirin. Dipyridamole is not used routinely at this time. In cases of total occlusion, the patients are maintained on Coumadin and dipridamole for 3 months, and then the Coumadin is stopped and aspirin added to the dipridamole for another 3 months (6 months total).

All patients should have a stress EKG preferably with thallium as close to the time of successful PTCA as possible to use as a baseline test for later comparison should angina symptoms return or at the time of routine post-PTCA treadmills, which should be performed 5–6 months after the procedure. Treadmill tests at yearly intervals following angioplasty are recommended.

"AD HOC" ANGIOPLASTY

"Ad hoc" angioplasty is defined as an angioplasty performed at the time of the initial diagnostic coronary angiogram. Extensive experience with this form of angioplasty has proven it to be a safe and efficient variation to use if the considerable logistics are possible in an individual cardiovascular center.

The initial experience with ad hoc angioplasty came in emergency settings, in which the patients were clinically unstable and underwent diagnostic angiography. They were deemed too unstable to wait for a separate angioplasty procedure, and direct PTCA was carried out. Since this was demonstrated to be safe and efficacious, the ad hoc procedure was extended to elective cases.

It is estimated that somewhere between 20 and 50% of patients with angiographically documented coronary artery disease are candidates for angioplasty. This percentage varies with the expertise and philosophy of the practitioners involved. Since this obviously represents a large number of patients undergoing initial angiography, the savings in time and medical expenses in this group of patients can be enormous.

To have the capability of ad hoc angioplasty, the patients must have presigned consent forms for PTCA and emergency coronary bypass surgery and the capability of rapid film development must be present. "Ad hoc" surgical back-up of an appropriate nature must also be available. Once the initial coronary angiograms are performed, the films are developed and reviewed by the angiographer. It is important that the films be developed and thoroughly reviewed and that the TV or videodisc replay system not be trusted in this situation. Perhaps in some of the newer digital or VHS laboratories in the future, this will not be the case, but in most laboratories, 35 mm cineangiography remains the standard. This step is necessary to assure that no surprises are seen later on in the films that might change the strategy of the procedure. In this context, rapid film developing must be available.

If angioplasty is deemed the treatment of choice, this is then discussed with the patient, the family, and, if possible, the referring physician. If all are in agreement, the angioplasty can be carried out at the same time. If there is any hesitation on the part of anyone involved, then the procedure should be delayed until a firm decision can be made by all parties.

In choosing ad hoc angioplasty as a treatment strategy, the amount of contrast agent employed during the diagnostic study and a predicted amount of contrast agent needed for the continuation of the procedure must be considered. In this context, the age of the patient and the preprocedural evaluation of renal function must also be considered and appropriate decisions made with the patient's safety the determining factor. Fluoroscopy time is also a limiting feature, and this should be reviewed and considered before the final decision is made regarding proceeding with an ad hoc angioplasty.

It is necessary to obtain permits for everything needed for an angioplasty procedure prior to the initial angiography since the patient will already be sedated under for the initial angiogram and fully informed consent might be questionable in the premedicated patient. The necessary permits can be processed when the patient is admitted to the hospital. Fully informed consent of the patient and family for both the diagnostic angiography and potential angioplasty and emergency bypass surgery if necessary can be obtained, and the physician needs to be satisfied that the information imparted by him/her and other teaching aids to the patient and the patient's family have

supplied them with the necessary information with which to make a decision in the midst of the procedure regarding continuing with angioplasty. Obviously, if the diagnostic angiogram does not show any need for angioplasty, the permits for angioplasty and bypass surgery are disregarded.

The advisability of this approach must be individualized. Many patients come to our center because they are referred for the possibility of angioplasty and therefore are already familiar with the procedure. As angioplasty becomes more familiar to the patient population, the discussion of the potential for an ad hoc angioplasty seems in many cases to be a natural progression of the diagnostic procedure. If there is any hesitancy on the part of the patient or the patient's family when this potential approach is raised, it should not be utilized in that patient.

The logistic problem within the hospital sometimes precludes the potential for elective ad hoc angioplasty. If several catheterization laboratories are available within the laboratory suite, and surgery has the flexibility to be available on short notice, ad hoc angioplasty can be done successfully. If only one catheterization laboratory exists in an institution and is heavily scheduled, the disruption of the schedule by significantly lengthening a procedure on short notice is probably prohibitive for ad hoc angioplasty. If the surgeons, anesthesiologists, pump technicians, etc., as well as the surgical facilities are not readily available for back-up on short notice, obviously ad hoc angioplasty is not a possibility.

In my experience, ad hoc angioplasty does not diminish the success rate. The overall success rate of ad hoc angioplasty is 92%, and the need for emergency coronary bypass surgery is 1.6%. There was a subset of 3.6% of patients who had periprocedural myocardial infarctions. There were no deaths in the group of ad hoc angioplasties. The conclusion can therefore be drawn that ad hoc angioplasty is a reasonable approach in the proper logistic setting and is a safe alternative to performing two separate elective procedures on the patient.

5. Complex PTCA I: Multiple-Vessel Disease and Long Segmental Stenoses

Advances in technology and technique have allowed the original restrictive indications for PTCA to be expanded to include multiple-vessel angioplasty. In the early 1980s, a small number of patients undergoing coronary angioplasty had angioplasty performed on a single vessel in the presence of multiple-vessel disease. This is currently still considered single-vessel angioplasty. Multiple-vessel coronary angioplasty should be defined as angioplasty in two or more coronary arteries performed either during the same procedure or as staged procedures. If a patient is selected for multiple-vessel angioplasty, the goal should generally be to achieve as complete revascularization as could be achieved by coronary artery bypass surgery. Some exceptions to this rule exist and will be discussed below. Since multiple-vessel coronary angioplasty generally entails angioplasty on arteries that supply a significant amount of myocardium, the potential for complications is theoretically greater than when dealing with single-vessel disease; therefore, multiple-vessel angioplasty should be performed by experienced operators who have gained their initial expertise performing straightforward single-vessel cases.

STATISTICS AND BACKGROUND MATERIAL

In many large series of patients undergoing multiple-vessel coronary angioplasty, including an early series of 494 patients studied by my colleagues and me at the San Francisco Heart Institute in the mid-1980's, the initial patient success rate is between 90 and 95%, and the vessel success rate is between 85 and 90%. In most cases, in the selection of these patients for inclusion in published reports of multiple-vessel angioplasty, it was determined prior to the angioplasty attempt that all target lesions were amenable to treatment by angioplasty and that angioplasty would achieve as complete revascularization as could bypass surgery in these patients. Exceptions to this goal do exist in special circumstances, but such cases should not be included in one's statistical analysis of multiple-vessel angioplasty.

The difference between "patient success" and "vessel success" should be explained. In some cases, patient success is achieved in the sense that the lesions successfully dilated relieve the patient's symptoms and/or reduce or obliterate the amount of ischemia seen on thallium treadmill testing. Vessel success relates to the actual angiographic success rate in each vessel attempted. The difference between these two success rates is explained in part by the strategy involved in approaching many of these cases. This is expanded on in the strategy section to follow, but, in general, the more severe and most difficult lesions are attempted first, and in any given patient, a secondary or tertiary vessel attempted after initial success in the main target artery may not be successful. In such a case, the patient may be a symptomatic success because of the successful dilatation of the main problem artery, whereas all vessels attempted have not been dilated.

Complication rates in a large series of multiple-vessel coronary angioplasty are detailed in Table 5-1. The emergency bypass surgery rate of 2.8% is consistent with that of angioplasty, in general, in experienced centers as is the myocardial infarction rate of 3.0%. Two deaths (0.4%) have occurred in this subset. In total, 19 patients had one or more of these three serious side effects for a major cardiac event rate of 3.8%. Dividing a series of multiple-vessel angioplasty patients into two groups in an attempt to analyze the potential for failure in each group provides some insight into the problems encountered in multiple-vessel disease (Table 5-1). Patients included in group A have "straightforward" or "ideal" lesions in two or more coronary arteries with no complex disease present. Group B patients have at least one "complex" lesion (e.g., total occlusion, long segmental stenoses, bifurcation lesion requiring the kissing balloon technique, or bypass lesion) as least one of the multiple lesions in their coronary system. An analysis of these two groups demonstrated that the presence of a "complex" lesion in multiple-vessel angioplasty did not increase the risk of complication, nor did it predict initial patient success.

If complex disease is present, however, the strategy in approaching the case is altered somewhat. The complex lesion is generally attempted first, and, also in this comparative series, patients with at least one complex lesion were more likely to be staged than done sequentially at the same procedure. Analyses of recurrence in patients undergoing multiple-vessel dis-

47

TABLE 5–1. Multiple-Vessel Angioplasty Complications

Complication	No. among 494 patients studied (%)
EM/CABG	14 (2.8)
MI	15 (3.0)
Death	2 (0.4)
Major cardiac event	19 (3.8)

ease has yielded interesting data. Since the question of recurrence is often revolved around whether recurrence is due to a "lesion factor" or a "patient factor," it was hoped that analysis of recurrence in multiple-vessel angioplasty would shed some light on this comparative etiology of recurrence.

Those patients undergoing successful multiple-vessel angioplasty who subsequently recur can be divided into three groups. Group one consists of patients in whom all lesions dilated have recurred, group two consists of patients in whom some of the lesions dilated have recurred, and group three consists patients in whom all lesions dilated have remained patent. It should be emphasized that the true recurrence rate in any series or subset of patients cannot be accurately determined unless 100 angiographic follow-up is achieved. Once patients have been at risk for recurrence for 6 months postangioplasty or have returned for angiographic restudy earlier than 6 months because of recurrent symptoms or recurrence of documented ischemia on electrocardiographic or thallium treadmill testing, they can be included in a statistical analysis of this type. It must be kept in mind that "false positive" and "false negative" suggestions of recurrence exist if only the clinical analysis of the patient is undertaken.

Factors predicting recurrence were primarily clinical (diabetes, smoking, and hypercholesterolemia) in those patients who developed restenosis in all vessels dilated and primarily morphological (severity of stenosis of the lesion before PTCA and the "hardness" of the lesion) in those patients in whom restenosis occurred in one vessel but not in the others. This matter is described more fully in Chapter 10 (Recurrence Following Successful PTCA) dealing with restenosis.

SELECTION OF PATIENTS FOR MULTIPLE-VESSEL ANGIOPLASTY

In general, the goal of multiple-vessel angioplasty should be to achieve as complete revascularization as would be available to the patient if the patient chose to have coronary artery bypass graft surgery. Some colleagues have suggested that, in patients with multiple-vessel disease, only a major target artery need be treated with angioplasty, leaving the patient with other lesions untreated by angioplasty but which would have been bypassed had the patient undergone bypass graft surgery. The goal in selecting patients for multiple-vessel angioplasty should be to achieve complete revascularization except in several special circumstances, which will be described below.

In assessing the preangioplasty angiograms, each lesion should be individually analyzed and the selection of equipment made for each lesion as if this were the only lesion present in the coronary system. Once this assessment has been carried out and it is determined by the operator that all lesions are amenable to angioplasty, a full discussion with the patient and family should be carried out in detail and the advantages of angioplasty as well as the risks and benefits explained in each individual case. The cardiac surgeon should be fully involved in the decision-making process with particular emphasis on his/her assessment as to which vessels are indeed bypassable. Once the patient has been selected for a multiple-vessel coronary angioplasty, a distinct strategy in approaching the angioplasty must be determined.

STRATEGY IN MULTIPLE-VESSEL ANGIOPLASTY

As in all cases of angioplasty, the safety of the patient must be first and foremost, and the potential need for emergency bypass surgery must be recognized and planned for. If compromised left ventricular function is present, the use of the intraaortic balloon pump or supported angioplasty using a full cardiopulmonary bypass support technique should be considered.

The question of whether to perform multiple-vessel angioplasty as a sequential procedure (i.e., all lesions treated during the same procedure) or a staged procedure (i.e., all lesions treated in two or more separate procedures) should generally be assessed primarily with the safety of the patient as the primary consideration. If all lesions can safely and expeditiously be dilated during the same procedure, this would preferable from most standpoints. If, however, in multiple-vessel disease, in which the majority of the myocardium is at risk by the multiple dilatations, it is important to be certain that a satisfactory result has been obtained in the first and subsequent lesions before further lesions are dilated, placing the entire myocardium at risk. If previous myocardial infarction has occurred and left ventricular dysfunction is present in some segments of the left ventricle, angioplasty of vessels supplying the patient's remaining good myocardium should be undertaken, keeping in mind the potential for intraprocedural arterial closure and subsequent abrupt reclosure in the early postangioplasty period.

Another consideration that may have weight in determining whether to stage a procedure is the length of the procedure. The discomfort of the patient caused by lying on the table for a considerable length of time is sometimes a limiting factor. Another obvious limiting factor is the amount of contrast medium that the patient receives during the procedure. The patient's renal status should be kept in mind at all times, and if excessive contrast is used, postprocedural hydration and/or diuretic agents should be utilized. One advantage of multiple-vessel angioplasty is that the patient with compromised renal function need not be put at unnecessary risk from that standpoint since the procedure can be staged. Even though it is neat and impressive to carry out multiple-vessel angioplasty at one sitting, the safety of the patient and the comfort of the patient must be of prime consideration, and staged procedures in multiple-vessel disease are entirely acceptable. In reviewing the differences between group A patients and group B patients as described above, it was found that patients in group B, i.e., patients with a complex lesion as one of their stenotic areas treated with angioplasty, staged over a 1 or 2 day interval more commonly than did patients in group A. In our initial series, 93% of patients in group A were treated at one procedure and 84% in group B were treated in one procedure with 16% staged over 2 or more days. This difference relates to the difficulty of treating complex lesions and the longer time and more contrast involved in these procedures.

Order of Lesions Dilated

The success of multiple-vessel angioplasty depends not only on the selection of appropriate patients, but also on the selection of a strategy that will most likely ensure the safety of the patient and the overall success of the procedure. In general, the lesion dilated first should be the lesion that appears to be most technically difficult, the lesion that supplies the largest amount of myocardium, or the lesion that is clearly the symptomatic ischemia-producing lesion. In the best of all worlds, one lesion would fulfill all these criteria, but, in fact, often decisions need to be made compromising initial lesion selection. The question that should be asked in planning strategy is, "Is there

a lesion that, if angioplasty is not successful, will necessitate the need to go to surgery in order to achieve adequate revascularization?" The predetermined "most important lesion" should generally be dilated first. If this lesion also appears to be the most technically difficult, as is often the case, then the strategy of approach to lesions is simplified. If, however, there is a technically less difficult lesion that must be dilated in order to achieve a result that will keep the patient from needing bypass surgery, then this lesion should be tried first in order to have the best assurance of completeness of the procedure.

Generally, if a complex lesion is present, this lesion should be approached first. In the case of a total occlusion of a vessel, not only is it the least likely to be successful, but if antegrade flow can be reestablished through a totally occluded artery, the possibility of collateral protection to the other vessels to be approached by angioplasty as the procedure continues is also enhanced. If a lesion exists in an artery supplying collaterals to a totally occluded vessel, the successful initial PTCA of the totally occluded artery also decreases the amount of myocardium at risk when the second (collateral-supplying) artery is attempted. Other "complex" lesions should also be attempted initially since the more straightforward lesions will generally have a higher chance of ultimate success.

If the most technically difficult lesion or the lesion that supplies the most significant amount of myocardium is attempted first and cannot be successfully dilated for whatever reason, then the patient should be referred for bypass surgery in order to achieve the necessary revascularization. To dilate more technically ideal but less significant lesions in the face of the inability to dilate a lesion supplying a large amount of myocardium should not be an acceptable procedure.

Other Considerations

The selection of equipment in multiple-vessel disease generally does not differ from the strategy described in Chapter 2 (Coronary Angioplasty Equipment) on equipment selection. Each lesion should be approached individually, and the balloon sizing and guide wire selection should be chosen as though each lesion were an individual target vessel. One should be prepared for multiple changes of guiding catheters, balloons, and guide wires if necessary to perform multiple-vessel angioplasty in the appropriate order as described above. Compromise of the best strategic approach to each individual lesion in multiple-vessel angioplasty because of an easier method of use of the equipment should not be undertaken.

Special Circumstances and Exceptions to the General Rule in Multiple-Vessel Angioplasty

The statements made above regarding the selection of patients for multiple-vessel angioplasty and the need for achieving complete revascularization do have some exceptions. In certain cases, incomplete revascularization is acceptable. In elderly patients who could be identified as higher-risk surgical candidates, in whom one severe lesion is clearly the symptomatic vessel but less severe lesions exist in other arteries as well, dilatation of that target vessel in order to achieve symptomatic improvement and keep the patient from having to go to surgery is an acceptable exception to the rule of attempting to achieve complete revascularization. In other patients who are poor surgical risks because of concurrent noncardiac disease, incomplete revascularization to eliminate symptoms by dilating fewer than all the lesions that would be bypassed if the patient had undergone bypass surgery is also an acceptable exception to the rule.

COMPLICATIONS AND PITFALLS

The possibility of a complication in multiple-vessel angioplasty is obviously increased over that in straightforward single-vessel disease disease because more lesions are being dilated and more myocardium is at risk. Each lesion dilated carries its own independent chance of complication, so if three lesions undergo angioplasty dilatation, the same risk for complication in each of these vessels must be recognized. In the case of abrupt reclosure or spasm of the arteries, if multiple-vessel dilatation has been carried out, a larger amount of myocardium may be at risk, and if this untoward event occurs, the patient may be more unstable when presented to the cardiac surgeon for emergency bypass surgery than the patient in whom only one vessel has been dilated. A more liberal use of the intraaortic balloon pump in patients with multiple-vessel disease is a safety factor that should be encouraged. The use of full cardiopulmonary support with the heart lung machine during the procedure may also extend the application of multiple-vessel angioplasty to patients in high-risk groups. Closer post-angioplasty observation, i.e., observing the patient in the coronary care unit rather than in an intermediate care ward, is advisable. It is also important to try to achieve a high restudy rate in patients with multiple-vessel angioplasty, since, obviously, a larger amount of myocardium is at risk for recurrence. It is clear, however, that multiple-vessel angioplasty has been shown to be a very safe and effective alternative to bypass graft surgery with patients with multiple-vessel coronary artery disease when the procedure is performed carefully and thoughtfully by experienced practitioners of angioplasty.

TANDEM LESIONS AND LONG SEGMENTAL STENOSES

In patients presenting with "tandem" lesions in the same artery or long segmental areas of disease in a single coronary artery, the approach to angioplasty of that vessel is somewhat different. Whereas the term "tandem lesions" obviously signifies two lesions in the same artery, there may be three, four, or even more separate lesions in the same vessel that have areas of relatively normal artery seen angiographically between the discrete stenoses. Pathologically, of course, these vessels are diffusely diseases throughout their courses. In patients with tandem or more discrete lesions, the general approach is to try to cross all lesions initially with the guide wire and then to pass the balloon catheter across all lesions as well. The importance of attempting to do this relates to the initial balloon profile prior to inflations of the balloon, particularly at higher pressures. It is useful with many balloon systems to prep the balloon with the balloon sheath on to maintain the lowest possible profile in order to cross a series of stenoses. The possibility of extrusion of air distally during balloon inflations when the balloon has been prepared in this manner must be recognized and is usually easily dealt with in the laboratory. If all stenoses can be crossed, then back-dilatation toward the ostium, dilating the most distal lesion first and the most proximal lesion last, is the preferable approach. In some cases, however, it is not possible to cross all lesions because the proximal lesions may be so stenotic that the shaft of the balloon catheter will not advance because of friction in these areas. In these cases, dilatation of proximal lesions first will often free up the catheter and allow forward progression across the rest of the lesions. In these cases, difficulty in advancing the balloon catheter and its shaft diameter through the proximal lesion necessitates dilatation of that lesion in order to gain access to the more distal stenoses. Trying to dilate the more distal stenosis first is done basically to be sure that it is physically possible to cross all stenoses. In dealing the tandem or multiple discrete lesions, a lesion in the more distal aspect of the vessel may require a smaller balloon than those in the proximal areas. In this case, an exchange or extendible wire should be used initially so that the appropriate-sized balloon can be used at each lesion as if it were a discrete solitary stenosis.

It should be remembered that, with each balloon inflation in the artery with tandem or more discrete lesions, each area treated by angioplasty has an independent chance of recurrence. Therefore, it is theoretically likely at least that the recurrence rate would be higher in vessels treated with multiple balloon inflations at different sites in the vessel. If one or more areas recur, then certainly, as in single-vessel disease, repeat angioplasty is usually the treatment of choice.

In patients with long segmental disease, i.e., a long area of disease in the artery as opposed to discrete stenoses separated by areas of apparently normal vessel, the strategic approach is much the same. The entire segment of disease should be crossed with the guide wire and then an attempt made to get the balloon catheter to cross the entire area of disease and back-dilate through that segment. Preparation of the balloon with the balloon sheath in place again will achieve the lowest possible profile of the balloon segment of the catheter and enhance the ability to cross the entire area of disease. As noted above, with several discrete stenoses, the tightness of a long segment of disease in its proximal portion may preclude this ideal approach and it may be necessary to dilate in a forward manner through the area of disease. This approach, of course, does not ensure that the entire area of stenosis can be crossed and subsequently dilated. Multiple balloon inflations in an area of long segmen-

tal stenoses at least theoretically predispose to a higher chance of recurrence.

There are longer balloon catheters available, and these catheters are somewhat less maneuverable in terms of their ability to be advanced over a wire. If molding inflations with a longer balloon is thought to be advantageous, as is often the case, it may be necessary to dilate the area of long segmental disease initially with overlapping standard balloon catheters, and then once the severe stenoses have been relieved, the initial balloon can be removed and replaced over an extended or exchange wire with a long balloon and longer molding inflations made. The use of a perfusion balloon catheter to achieve longer time inflations in long segmental disease may prove beneficial in terms of initial success and recurrence, but in series so far reported, this has not shown to be true. Theoretically, at least this approach has some application.

In many cases, angioplasty of long segmental disease or multiple areas of discrete stenoses amount to an internal endarterectomy by balloon of the artery. Certainly, a higher recurrence rate is seen in these cases, and this should be remembered in their selection and fully discussed with the patient and the patient's family. Recurrence often occurs only in isolated segments of previously dilated artery, and a second angioplasty is often very successful in treating these less complex recurrent lesions.

6.   Complex PTCA II: Total Occlusions

This chapter deals with PTCA in patients with an angiographically documented total occlusion of a major coronary artery. Among this series of patients, all presented at the time of angioplasty with an angiographically documented total occlusion of a major epicardial coronary artery *not* in the setting of an acute myocardial infarction. Unstable patients during acute myocardial infarction or patients having PTCA in combination with pharmacologic revascularization are excluded from this chapter's discussion. These patients are, however, discussed in Chapter 9 (Direct PTCA in Acute Myocardial Infarction), describing direct PTCA in acute and evolving myocardial infarction. Also excluded in these discussions are patients with so-called functional total occlusion. This term has been used by some investigators, and patients in this category have been included in some series along with other patients with true totally occluded coronary arteries. For purposes of this chapter, the patients discussed have an absolute total occlusion of the coronary artery with no antegrade flow through the main channel of the vessel for the length of the total occlusion.

An early series of 264 patients who underwent attempted angioplasty of a totally occluded major epicardial coronary artery was reported by my colleagues and me at the San Francisco Heart Institute. Other groups have previously and subsequently reported their series of angioplasty attempts in patients with totally occluded coronary arteries (see Bibliography). The data on the early series of patients through 1986 provide insight into the general problem of total occlusions and can prove instructive to review. Clinical data on these patients are outlined in Table 6–1. The age range in this series of patients is 31–85 years, with a mean of 54 years. Eighty percent of the patients were male.

Sixty-five percent of the patients in this total occlusion series had the totally occluded coronary artery as their only significant lesion. Thirty-five percent of the patients had the totally occluded coronary artery in combination with lesions in other vessels that were judged appropriate for treatment by angioplasty in order to achieve complete revascularization. The strategy in dealing with patients with total occlusions in combination with other lesions is discussed later in this chapter.

The target vessels in this series are also depicted in Table 6–1. The left anterior descending coronary artery was the most frequent target vessel, with the right coronary artery second. Three patients had total occlusions of the saphenous vein bypass grafts. All patients had collaterals demonstrating the distal vessel, and in 90% of the patients, the left ventricular ejection fraction was greater than 45%. This indicates that these patients had not suffered full-thickness myocardial infarction and, in fact, had functioning myocardium in the distribution of the totally occluded artery, thereby fulfilling the selection criteria of ischemic myocardium in the distribution of the vessel to be approached by angioplasty.

In analyzing the likelihood of success or failure in this group, the most important determinant was shown to be the length of time of total occlusion. This can be calculated either by a clinical event dating back to the onset of or change in the patient's symptomatology to indicate that the total occlusion occurred or, in some cases, to a previous angiogram that showed the artery to be subtotally occluded, with a subsequent angiogram that demonstrated total occlusion of the vessel. In our series, at the time of the initial angiogram, 179 of the patients had totally occluded coronary arteries, and 85 had a subtotal occlusion of the target coronary artery. At the time of angioplasty attempt, all patients had total occlusions of the coronary artery. Therefore, in 33% of the patients, the length of time from total occlusion to PTCA attempt could be more accurately judged because of the previous angiograms in which the vessel was patent than in the other 67%, in whom reliance on clinical facts was necessary to estimate the duration of the total occlusion.

Initial success was achieved in 71% of the 264 patients. Success is defined as at least a 35% reduction in the initial percent diameter stenosis and a post-PTCA gradient of less than or equal to 15 mmHg, with no complications necessitating a coronary bypass procedure or resulting in myocardial infarction. In the 29% of patients in whom primary success was not achieved, the failure was due to the inability to cross the total obstruction with the wire in 21%. In the other 8% of unsuccessful cases, the wire crossed the lesion, but no balloon catheter could be forced across the stenosis. Discussions of current ways to improve these statistics will be presented later in this chapter.

TABLE 6–1. PTCA: Total Occlusions (N = 264)

	Years	Mean
Age	31–85	(54)
Sex	210 M	(80%)
Vessel		
LAD		112
RCA		103
LCX		45
SVG		3
LM		1
LVEF	> 0.45	(90%)
Collaterals	264	

Clinical and procedural aspects were analyzed in an attempt to determine factors that might predict success in this group of patients. These factors are listed in Table 6–2. The age and sex of the patient were not statistically significant in determining success. The only clinical factor demonstrating significance was the duration of symptoms (from the time of onset of symptoms to the angioplasty attempt). Those patients undergoing successful angioplasty had a mean symptom duration of 14 ± 21 weeks, whereas those in whom angioplasty was not successful had a mean symptom duration of 27 ± 34 weeks. This is a statistically significant finding.

The target artery in which angioplasty was attempted did not predict success or failure. The percent diameter stenosis pre- or postangioplasty, the pressure gradient pre- and postangioplasty, and the inflation time and pressure were not of statistical significance in predicting success. In the 85 patients who had a subtotal occlusion at the time of the initial angiogram, and whose lesions progressed to a total occlusion at the time of angioplasty, the interval from the first study to the total occlusion was, indeed, a predictor of success. In patients whose time to total occlusion was angiographically documented to be less than 8 weeks, 87% were successfully treated. If the time to total occlusion was greater than 8 weeks, only 28% of patients had successful dilatation of the totally obstructed segment. This is also statistically significant to the $P = .001$ level. Therefore, the time from total occlusion to angioplasty attempt, either by clinical syndrome or by angiographic documentation, remains the single most important predictor of success in this group of patients and should be kept in mind in the selection of patients for angioplasty.

TABLE 6–2. Total Occlusion: Analysis of Success Factors

Parameter	P
Age	NS
Sex	NS
Artery dilated	NS
PDS (pre and post)	NS
Gradient (pre and post)	NS
Inflation time and pressure	NS
Symptom duration	< .001
Angiographic time to total occlusion	< .05

SELECTION OF CASES AND STRATEGY

Patients with angiographically documented totally occluded coronary arteries should be selected for angioplasty based on the following criteria:

1. All patients should have persistent angina pectoris relatively refractory or unresponsive to medical therapy. As indicated above, all patients will likely have good collaterals such that the distal vessel could be identified and all will have reasonably well-preserved left ventricular function, based on left ventriculography and noninvasive assessment. These findings would indicate the presence of viable myocardium in the distribution of the totally occluded coronary artery that is kept alive by the presence of collaterals, which in many cases are not adequate to allow the patient the quality of life that he/she desires with medical treatment. These patients would obviously be candidates for bypass surgery, were angioplasty not available.

2. All patients should have angiographically documented ipsilateral or contralateral collaterals that provide visualization of the distal vessels so that the route of the guide wire, once across the total occlusion, could generally be ascertained. This presence of visualization of the distal artery is necessary for the safe maneuvering of the guide wire into the distal vessel to provide a tract across which the balloon can be passed. It should be pointed out that, in many cases of total occlusion, the distal vessel is not seen with the clarity that a full antegrade flow of contrast would provide. Often, the distal vessel is larger than anticipated before angioplasty because of the diminished flow of contrast into the distal vessel via the collateral route. It is also important to recognize that unsuspected secondary (tandem) lesions are often seen in the distal vessel following the reestablishment of antegrade flow. It is imperative, however, for the physician to recognize the importance of coronary artery spasm in these distal segments and the marked prevalence of spasm in cases of previously totally occluded vessels in which higher-pressure antegrade flow is reestablished. Dr. Tim Fischell has brilliantly described this phenomenon, and the major importance of its recog-

nition is that if spasm occurs after antegrade flow is reestablished, it can be treated with nitroglycerin and need not be treated with distal balloon inflations. The differentiation between reflex spasm or fixed obstruction is of paramount importance in the appropriate and successful completion of the transluminal treatment of the diseased artery. When an artery is totally occluded and the distal is filled via low-pressure collaterals, that distal vessel becomes accustomed to a lower filling pressure. When antegrade flow is reestablished and filling pressure is higher, a reflex spasm occurs often segmentally and many times diffusely. Intracoronary nitroglycerin should be administered in such cases and then repeat angiography performed 3–5 min later to see if the apparent distal lesions have, in fact, disappeared following relief of the reflex spasm by nitroglycerin administration. If distal lesions are still obviously present, then these downstream obstructions should be so identified and appropriately dilated. Digital subtraction angiography is particularly helpful in visualizing the distal vessel, which is generally underfilled with contrast. "Matching" views of the proximal stump and the collaterally filled distal vessel can be combined in one digital image using the ADAC program to provide a complete vessel view that is dramatically helpful in angioplasty of total occlusions.

3. These patients will have well-preserved left ventricular function and demonstrated reversible myocardial perfusion defects by thallium exercise testing in the distribution of the totally occluded artery.

The general procedure of angioplasty in patients with totally occluded coronary arteries is similar to the standard technique. Prior to the angioplasty attempt, each patient is premedicated with a calcium channel blocker, and immediately prior to the angioplasty, selective coronary angiography is performed to elucidate any changes from the control study and to provide videodisc and digital subtraction recording maps. Intracoronary nitroglycerin should be administered to determine if any antegrade flow can be reestablished by relief of superimposed spasm at the site of obstruction. Ten thousand units of heparin is administered following the achievement of arterial access and prior to the introduction of the angioplasty equipment. Additional heparin is administered during a prolonged procedure, generally 5,000 units per hour.

A multipurpose pacing catheter is positioned in the right heart through venous access, and pacing mechanism is established prior to the angioplasty procedure in all cases. If transstenotic pressure gradients are measured, they can be expected to be somewhat lower than usual because of the presence of significant collaterals in all cases. By definition, the percent diameter stenosis prior to angioplasty is 100%; after angioplasty, the mean diameter stenosis should be calculated and recorded in the usual manner.

Balloon inflations tend to be at higher pressures and for longer periods of time than in the general angioplasty series. The presence of collaterals in all of these patients allows for longer balloon inflation times to be tolerated, even without perfusion balloon catheters. The initial balloon inflation should be performed at a pressure adequate to achieve full inflation of the balloon, and subsequent balloon inflations may be performed at lower pressures to remodel the area for longer periods of time.

It is important to emphasize that patients with totally occluded coronary arteries should have full surgical back-up coverage, the same as patients with nontotally occluded arteries. One might theorize that since the artery is completely occluded to begin with, no harm could be done that would necessitate emergency bypass surgery, but this is simply not true. For various reasons, in some patients, when the totally occluded artery is opened and then subsequently does not remain opened, either by dissection of thrombus, the patient enters into a clinical syndrome of acute myocardial infarction and must go immediately to the operating room. This may well be due to distal emboli of the material that is causing the total occlusion, subsequently finding its way into the small collaterals and occluding these protective vessels, thereby depriving the patient of his/her collateral supply. Another obvious problem that could necessitate emergency bypass surgery in these patients is damage to the proximal vessel, particularly by the guiding catheter. In many cases, considerable force is necessary to get either the wire or balloon to cross an area of total occlusion, and in doing so, a power position of the guide may be used, presenting the possibility of deep-seating the guide in the proximal right coronary artery or left main coronary artery and the potential for trauma to those proximal vessels exists. Obviously, if a left main coronary artery were to be dissected by the guiding catheter, the possibility of emergency bypass surgery on a very urgent basis must be immediately available.

In this series of patients, the postangioplasty medical regimen differs from the general series in that patients are usually kept on heparin until adequate anticoagulation with warfarin is achieved. This prolongs the hospital stay from an average of 2 days, in patients not treated with warfarin, to 4 days in patients so treated. In some cases, this can be carried out on an outpatient basis if the angioplasty physician is convinced that adequate monitoring can be obtained.

It is preferable to discharge these patients from the hospital on warfarin, a calcium channel blocker, a long-acting nitrate if tolerated, and dipyridamole. The warfarin is continued for 3 months, and then aspirin is started and continued for an additional 3 months. Dipyridamole is continued for 6 months postangioplasty. Following the 6-month recurrence concern interval, the patients then can be treated as patients with nontotal occlusions and weaned from their calcium channel blockers and nitrates and kept long term only on a small aspirin dosage.

In patients with a total occlusion as the only significant coronary lesion, the approach is obviously to reestablish antegrade flow in that vessel and check the distal vessel for secondary lesions not visualized by the collateral filling of the distal vessel. Again, it should be kept in mind that reflex spasm often occurs in these distal vessels and should always be considered, treated with intracoronary nitroglycerin, and then reevaluated after an appropriate time interval (3–5 min) to see if the apparent distal lesions were real or, in fact, spasm. In patients with the totally occluded coronary artery as only one of two or more significant coronary lesions, the strategy of approach becomes somewhat different.

In general, the totally occluded vessels should be attempted first. In most large series of patients, the success rate is lower in total occlusions than in any other group and, therefore, should be considered the least likely to be successfully treated in a case of multiple-vessel angioplasty. If the patient has well-preserved left ventricular myocardium and documented reversible defects in the distribution of the totally occluded coronary artery, then, if that artery cannot be opened by angioplasty, complete adequate revascularization probably cannot be achieved. Therefore, in general, the totally occluded coronary artery should be tried first, and if that is successful, the second or subsequent lesions can be approached either at the same sitting or as staged procedures. In some cases, the procedure may be staged over a few days so that the patient can be returned to the laboratory sometime after the initial opening of the totally occluded artery and that vessel checked angiographically to assure its patency before the second or subsequent vessels are tried. If the angioplasty of the totally occluded artery is accomplished quite rapidly, then sequential angioplasty rather than a staged procedure of the other vessels can be reasonably considered.

In patients with multiple lesions in the coronary vessels, including a totally occluded artery, the criteria for attempting a total occlusion can sometimes be widened. If the patient has had a previous infarction and has a totally occluded coronary vessel with a scar in the distribution of that vessel and no significant reversible thallium defect, but with collaterals going to that vessel from another major epicardial coronary artery that itself has a significant lesion, the total occlusion should be opened first to provide antegrade flow through that vessel and also to provide the possibility of collateral flow to the other vessel undergoing angioplasty in the event of a dissection, spasm, or abrupt reclosure of that second vessel during the procedure. This is a protective mechanism for the second artery involved, and although the amount of functioning myocardium in the distribution of the totally occluded artery may not be great, the insurance that reestablishment of antegrade flow through the totally occluded vessel provides during the angioplasty attempt of the second vessel is significant and may ensure the ability to present the surgeon with a stable patient if a problem develops during the PTCA attempt in the second vessel. In the case of a totally obstructed major epicardial coronary artery that receives its collateral supply from another diseased major artery (i.e., a totally occluded LAD with collaterals from a dominant right coronary artery that has a 90% lesion), establishing antegrade flow through the totally obstructed artery first is necessary so that dealing with the lesion in the other artery does not jeopardize essentially two-thirds of the myocardium should a problem develop during the procedure (i.e., a left-main equivalent in terms of myocardial supply). Cases presented in Appendix I demonstrate some of these theories advanced above.

EQUIPMENT AND TECHNIQUE

PTCA of totally occluded vessels can be done by either the brachial or femoral technique. The technique should first be selected based on the experience of the practitioner with the approach route. If equal experience with both techniques is available, the technique that would most likely provide the best back-up platform from the guiding catheter to assist the passage of the wire and balloon across the area of total obstruction should be chosen. One advantage of the brachial technique over the femoral technique is the ability to deep-seat the guiding catheter in the proximal third or half of the right coronary artery and to selectively position the tip of the guiding catheter in either the left anterior descending or circumflex coronary arteries in order to achieve more powerful back-up to cross total occlusions. It must be kept in mind, however, that these techniques represent some danger of dissection of the proximal artery and should only be attempted by practitioners who are very experienced in handling brachial catheters.

In the early series of patients noted above, in the 29% of patients in whom initial success was not achieved, 70% were tried by the femoral route and 20% by the brachial route. Ten percent were tried by both approaches. The second approach was used in these dual cases with the expectation that better back-up could be achieved.

If the brachial approach is to be used, the initial guiding catheter is predominantly a 3 inch medium-style brachial guide. If a small aortic root is present, a 2 inch medium guide is often satisfactory. Not infrequently, the "bent tip" Amplatz-style brachial catheter is needed to provide the back-up pressure necessary to force the dilatation catheter system across the total occlusion. In the right coronary artery, in particular, the total occlusion of that vessel may cause damping of the brachial guide when it is inserted into the right coronary ostium. This should be avoided, and adequate pressure and flow can be accomplished and maintained throughout the procedure by either changing to an 8 French (as opposed to the commonly used 8.3 French) catheter or using a catheter with side holes to provide antegrade flow into the proximal portion of the vessel while attempting the angioplasty. This is generally not a problem in the left coronary system, since either the left anterior descending or circumflex vessel is usually open if the other vessel is totally occluded.

From the femoral approach, when the right coronary artery is the target vessel, it is generally appropriate to start with a standard FR4 Judkins-style guiding catheter. Not infrequently, this catheter will wedge in the proximal stump of the totally occluded right coronary artery, and if this happens and pressure damping occurs with dye injections hanging up in the proximal stump and its side branches, then a catheter with prepared side holes should be used to achieve antegrade flow in the proximal part of the vessel, which usually has numerous side branches, often including the SA nodal branch, that do not tolerate occlusion for the long period of time sometimes necessary to cross total occlusions. The Judkins-style catheter, however, may not provide adequate back-up to force the balloon across the total occlusion. If the lesion is in the middle or distal segment of the right coronary artery, then sometimes a Judkins-style catheter can be advanced over the wire into a deep-seated position in the artery to achieve better back-up force for advancement of the balloon catheter system. If this deep-seating is possible, further advancement of the guide

with a forward push from its femoral insertion site may provide additional back-up support by forcing the body of the guide against the opposite side of the aorta. This maneuver is possible once the tip of the guide is firmly entrenched in the proximal vessel. This technique again presents the potential danger of trauma to the proximal vessel and should be used with care and only attempted by skillful and very experienced practitioners. If the lesion is proximal or if the vessel is small, this deep-seating often cannot be accomplished. An Arani-style catheter will often provide a very similar type of back-up support. The selection of the Arani-style catheter will be determined on the angle of takeoff of the origin of the right coronary artery, and the shorter or longer tip length also can be appropriately selected. Often, the information needed to select these variations of catheters is provided by the experience and sensation gained by starting with the familiar standard Judkins-style guide. Amplatz-style guiding catheters can also be used to provide better back-up than that of Judkins-style catheters in the right coronary artery. I have found that the Amplatz right 1- and 2-style catheters often do not provide good back-up because of the shortness of their tip and shaft curve. An Amplatz left 1 or 2 catheter positioned in the right coronary artery will often provide excellent back-up support. El Gamal model catheters are also often useful to provide back-up support, particularly in cases with a wide aorta.

The ultimate balloon size should be predicated on the size of the artery just as it would if the artery were not totally occluded. Because of the smaller appearance of hypoperfused distal vessels receiving their supply by collaterals, the initial assessment of balloon size may need to be revised upward once the artery is open and antegrade flow reestablished, again making sure that distal spasm is not present. A much larger caliber vessel may be seen and upsizing of the balloon may be necessary. This phenomenon, of course, is very familiar to surgeons who for years have commented that collaterally filled arterial segments appear much larger "in person" than they do angiographically. However, in many instances, it is necessary to start with a smaller balloon to achieve initial passage across the total occlusion and, then using an extendible or exchange wire, pass a larger balloon across the opened total obstruction to achieve the ideal size required in that vessel. I have found it helpful to prepare the balloon with the balloon sheath still over the balloon segment to maintain the extremely low profile that is present before actual balloon inflation. Even minimal "winging" or "flagging" of the balloon segment can thwart the ability to pass the balloon segment across a wired total occlusion, particularly if the back-up support from the guide is somewhat less than ideal. If this method of balloon preparation is used, the balloon in the sheath should be maintained on constant 4–6 atm for a considerable time, then returned to neutral. Negative pressure should be applied only just before lesion crossing is attempted. If the initial balloon inflation at the lesion demonstrates the pressure of air, this may be diffused downstream during the balloon inflation and some pain and ST segment changes may persist following balloon deflation. Forcefully injecting contrast through the guiding catheter will usually clear the vessel of the small amounts of air and relieve the symptomatic and electrocardiographic evidence of persistent ischemia. Subsequent balloon inflations usually show complete filling of the balloon with contrast with no air present. This phenomenon, the price for a nonwinged balloon to cross a tight stenosis, varies in different balloon types.

If the total occlusion is quite recent (within 2 months), the chances of being able to pass the appropriate-sized balloon across the total obstruction initially are quite good. In the case of a very old total obstruction, these chances lessen, and in those cases, it is wise to begin with the lowest-profile, stiffest balloon catheter available to open a small channel and then, using either the extendible or exchange wire, insert the proper-sized balloon for the target vessel. As always, the anatomy of the artery proximal to the lesion must be considered. If considerable tortuosity is present, the ability to provide force at the site of total occlusion is diminished and may thwart the success of the procedure. As discussed in Chapter 2 (Coronary Angioplasty Equipment), dealing with angioplasty equipment, some of the low-profile balloons have a stiffer shaft than others, and, in general, for total occlusions, the stiffest shaft is necessary to cross the total occlusion, particularly if it is older than 2 months.

The selection of guide wires in total occlusions is, of course, of great importance in achieving success. It must be kept in mind that even with a total occlusion the safety of the wire within the vessel must be a prime consideration; I generally prefer to use a 0.014 wire and in my experience have found that going to a stiffer 0.016 wire has only rarely been successful. I generally start with either a 0.014 USCI, flexible steerable wire or a 0.014 ACS High-Torque Floppy II wire. If, with manipulations described below, these wires will not cross the total occlusion, then I prefer to switch to a 0.014 ACS intermediate wire. This currently seems to

be the "magic" wire to cross total occlusions, and in many cases of total occlusions, that is the initial wire that I select. If 0.016 steerable or stiffer wires are used, the increased chance for success is low, but certainly the potential for damage and dissection of the artery is higher than with the 0.014 wires.

In selecting the initial wire, the proximal vessel prior to the total occlusion should be kept in mind. If tortuosity or diffuse disease is present, then the use of a 0.014 flexible steerable or High-Torque Floppy II wire to at least get the equipment to the level of total occlusion is preferable.

The wire I usually start with is either the 0.014 ACS High-Torque Floppy II wire or the 0.014 flexible steerable 98% Teflon-coated or fully silicone-coated USCI wire. In general, the wire is passed into the vessel and up to the total obstruction by itself. An attempt is then made to cross the total occlusion with the wire alone. In some cases, the mandril in these wires will buckle once the tip of the wire has reached the total occlusion, and the power necessary to cross the total occlusion cannot be transmitted to the tip of the wire. In these cases, the balloon can be passed over the wire so that the dip of the dilatation catheter advances to the level of the mandril and thus prevents the mandril buckling. This, in essence, makes the system similar to the old G or DG systems, but this maneuver is often just enough to allow these very gentle wires to be forced across the area of total obstruction. If this stiffening of the wire with the balloon does not work, then changing to a 0.014 steerable wire or, preferably, the 0.014 ACS intermediate wire often provides just enough increased stiffness that the wire will successfully cross the total obstruction. This is usually done with the balloon left in its position in the artery so that the proximal portion of the artery does not have to be traversed with the wire again. Another advantage of leaving the balloon in this position is that, if accentuated tip curves of the wire were necessary to negotiate the proximal vessel, a straighter or minimally curved tip can then be used to try to advance across the total occlusion that usually does not have any troublesome curves in it. Once the total obstruction is crossed, it is of utmost importance that the physician maneuvering the wire be certain that the tip of the guide wire is free and turning nicely, since this is a prime indication that the wire is in the true lumen of the vessel. If the tip does not turn freely and will not advance easily, then either a small side branch distal to the total obstruction may be engaged or the tip may be in a false lumen and should not be advanced. In some cases, the tightness of the area of total obstruction crossed may preclude easy wire-tip rotation, but some turning of the tip of the wire should be possible if it is in the true lumen.

In a large series of patients, in those patients in whom we could not achieve initial success, two or three wires were used in 42% of the cases. In the successful cases, 92% success was achieved with the primary wire, 6% with the second wire, and 2% with a third wire.

Once the tip of the wire is across the total obstruction and moving freely, the wire should be passed as far distally in the vessel as possible to provide a good back-up stent for the balloon to track across the area of total obstruction. The balloon catheter is then advanced to the total obstruction and the tip engaged, and with as much back-up as necessary from the guiding catheter, the balloon is passed across the total obstruction. It is generally advisable to pass the balloon as far distally as possible in the length of total obstruction, to be sure that the entire length of the complete stenosis can be crossed. Once this is achieved, the balloon should be slowly inflated to adequate pressures, usually 7–9 atm, to achieve full balloon inflation without indentation. If the total obstruction is long, then the distal part of the total obstruction should be dilated first, and then balloon inflations carried out in the proximal part of the total obstruction. In some cases, the balloon will not cross the entire length of the total obstruction due to the severity and length of the lesion. If partial crossing can be achieved, antegrade balloon inflations will often allow forward progress of the deflated balloon as the overall obstruction is lessened. Total crossing of lesions in this manner is often the only way that a lengthy total obstruction can be traversed. Once this has been achieved, the balloon could be withdrawn into the guiding catheter and injections made to visualize the lumen molded by the balloon inflations. For these injections to be adequately made, if the guiding catheter has side holes, the balloon catheter tip must be withdrawn proximal to the side holes to achieve best visualization.

Once this has been done, the adequacy of the lumen formed can be evaluated, and the presence or absence of any distal lesions can also be ascertained. Intracoronary nitroglycerin will differentiate between reflex distal spasm and true fixed obstructions, as discussed above. If obstructive distal lesions are present, they should be dealt with on an individual basis with the wire still across the entire length of the artery. This may necessitate extending the wire and using smaller balloons in distal segments of the artery. If a larger balloon is needed to achieve an adequate lumen at the site of total obstruction, then either the extendible or an exchange guide wire should be used, leaving the tip of the guide wire across all lesions.

As in other vessels, if the dilatations have been carried out in the proximal part of the artery near the ostium (particularly in the right coronary artery), the safety of postangioplasty angiography must be of considerable concern. One must be careful not to allow the tip of the guide or a diagnostic catheter to seat in the area of balloon inflations, a situation that courts dissection and failure while attempting to obtain good visualization of the vessel postangioplasty. In many cases, the final angiographic injections should be achieved with the wire still in the vessel and, particularly if digital subtraction equipment or excellent quality videodisc replay is used, will provide adequate postangioplasty angiograms to assess the results.

COMPLICATIONS AND PITFALLS

Perhaps the greatest pitfall in this group of patients would be to assume that because the artery is totally occluded to begin with there could be no complications. As can be seen in Table 6–3, there is a 2% emergency surgery rate and a 3.2% myocardial infarction rate. As discussed previously, this may relate to proximal dissection of artery or dislodgement of the material totally obstructing the vessel, causing distal embolization that may shut off collateral supply. It is imperative that these patients have full cardiovascular surgery back-up as with other patients undergoing angioplasty. One complication of more concern in this series than in either subsets of native artery subtotal blockage is that of distal embolization. One must remember that the artery is totally occluded and that the wire and balloon are being pushed through that area of total occlusion. In making the initial hole, certainly one must theorize that small amounts of debris are pushed distally in many cases. This distal embolization can provide occlusion of very small distal vessels result-

TABLE 6–3. PTCA: Total Occlusions (N = 264)—Complications

	Percent
EM/CABG	2
Q wave	0.7
"Pruning"	1.9
Death	0

ing in chest discomfort and ST elevations, which may last for a few hours with no important sequelae. However, large distal vessels may also be obstructed, and in one such case, the patient was taken to surgery because of significant amount of myocardium that would have been lost had that distal vessel not been reopened. The closure of collateral routes is also a distinct possibility.

The threat of arterial perforation is theoretically higher in the subgroup. Both at the level of the total obstruction and in the distal vessel that has not been optimally visualized, the manipulation of the guide wire must be undertaken with extreme care, and it should be remembered that advancement of the guide wire should never be forced.

In the initial series of patients referenced in this chapter, emergency bypass surgery was required in three patients (1.7% of the total series) (Table 6–3). One patient had unremitting spasm, a second had distal embolization to a major distal branch, and the third went to surgery because the guide wire appeared to have extruded into the pericardium (but, in fact, at surgery it was demonstrated to be in a very small side branch not angiographically obvious). Q wave infarction was seen in 0.8% of patients, and a significant elevation of the CPK-MB was present in 3% of patients. "Pruning" of distal vessels, not considered clinically significant, was nevertheless angiographically demonstrated in 1.9% of the patients. There were no deaths in this series. Allowing for duplication in the above subset of complications, there were significant complications in 2.3% of the series. Interestingly, three patients in this series suffered abrupt reclosure in the early hours following angioplasty. One would think that such events would be "silent," but the sudden onset of severe chest pain and striking EKG changes—and in one case complete heart block—heralded the abrupt reclosure. These patients had all been perfectly stable with a totally occluded artery hours before, but when it reoccluded, obviously the collaterals were not available to perfuse the affected myocardium. Distal small embolic debris may have compromised the collateral flow. All patients were returned to the catheterization laboratory, and the recurrent total occlusion crossed with a gentle wire and the artery reopened. None of these patients went to bypass surgery.

RECURRENCE

Recurrence in angioplasty, in general, is discussed in detail in Chapter 10 (Recurrence Following Suc-

cessful PTCA) in this book and in more detail elsewhere (see Bibliography to Chapter 10). Without 100% angiographic restudy, the true recurrence rate in any subset of patients cannot be determined. In this initial series of patients, an angiographic restudy rate of 42% was achieved. An analysis of the restudied patients in this group illustrates the imperfection of relying on any parameter other than angiographic restudy as an indicator of significant recurrence. Of the 79 patients restudied, 39 total or partial recurrences were seen. Twenty-five patients demonstrated a total recurrence on angiographic restudy, and 14 patients demonstrated a significant partial recurrence. Of these 39 patients, 10% were asymptomatic, and therefore, had symptoms alone been depended on to indicate patency or recurrence, these patients would be considered "patent."

Conversely, of the 79 patients restudied, 40 were demonstrated to have full patency of the previously dilated, totally occluded segments. Of these 40 patients, 60% were symptomatic, and therefore, had clinical symptoms been used to predict recurrence, these patients would have been considered to have reoccluded when, in fact, the segment was angiographically patent.

Table 6–4 demonstrates the parameters that were statistically analyzed in this group in an attempt to predict recurrence in patients with total occlusions undergoing successful initial PTCA. No clinical factor, including age, sex, lipids, and the presence of diabetes, proved to be a predictor of recurrence. The percent diameter stenosis pre- or postangioplasty, and the pressure gradient pre- and postangioplasty, as well as the occlusion duration (which has previously been documented to be a predictor of *success*) did not prove to be statistically significant as a predictor of recurrence.

However, in those patients in the subgroup who recurred, two intraprocedural factors proved to be statistically significant as predictors of recurrence. The higher the balloon inflation pressure needed to achieve a satisfactory result and the more balloon inflations needed to achieve this result, the more likely was the chance of recurrence. Table 6–5 shows the

TABLE 6–4. PTCA: Total Occlusion—Recurrence

Parameter	P
Higher balloon inflation pressure	$< .05$
More balloon inflations	$< .05$
Age, sex, lipids, diabetes, PDS, $^{\Delta}$, occlusion duration	NS

TABLE 6–5. Predictors of Restenosis (Mean Values ± SD for Patent and Recurred Patients)

Predictor	Groups		Significance (P vs. R)
	Patent (P)	Recurred (R)	
Balloon inflations	4 ± 1.1	6 ± 1.6	i = 293 P < .01
Inflation pressure	7 ± 1.4	9 ± 1.5	i = −1.97 P < 1.05

mean values for patients demonstrated angiographically to be patent or to have had recurrence in terms of numbers of balloon inflations and the maximum inflation pressure uses. In those patients with demonstrated continued patency, the mean number of balloon inflations was four, whereas in those patients with recurrence, the mean number of balloon inflations was six. The maximum inflation pressure used in patients with demonstrated continued patency was 7 atm, and in those patients who recurred, the mean inflation pressure was 9 atm. These differences are statistically significant.

Of those patients with demonstrated significant recurrence, 70% were treated with a second angioplasty with a good long-term result and 10% had elective coronary bypass surgery. Twenty percent of patients decided to continue on medical therapy as their only treatment.

CLINICAL IMPLICATIONS: EFFICIENCY OF PTCA IN TOTAL OCCLUSIONS

In the initial series of patients referred to above, 71% had primary success. A higher primary success rate can now be expected because of further improvements, particularly in wire technology and also lower-profile and stiffer balloon catheters to deal with total occlusions. The place of laser angioplasty in dealing with total recurrences is not yet clear in the coronary system. The current status of lasers in total occlusions is described in Chapter 13 (New Technologies for the Treatment of Obstructive Arterial Disease). At some point in the future, it may be an appropriate part of the interventional armamentarium to have a hot tip or direct laser available in order to open total occlusions. Once this has been accomplished, a gentle wire can be used to cross the reopened channel and subsequent balloon angioplasty performed to achieve the adequate lumen size desired. It is clear that if a symptom duration of less than 4 months is the criterion for selection of patients, the overall efficiency rate of success can probably rise into the 80% range. Although success rate is lower in older total occlusions, some very old (up to 10 years) total occlusions have certainly been successfully crossed and dilated, and although each individual case must be judged on its own merits, attempting angioplasty in very old total occlusions is certainly warranted in selected cases.

7.   Complex PTCA III: Bifurcation Lesions

In the early years of coronary angioplasty, bifurcation lesions involving a major side branch were considered a specific contraindication to angioplasty because of the concern over the loss of the side branch during the angioplasty procedure. A major side branch would be considered one that was large enough to bypass and that supplied a significant amount of myocardium such that loss of that myocardium would cause substantial damage to the overall myocardial function. It has been reported that the possibility of loss of the side branch is approximately 14% if the side branch itself is involved with the lesion and has a lesion at its origin or in its proximal portion. That potential closure rate drops to 5% if the side branch originates from the area of disease in the major vessel, but does not have a lesion at its origin. Either of these statistical threats of vessel closure is an unacceptable additive risk to the procedure of angioplasty since the occlusion of these side branches would most likely result in a significant periprocedural myocardial infarction.

Figure 7–1 demonstrates four different anatomic variations of bifurcation lesions and also indicates the philosophy regarding the need for the "kissing balloon" technique in each case. In general, if the artery designated as a major side branch would be large enough for the surgeon to bypass if the patient undergoing elective coronary artery bypass graft surgery, then one must be concerned regarding the amount of myocardium that would be lost if side branch occlusion should occur during angioplasty.

The procedure of kissing balloon angioplasty was first described by Gruentzig in the internal-external iliac system, and in his original procedure two angioplasty balloons were inflated simultaneously to prevent the iatrogenic loss of either branch during the angioplasty procedure. Kissing balloon angioplasty has been described in numerous vessel systems, including the renal arteries, and is now an important technique allowing patients with bifurcation lesions to be considered candidates for angioplasty without the higher potential incidence of myocardial infarction from side branch occlusion during angioplasty that would occur without the protective presence of a second wire or balloon catheter system. The early experience with balloon angioplasty of coronary bifurcation lesions has been reported in the literature. An early series with my colleagues at the San Fran-

cisco Heart Institute of patients undergoing angioplasty by the kissing balloon technique indicated a very high initial success rate (65 of 66 patients successful) without any significant complications. There were no differences in this subgroup from the general series of patients as far as age, sex, or clinical factors were concerned that would allow prediction of success or failure at the time of angioplasty. The incidence of myocardial infarction in this subset of patients was 1.5%, and the incidence of emergency coronary bypass graft surgery was 1.5%. There were no deaths in the initial series, and the "major cardiac complication" incidence was 1.5%. These figures indicated that the kissing balloon technique to preserve major side branches in patients with bifurcation lesions could be done safely by experienced angioplasty physicians without any excessive risk to the patient.

A definite figure for recurrence in this group could not be ascertained because of reasons indicated in the chapter on recurrence, namely, the absence of 100% angiographic follow-up data (see Chapter 10, Recurrence Following Successful PTCA). A restudy rate of only about 36% was achieved in this subset of patients, and as stated above, the true restenosis rate cannot be accurately defined if 100% angiographic follow-up is not achieved. There are false negative and false positive indicators of the presence or absence of recurrence on clinical grounds, and although exercise testing and nuclear scintigraphy give some objective evidence of the state of vessel patency, it is clear that an accurate assessment of restenosis cannot be achieved without 100% angiographic follow-up. Of the 24 patients restudied in the initial series of 66 patients, 13 had signs of recurrence. Of the patients who recurred, ten were treated with repeat angioplasty and three underwent elective coronary artery bypass graft surgery rather than undergo a second procedure.

In the analysis of factors that might warn of the potential recurrence, the only clinical or anatomic factor that proves significant on multifactorial analysis of patients and vessels involved using the φ^2 and logistic regression analyses methods was the percent diameter stenosis prior to the angioplasty. If the percent diameter stenosis was 90% or more prior to balloon angioplasty, the chance of recurrence was greater in this subset of patients.

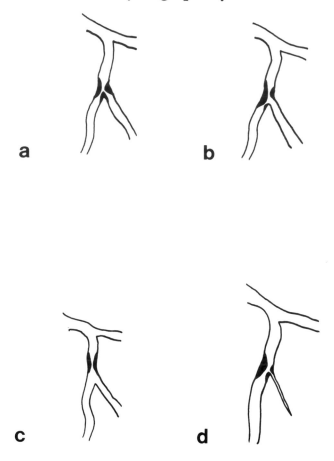

Fig. 7–1. Four types of major and side branch bifurcation stenosis. **a:** Ostial stenosis of large side branch that is involved in major branch stenosis (classical "kissing balloon" indication). **b:** Large side branch free of stenosis but balloon inflation position in the major branch will "override" the side branch (possible "kissing wire or balloon" indication). **c:** Lesion in major branch proximal to uninvolved side branch (single ballon indication). **d:** Stenosis of major branch also involves origin of the side branch that, however, is very small and would not be considered surgically bypassable (single-balloon indication).

SELECTION OF CASES AND STRATEGY

As indicated above, patients selected to undergo angioplasty by the kissing balloon technique should have a significant occlusion of a major vessel as well as a significant side branch originating from that area of disease. These may be the only coronary lesions to be approached from an angioplasty standpoint or may occur in combination with other straightforward or complex lesions in other vessels. If a major side branch arising from the area of disease in a major epicardial coronary artery is deemed suitable for bypass surgery or angioplasty, then protection of that side branch utilizing the kissing balloon or kissing wire technique should be utilized.

The strategy of approaching the two vessels depends on the amount of myocardium supplied by each. In most cases, the largest amount of myocardium will be supplied by the major vessel with the smaller amount of viable myocardium supplied by the side branch, but in some anatomic situations, the reverse is true. For example, in an LAD system with a small continuing LAD and a large diagonal branch, the diagonal branch may, in fact, supply more myocardium than does the continuing LAD. In any case, the greatest concern must be for the vessel supplying the largest amount of myocardium and that vessel is usually dilated both first and last during the kissing balloon procedure if sequential balloon inflations are employed.

In the early cases of kissing balloon angioplasty, the balloons were inflated simultaneously at some point during the procedure. Initially, in the coronary system, it was thought wise to undersize the balloons for each vessel so that simultaneous inflations could be carried out without the chance of disruption of the segment of vessel in which the two balloons would be side by side. An extension of this concept is currently used in large grafts and large coronary arteries where two balloons of an appropriate additive size are positioned at the area to be dilated and inflated simultaneously in order to achieve a larger lumen than would be possible with the commercially available balloon sizes (hugging balloon technique).

In the bifurcation lesion situation, the technique of undersizing balloons to prevent overdilatation of a segment of artery resulted in some less than satisfactory hemodynamic and angiographic results as well as an apparent higher recurrence rate. Therefore, the current strategy is to size the balloons individually for each vessel as though it were the only vessel to be treated by angioplasty and to employ sequential inflations so that additive balloon size would not damage the segment of artery where portions of the balloons are, in fact, side by side.

In general, the vessel thought to be most difficult to wire should be wired first. This assessment is made from preangioplasty angiographic evaluation and may involve the severity of the lesion, the angle of the origin of the side branch, or the tortuosity of the vessel involved. Once the presumably more difficult vessel is wired, then the second wire is placed into the other vessel, and both wires are comfortably held across the area of the disease. (The use of guiding catheter systems is discussed fully in the next section in this chapter.) At this point, the strategy is to treat the major vessel first with balloon angioplasty (major vessel again implying the amount of myocardium supplied by either artery). The balloon is passed across the area of stenosis in the major artery, and balloon angioplasty carried out in the usual fashion. During this procedure, the side branch or minor vessel is protected by a wire in place. If pressure gradients are measured, it should be understood that the presence of additional equipment in the coronary system may produce artifactual high gradients during and following balloon angioplasty in either vessel. Once an adequate angioplasty has been performed in the major artery, as seen by hemodynamic and angiographic assessment, the balloon catheter is then either advanced forward in the vessel beyond the area of second branch origin (if two guiding catheters are used) or more commonly is withdrawn into the guiding catheter before the second vessel is approached. The balloon catheter system selected for the second vessel (usually smaller) is then passed into that artery and balloon angioplasty carried out as though this were the only lesion being treated. Once an acceptable result has been achieved in this vessel, then contrast injections following balloon withdrawal into the guiding catheter can be used to assess the area of stenosis and the patency of the bifurcation. If the bifurcation is preserved and the flow into both vessels is deemed excellent, the balloon catheter should be advanced again into the major vessel and a molding inflation carried out at low pressures (1–2 atm) to remodel the area in the major vessel following the more recent angioplasty in the side branch. This remodeling ensures patency in the vessel supplying the larger amount of myocardium. Another technique that can be used at this point is to leave the balloon catheter system in the side branch at the time of this last molding inflation to provide a somewhat larger stent than the wire itself would provide in the side branch during the molding inflation. With this technique, the balloon is not inflated simultaneously.

If the bifurcation seems to be disrupted or still compromised, both balloons can be positioned at the bifurcation and simultaneously inflated to very low pressures (1–2 atm) to remodel in the in-flow into both major and minor vessels. Once this has been achieved, both balloons should be withdrawn into the guiding catheter system, and an injection of contrast carried out to reassess the patency of the bifurcation. Following an appropriate time interval, the wires can be removed and postangioplasty angiogram performed to give an accurate assessment of the results. If there is question, the balloon catheters can be removed from the guiding catheter system, both wires left in place, and an injection made through the guiding catheter that will usually provide better flow of contrast to assess the results.

In some cases, while the final balloon inflation is being carried out in the major vessel, the balloon catheter can be left in place in an uninflated state in the side branch, and the balloon in the major vessel inflated using the uninflated balloon system as a stent to

preserve the origin of the secondary vessel. This is essentially kissing balloon angioplasty with only one of the balloons inflated.

A natural evolution of the original simultaneous kissing balloon technique is the most commonly used method now, the "kissing wire" technique, in which a major side branch is not involved directly with the disease process and does not have any significant luminal narrowing at its origin, but does arise from the area of a major vessel in which the balloon will be inflated during the angioplasty attempt. The likely incidence of closure in this type of side branch is approximately 5%, and that additive percentage is an unnecessarily high potential for myocardial infarction in this group of patients. In these cases, the second balloon system (usually a different size) can be set up exactly, as in the true kissing balloon technique, and, with both wires across the lesions, the major artery treated first with angioplasty; then if any disruption of the secondary branch is seen, the appropriate balloon can be passed over the wire already in place in this side branch.

EQUIPMENT

The kissing balloon technique can be performed using two guiding catheters or, more commonly, a one-guiding-catheter system. If two guiding catheters are used, it can be done by the brachial-femoral approach, the femoral-femoral approach, or the brachial-brachial approach. The utilization of one large lumen guiding catheter from the femoral approach is the most common technique used today.

The majority of the early cases were performed using the brachial-femoral approach. This did have some advantage over a bifemoral approach in that when the brachial and femoral systems are introduced into the ascending aorta they approach the left main ostium from different directions (the brachial guide from below and the femoral guide from above). This different anatomic orientation allows the two guiding catheters to get out of each other's way as the procedure unfolds. There is certainly less competition for positioning in the left main coronary artery utilizing this technique. If two femoral guiding catheters or two brachial guiding catheters are used, then the orientation of these guides to the coronary orifice will be identical, and in some cases, the ease of manipulation is compromised.

In using the brachial-femoral approach, the individual guiding catheter should be selected as though the cannulation of the coronary ostium were being carried out only by each individual guiding catheter system. The entrance to the branchial or femoral artery is by the standard approach: A pacing catheter in the right heart is advised and can be placed either through the brachial cutdown site or via puncture of the femoral vein.

In using the one-guiding-catheter/two-wire technique, a large lumen guide is necessary. A special "Y" connector with dual hemostatic valve ports is used, and the initial maneuver is usually to pass a "bare" wire through the guide and across the lesion into the secondary branch. The balloon and wire system to be used in the major branch is then advanced through the duostat adaptor and advanced to the tip of the guiding catheter. Advancing the balloon with no leading wire can lessen the chance of wrapping the two wire systems within the guiding catheter shaft. Once the balloon tip is at the end of the guiding catheter, and the wire from the first system seated across the lesion and in the secondary branch, the major vessel should then be wired, again taking care to avoid wrapping of the two wires now in the coronary artery. To-and-fro movements of the wire tip should be used rather than large circumferential turns, since this lessens the chance of wire wrapping. Once the major vessel has been wired, the balloon catheter can be positioned at the lesion and appropriate inflations carried out. This balloon catheter can then be withdrawn into the guiding catheter and injections made through the guide to assess the patency and the necessity for treating the secondary branch with balloon angioplasty. If that appears to be necessary, the balloon over the wire in the major branch should then be withdrawn from the guiding catheter system over an extended wire and either that same balloon or an appropriately sized balloon advanced over an extended wire into the side branch and inflations carried out. Although somewhat tedious, it is then often advisable to remove this secondary balloon catheter system and reintroduce the balloon in the major vessel for the final low-pressure molding inflation. Although I favor using extendible wires in this circumstance so that the extendible portions can be removed and taken from the field during the procedure, the initial use of two long exchange wires is also an appropriate alternative to use. the use of a monorail system may also prove to be efficacious in this setting.

If the brachial-femoral or bifemoral approach is used with two guiding catheters, the preliminary angiographic pictures can be obtained using either guiding catheter system. Once these have been obtained, it is wise to position both guiding catheters in readiness for the procedure as the next step. Both balloon and guide wire system should be prepared prior to any insertions, and then both the systems should be inserted into the dual guiding catheters and advanced to the tip

of the guiding catheter, ready to cannulate the coronary artery before either is advanced into the coronary artery system. This enhances rapid progression of the procedure once the coronary artery has been entered and is an important aspect of the dual guiding catheter technique because of the potential for relative myocardial ischemia once the catheter system is in place. If any undue delay in getting the second dilatation catheter system occurs, myocardial ischemia and patient discomfort can be significant from the first balloon catheter system already in place.

As stated above, balloon catheters should be selected for each individual lesion and should be sized according to that vessel. If the tortuosity of either vessel appears to be a problem, the balloon catheter selected should have maximum trackability. If the stenosis is particularly tight, the stiffness of the shaft of the catheter may influence selection of the system used (see Chapter 2, Coronary Angioplasty Equipment, on equipment for the various qualities of balloon catheters).

Guide wire selection should again reflect the anatomy of each individual artery. If a lesion is particularly tight and upsizing of the balloon thought to be potentially necessary, the use of an exchange wire initially or the availability of an extendible wire is certainly important. This strategy again reflects the theory that each lesion should be approached individually, and the equipment selected appropriate for that lesion viewed as an independent solitary challenge. The tortuosity of the vessel proximal and distal to the lesions may provide a clue for the selection of the wire. In the case of the major side branch, an acute angular origin may be encountered. The tip of the guide wire selected for that vessel may need to have an accentuated curve in order to cannulate the origin of the vessel selectively. This is sometimes of extreme technical difficulty, because the origin may originate from an area of stenosis and that stenosis may direct the tip of the wire in a direction away from or not consistent with the origin of the major side branch. For this reason, it is frequently advisable that the major side branch, if deemed to be the most difficult to cannulate, is wired first. If an accentuation of the angle at the tip of the guide wire is necessary, manipulation of this wire first will also lessen the chance of wrapping of wires once both are in the artery since the second wire could potentially have a less angled tip and therefore carry less possibility of twisting around the wire already existent in the vessel.

If a dual guiding catheter system is utilized, both guiding catheters should be positioned in the ascending aorta, ready to cannulate the coronary ostium, and both balloon and guide wire systems advanced to the tip of the guiding catheters. The guide carrying the balloon sized for the branch deemed most difficult to cannulate is then positioned at the coronary orifice. At this point, the wire is advanced into the first vessel to be cannulated and the distal vessel wired. The guiding catheter of that system is then withdrawn from the coronary orifice to allow the second guiding catheter to be advanced into position. The second balloon catheter and wire system is then advanced into the next branch to be cannulated and the wire passed across the lesion and into that distal vessel. That guiding catheter is then withdrawn from the coronary orifice, and at this point in the procedure, with both vessels wired, strict attention should be paid to the presence of myocardial ischemia (as evidenced by EKG changes or patient complaints) that may be induced by the presence of the two wires in the coronary arteries. This is also true of the one-guide, two-wire technique since just the profiles of two wires in a severely stenotic area of the coronary artery may induce considerable myocardial ischemia. In general, 0.014 wires are used, but even their additive diameters may be sufficient to produce ischemia. The balloon should then be advanced rapidly and smoothly into the major vessel and balloon angioplasty carried out. Following a good result in this artery, the balloon segment of the dilatation catheter should be removed from the area of stenosis, either by advancing it into the distal vessel or, more commonly, by withdrawing it into the guiding catheter. If it is withdrawn into the guiding catheter, the guide can then be withdrawn from the coronary orifice and the second guide positioned with subsequent advancement of the second dilatation catheter system into the next vessel. The angioplasty is then carried out in the secondary vessel, and following an appropriate result, the balloon catheter system is generally withdrawn into the guide, as noted above. The major vessel that first underwent angioplasty is then reentered with the balloon catheter and inflation carried out at low pressures (1–2 atm) to remodel that area. If there is any question about the patency of the bifurcation, when dual guiding catheters are used, both balloons can be positioned at the bifurcation and simultaneously inflated at low pressures.

With the one-guide, two-wire system, true "kissing balloon" angioplasty cannot be carried out unless the dilatation catheters used are "balloon-on-wire" systems. Utilizing a large lumen guiding catheter, two of these catheters can be advanced through the guide and both the major and minor branches wired, and the potential for either sequential or simultaneous balloon inflation exists. Other than the potential simultaneous balloon inflations, there is no advantage to use the

balloon on wire equipment over the one-guide, two-wire, single-balloon sequential technique.

It should again be emphasized that in advancing the second wire into the coronary system after the first wire is in place, very little torquing of the second wire should be undertaken. If excessive torque manipulation is needed, the chance of the wires wrapping around each other in the proximal vessel is enhanced, and this wrapping makes it very difficult to advance either balloon catheter system into the target vessel. Viewing of the position of the wires in at least two angiographic angles will confirm or disprove the presence of any wire wrapping.

Following the procedure, postangioplasty angiogram should be undertaken with the guiding catheter, and all systems should be kept sterile and available for reentry should any problems be shown on the formal postangioplasty angiograms. With the one-guide, two-wire system, removal of the balloon and injections made through the guide with only both wires in place generally gives excellent angiographic evaluation of the area. If the result appears satisfactory, then the wires and the guiding catheter systems are removed by standard techniques.

In the initial days of the kissing balloon technique, the procedure was very cumbersome. One of the difficulties was the amount of hardware needed for the procedure. Two guiding catheters, four manifolds, and two balloon catheter systems, complete with balloon inflation devices, composed considerable equipment that can be confusing to the practitioner. With the development and popularity of the one-guide, two-wire, one-balloon technique, a lot of this clutter has been removed and the technique simplified greatly. It is, however, a very complex procedure and should be attempted only by physicians possessing extensive experience gained in dealing with straightforward lesions. The complexity of the procedure and the necessity of insertion and removal of equipment is, in my opinion, better handled by having two experienced practitioners working together. This certainly enhances the ease of the procedure and decreases the risk to the patient.

COMPLICATIONS AND PITFALLS

As stated above, the major complication rate in this series of patients is about 1.5%. This includes 1.5% emergency bypass graft surgery and 1.5% myocardial infarction. Despite the complexity of the technical aspects of the procedure, there is no increased periprocedural risk in this subset of patients. It is also obvious that in this subset of patients, were the kissing balloon technique not used, the risk to the patient would be dramatically increased by up to 14% chance of significant myocardial infarction during the procedure.

The unique procedural pitfalls that must be avoided revolve around the amount of hardware being introduced into the coronary system during this technique. In a case of a very severe stenosis, the additive diameter of the two guide wires may be enough to produce ischemia, and in this case, the rapidity with which the angioplasty is carried out is of major significance. The presence of two experienced operators reduces the risk of this aspect at the procedure. Care must be taken during the procedure to be aware of the position of the guiding catheter or catheters so that obstruction of the main coronary orifice does not occur. If great care is not taken, it is particularly easy for this to happen during the procedure because of the introduction, removal, and reintroduction of various catheter systems that can cause movement of the guiding catheter tip during those maneuvers.

Compared with lesions of the left anterior descending/left anterior descending diagonal coronary artery (most frequent) and the left circumflex coronary artery, usually involving the main circumflex artery and an obtuse marginal branch, the incidence of kissing balloon angioplasty in the right coronary artery is dramatically low. Kissing balloon angioplasty in the right coronary artery is extremely difficult, because an appropriate lesion in the right coronary suitable for kissing balloon angioplasty generally occurs at the terminal bifurcation of the right coronary artery and the posterior descending and posterolateral branches. The length of the main coronary artery that must be traversed before this bifurcation is reached is usually considerably greater than is the proximal length of coronary artery in either the LAD/LADD or the LCX/OM systems. This increased length of proximal vessel in the right coronary artery leads to greater difficulties with wire-wrapping and often precludes the successful passage of the dilatation catheters to the point of obstruction. It is certainly easier to use the one-guide, two-wire, one-balloon system in this case since the presence of two-balloon catheter systems in the proximal right coronary artery for the usual long length of that vessel results in a very large additive diameter of considerable length, which can produce myocardial ischemia of significance during the procedure. Patients with bifurcation lesions in the right coronary artery should, therefore, be carefully selected, and it should be understood that the proximal right coronary artery must be of quite large diameter to accommodate the systems. Distal right coronary bifurcation lesions are most appropriately treated using the one-guide, two-wire technique.

Kissing balloon angioplasty for bifurcation lesions is now a well-developed technique that is entirely acceptable for dealing with bifurcation lesions. It lessens the risk of the procedure and in experienced hands can produce dramatic and excellent results. In the early days of development of this technique, it was somewhat limited by the fact that most cases were done utilizing two guiding catheters and that familiarity with the brachial technique was often a great advantage in performing the procedure. With larger lumen femoral guides and dual port "Y" adaptor valves, the technique has been greatly simplified, and although the true "kissing balloon" feature is no longer commonly used, the two-wire technique to protect the side branch is certainly a striking advance in the techniques of angioplasty. It extends the possibility of angioplasty to patients having this type of lesion and allows them to be treated safely and effectively by angioplasty.

8. Complex PTCA IV: Bypass Grafts

BACKGROUND AND STATISTICS

Since bypass graft surgery began in the late 1960s, the use of the reverse saphenous vein and the internal mammary artery as conduits to mechanically revascularize areas of ischemic myocardium by direct anastomosis to vessels distal to severely stenotic areas has been extensively used. Now that long-term follow-up of these conduits is available, it is obvious that, particularly in the case of the saphenous vein bypass graft, a high incidence of significant deterioration and stenosis of the grafts may occur several years postsurgery. Angiographic restudies have demonstrated that, in over one-third of the patients who have undergone bypass surgery 10 or more years ago, significant occlusive disease, either at the proximal or distal anastomotic site, or in the body of the bypass graft, has developed. Since nearly three decades have passed since the initiation of this surgical treatment for ischemic coronary artery disease, a large number of patients are now being reevaluated for recurrence of their symptoms because of either lesions in the grafts or progression of the disease in the native coronary arterial system.

Initially, the treatment for graft stenosis or occlusion was either the addition of substantial medical therapy or repeat bypass graft surgery. It is obvious that statistically there is higher morbidity and mortality associated with a second or third major chest surgery, and since the surgery is often technically more difficult, the revascularization achieved by repeat surgery is frequently incomplete. With the improvement in technology and increased operator experience, PTCA is now a reasonable technique for mechanical revascularization in patients with stenotic saphenous vein or internal mammary bypass grafts who are not significantly responsive to medical therapy and face the increased risk and discomfort of repeat coronary artery bypass graft surgery. The development of new lesions in native coronary arteries downstream from the distal anastomosis of a patent graft also presents an acceptable challenge to the experienced practitioner of angioplasty.

In my series of patients with stenotic lesions in bypass grafts, the majority of patients treated have lesions in the saphenous vein bypass grafts, but 5% of these patients developed problems with internal mammary bypass grafts. Angioplasty was technically suc-

cessful in 85% of patients, 86% of grafts, and 85% of the sites attempted. The mean time from bypass surgery to angioplasty was 51.2 months. The mean preangioplasty stenosis diameter of 77% was reduced to a postangioplasty diameter of 27%. Emergency bypass graft surgery was necessary in less than 2% of patients, and myocardial infarction occurred in 3.6% of patients. There were no deaths in the series. This experience is reported in more detail in the literature.

Statistical analyses were undertaken in an early group of patients by my colleagues and me at the San Francisco Heart Institute to attempt to predict success in this group of patients. The only statistically significant predictors of success were higher measured balloon-graft ratios, smaller diameter grafts, and shorter lesion lengths in the grafts.

The term "measured balloon-graft ratio" refers to the ratio of diameters actually measured of the inflated balloon documented angiographically during the procedure and the bypass graft measured in a segment deemed to be "normal" near the area of stenosis. It should be kept in mind that these "normal" areas of vein grafts in particular are probably diffusely diseased, although may appear smooth angiographically. A second ratio, which differs from the measured balloon-graft ratio, is the "expected balloon-graft ratio," which is derived from the commercially listed balloon size and the measured graft diameter, as described above. Measurements should be performed using a caliper computer and precise pre- and postangioplasty measurements of percent diameter stenosis, and lesion length should be calculated in three angiographic views with the computer calculating the mean of these results.

It should be kept in mind that with balloons made of polyvinyl chloride and other materials it is known that these materials have a compliance characteristic that allows for larger balloon diameters at higher inflation pressures than are indicated by the commercially "expected" balloon size. Therefore, the measured balloon size will often differ from the expected balloon size (see Appendix II–E).

It is interesting that analysis of the clinical factors in patients developing stenoses in bypass grafts reveals that insulin-dependent diabetes was found in about 20% of patients, elevated triglycerides, in 35%, and elevated cholesterol, in 22% and that fully 65% of the patients who developed significant problems with bypass grafts necessitating reintervention continued to smoke cigarettes after their bypass graft surgery and were smoking at the time of angioplasty.

The mean period of time in these patients since bypass surgery was 51.2 months with a range of 2–144 months. The majority (over 60%) had had their bypass surgery 12 months or more prior to angioplasty. The mean time from reonset of symptoms to the time of angioplasty procedure was 6.7 months (range 1–60 months). As stated above, a success rate of about 85% was achieved in this group of patients. This includes technical success in patients, and grafts and of sites attempted. The predictors of angiographic success were a higher measured balloon-graft ratio, a higher expected balloon-graft ratio, a smaller graft diameter, and shorter lesion length. This suggests that in bypass grafts, at least, the balloon should be slightly larger than the diameter of the vessel, and it is also noteworthy that the measured ratio of over 1.1:1.0 was associated with the lowest residual percent diameter stenosis after angioplasty.

In this series of patients, distal embolization or abrupt reclosure resulting in myocardial infarction produced a 3.6 major cardiac event rate. There were no deaths in these patients. In analyzing this group of patients for predictors of complications, the only predictor was the presence of diffuse atheromatous disease in the grafts. In those patients having complications, all grafts were older than 4 years. In an initial series of patients where 70 cases were performed with initial success, 26 patients had angiographic restudy at a mean of 7.9 months after angioplasty. Of these 26 patients, 16 had all lesions dilated patent, and ten had evidence of recurrence at at least one site. It should again be emphasized that in the overall series the recurrence rate cannot be determined with out percent angiographic follow-up. In the ten patients with recurrence in the early series, seven had no change in clinical classification and their exercise testing abnormalities were similar to their preangioplasty state at the time of suspected recurrence. The other three patients with recurrence had improvement in both clinical classification and in their exercise testing results.

Age, sex, anginal class or duration, presence or absence of diabetes mellitus, hypercholesterolemia, hypertriglyceridemia, smoking history, graft age, graft diameter, and native vessel grafted as well as percent diameter stenosis before or after angioplasty were not statistically significant predictors of restenosis, as has been suggested in other series. The only significant predictor of recurrence was the percent diameter stenosis immediately after balloon dilata-

tion. A low measured balloon-to-graft ratio was present in most of these cases and was also thought to be a strong predictor of recurrence.

SELECTION OF EQUIPMENT AND STRATEGY

Guiding catheters should be selected to appropriately coaxially cannulate the origin of the graft to be dilated, and it should be remembered that a power position of the guiding catheter may well be necessary, particularly if the lesions are in the middle or distal portion of the grafts, since a long distance may have to be traversed before the balloon is in position to be advanced across the lesion. Several guiding catheters labeled as graft guides are available, but often standard coronary catheters will suffice or even provide better back-up. In the case of the right coronary artery bypass graft, the angle of origin of the graft from the aorta is of importance in selecting the guide. If a diagnostic Judkins-style catheter is seated in a coaxial manner during the diagnostic angiogram, it may well provide excellent back-up during an angioplasty attempt. If the angle of the origin of the aortic anastomosis is more acute, that is, straight down, then a King or a multipurpose catheter may cannulate the proximal graft better. Amplatz-style catheters will often also provide good back-up in right coronary grafts. In the case of left bypass grafts, the height of the aortic anastomosis away from the aortic valve will often determine the type of guide needed. Again, in a significant number of cases, a standard right coronary Judkins-style guiding catheter will cannulate many of these left-sided grafts. Left coronary artery guiding catheters are rarely successful, but Amplatz-style guides will often cannulate the origin of the graft very suitably. In the case of left-sided venous bypass grafts placed high on the aorta, an approach from the right brachial position may solve back-up problems. With internal mammary bypasses, there are several angulated styles of catheters available, and generally one of these will intubate the origin of the left internal mammary or right internal mammary artery from its subclavian or innominate takeoff. It should be remembered that these guides can cause damage at the friable origin of the internal mammary artery, and "soft-tip" guides are usually preferable in these cases.

Although in some cases considerable back-up is needed because of the length of vessel to be traversed prior to the lesion, the lesions in the bodies of the grafts are often very soft and therefore strong back-up pressure is sometimes not necessary. As stated above, in internal mammary conduits, great care must be taken in the positioning of the guiding catheter at the origin of the internal mammary artery. This should be done with gentle finesse because the origin of this artery is notably friable and damage can occur from the guiding catheter either at the time of placement of the guiding catheter or during the attempt to advance the guiding catheter down the internal mammary artery to gain a more favorable power position. This potential danger should be emphasized strongly; it is a significant source of complications in patients with internal mammary bypass grafts. Dissection of the origin of vein bypass grafts is also a potential source of complication since these are often friable and many times contain areas of disease not readily discernible by angiography.

If a dissection of the proximal portion of the internal mammary artery or vein bypass does occur, then an attempt to "tack back" the dissection with a balloon of sufficiently large diameter is the initial treatment of choice. If this is not successful, and flow through the graft is compromised, then repeat surgery may be necessary.

As indicated in the data presented above, the balloon catheter selected for lesions in bypass grafts should be slightly larger than the exact size of the vessel, as precisely measured by calipers and caliper computers. A 1.1:1 ratio of the measured balloon diameter to the graft to be dilated is a positive factor for good long-term result without restenosis. Less than a 1:1 ratio is likewise implicated either in a poor initial result or in restenosis.

The most commonly used femoral guiding catheters in my series are the right Judkins catheter or a left 1 or 2 Amplatz guiding catheter for most vein grafts. A left internal mammary guiding catheter is the initial catheter of choice for internal mammary artery grafts. A brachial-style catheter from the femoral approach or an Arani-style catheter for saphenous vein grafts to the right coronary artery can also provide an excellent back-up platform. Guiding catheter selection should be determined by the configuration and orientation of the graft and the diameter of the ascending aorta. If the brachial approach is used, the catheter configuration that will selectively cannulate the graft is dependent on the size and shape of the ascending aorta and the positioning of the graft. In the case of a left internal mammary artery graft, approach from the left arm is advisable, and a femoral-internal mammary guiding catheter or a brachial guiding catheter may be used from this left brachial approach. A right internal mammary bypass graft is easily approached from the right arm. Both right and left internal mammary origins can be reached and cannulated using the femoral approach.

Selection of the guide wire depends on the area to be traversed both proximal and distal to the lesion in the graft. It must be kept in mind that the lining of bypass grafts is usually very friable, particularly if the graft is older than 5 years. "Unroofing" of the lining of the graft can occur as the wire is passed down the vessel with resultant embolization of debris or the raising of an occlusive flap within the graft. An example of this type of complication is demonstrated in Figure 3–5 Case A. The softness and flexibility of the tip, therefore, are extremely important, and since there are very few side branches in most grafts that will snare the tip of the wire, if the tip seems to be caught at any junction of passage down the graft, it should be immediately slightly withdrawn and turned until ease of forward advancement is present. A "caught-tip" in a graft should be considered to be a tip of wire that is underneath an irregular protrusion lining the vessel. If the tip of the guide wire is not free, this may indicate that it is beneath a piece of grumous material in the graft that might become dislodged and could cause dissection of the body of the graft or distal embolization into the native coronary system.

In cases of diffusely irregular grafts leading to the area of stenosis, I have tried to accentuate the tip curve of the wire nearly into a "U" configuration. This must be done carefully so as not to fracture the tip of the wire, but once accomplished, it allows the wire to be advanced through an irregular area of graft with a leading "U" tip that will bounce off any protruding irregularities. This type of wire may become commercially available in the future. Although the use of this configuration of wire is extremely safe in the proximal portion of bypass grafts, once the area of stenosis has been reached, it is then counterproductive and usually will not be the proper curve to cross the stenotic segment. The entire technique is to then pass the balloon catheter down the large segment of proximal irregularity over the "U" wire to the area of stenosis and then remove the "U" wire and replace it with a wire whose tip is appropriate to cross the area of stenosis and continue into the native coronary system. This makes the procedure a bit more complicated and lengthy, but does enhance the safety of the passage of the equipment in the proximal portion of grafts. In a very small graft, obviously, this technique is not appropriate if the "U" configuration of the tip of the wire would be bigger than the graft itself.

Another procedure performed in patients who have undergone previous coronary bypass graft surgery is to go through the graft (either vein or internal mammary) into the bypass native vessel in order to dilate a new lesion in the native vessel that is beyond the distal anastomosis of the graft. With proper selection of the guiding catheter, the wire is usually quite easily passed through the graft, into the native vessel, and then across the lesion. Since some considerable length of graft must be traversed in most cases, the steerability of the tip of the wire is enhanced by sequentially advancing the balloon catheter over the guide wire as it has passed through the graft, thereby giving more support to the wire and making the steerability of the tip much easier. Once the lesion in the native vessel has been crossed by the wire, the balloon should then be advanced across the lesion and inflated at the area of stenosis to achieve angioplasty. The balloon should be sized to dilate the native vessel appropriately.

COMPLICATIONS AND PITFALLS

The potential complications are mentioned above, and in this subset of patients in particular, distal embolization of debris from the lining of the graft is an area of concern. In very old grafts, this friable lining is most certainly present, even though the lumen appears to be quite smooth angiographically, and great care in manipulation of the guide wire as it passes through the graft should be taken. With any failure of the tip of the guide wire to advance easily, it should be withdrawn, turned, and then advanced only in a smooth fashion so that a flap is not raised or debris is not dislodged to become the source of distal embolization. The modified wire described above can lessen the chance of this happening. Figure 3–5 Case A demonstrates a case of a flap raised during wire advancement and subsequent healing of that flap. In this case, the area was "tacked back" using standard balloon techniques. In Case 17 in Appendix I, another method of treatment of graft body of flaps is described. This utilizes the perfusion balloon catheter, and prolonged

balloon inflations may enhance the ability to correct this complication.

Figure 3–5 Case B demonstrates distal embolization that occurs during balloon inflation. In this case, the initial balloon inflation opened the stenotic area of the bypass graft, but the immediate presence of ST changes of ischemia and chest pain indicated that distal emboli of the debris lining the graft had occurred. Another sign that this has happened is slow flow through the graft with contrast injection indicating that the plugged small distal vessels do not allow adequate runoff. If this complication occurs, emergency surgery is not advisable since the bypass is opened, but the ischemia is coming from embolic occlusion of very small distal vessels that are certainly not bypassable. In these cases, the occurrence of some degree of myocardial infarction must be accepted.

A higher chance of restenosis and a lower chance of initial technical success are present if a large enough balloon is not selected. The ideal ratio in grafts seems to be about 1.1:1, and if the ratio falls below 1:1 of a major balloon graft ratio, the chance of technical success decreases and the chance of restenosis increases. Careful measurement and selection of balloon size is therefore of paramount importance in the dilatation of bypass grafts. However, it should be cautioned that selecting balloons that are larger than a 1.1:1 ratio enhances the chance of dissection or disruption of the graft segment dilated and can, itself, cause significant complications.

Angioplasty of coronary artery bypass grafts now appears to be a feasible and, in fact, an excellent procedure to approach stenotic lesions in bypass grafts. It should be kept in mind that the process by which stenotic lesions occur is most likely different from the disease and the native coronary arteries. When carefully performed, however, angioplasty of the grafts can be carried out in a safe manner and as a satisfactory alternative to repeat bypass graft surgery in carefully selected patients.

9.   Direct PTCA in Acute Myocardial Infarction

Reperfusion therapy of evolving myocardial infarction limits myocardial damage, reduces in-hospital death, and improves long-term outcome. Although agreement on the advantages of early reperfusion in acute myocardial infarction is nearly uniform, different strategies of reperfusion, including pharmacologic, mechanical, surgical, and combination therapies, are available. For the past 10 years, the approach to acute infarct reperfusion practiced by the authors at the Mid America Heart Institute (MHI) has been direct infarct angioplasty *without* antecedent thrombolytic therapy (1). In this chapter, the technique, rationale, and results of direct infarct angioplasty will be reviewed and compared to thrombolytic therapy.

TECHNIQUE

Upon confirmation or strong suspicion in the emergency room of an evolving myocardial infarction due to the presence of chest pain and ST segment elevation, patients receive 10,000 units heparin intravenously, 160 325 mg of chewable aspirin, and a lidocaine bolus followed by a continuous infusion. The greatest benefit is anticipated in patients treated early in their course with at least partial preservation of R wave forces. However, patients as late as 24 hr from symptom onset are also studied if stuttering or persistent chest pain and ST segment elevation are present. Patients are then transported to the catheterization laboratory as quickly as possible, usually within 30 min of arrival in the emergency room. An additional 5,000–10,000 units of heparin are also given on arrival in the laboratory. Intravenous verapamil 5 mg or sublingual nifedipine 10 mg is also given unless conduction disturbances of hypotension are present. We have not routinely inserted femoral venous sheaths of temporary transvenous pacemakers during infarct interventions unless conduction disturbances have developed. In the setting of cardiogenic shock, an intraaortic balloon pump is inserted prior to cardiac catheterization. Arterial access is obtained, and left ventricular pressures are measured followed by a ventriculogram. This is omitted if circulatory collapse is present, but was possible in 91% of our first 500 patients (1). Based on left ventricular function and end-diastolic pressures, 100–500 cc intravenous dextran may be given for greater antiplatelet effects, particularly in patients not previously on aspirin. The suspected noninfarct artery and uninvolved bypass grafts, if present, are generally visualized with a diagnostic catheter, obtaining sufficient views to appreciate the anatomy. A guiding catheter is then used to inject the suspected infarct vessel that is usually completely occluded, often with the appearance of thrombus and dye staining, and is in a location concordant with the electrocardiographic and ventriculographic site of infarction. Initially, over-the-wire catheters accepting a 0.018 inch guide wire were used. More recently, over-the-wire systems with 0.014 inch guide wires have also been used successfully. A floppy-tipped guide wire is selected initially and can usually be used to cross the site of occlusion. Rarely stiffer guide wires are needed to punch across tight lesions underlying the thrombotic occlusion. Care must be taken at all times to gently steer the guide wire across the infarct site so as to avoid raising intimal flaps. Difficulties in crossing lesions with a guide wire or very hard lesions should prompt a reconsideration of the suspected infarct artery. A chronic total occlusion may masquerade as the infarct vessel, when in reality, a branch artery is the actual site of recent occlusion. In general, the initial balloon size is selected to match 1:1 with the luminal diameter just proximal to the site of occlusion. If there is uncertainty about the arterial diameter at the site of occlusion due to absent antegrade and collateral flow, a balloon judged to be slightly undersized may be selected for initial inflations. If appropriate, a larger balloon would subsequently be used to avoid underdilating the infarct zone. Typically, three to five inflations are performed for 45–120 sec with graded inflation pressures just sufficient to achieve full balloon expansion. Thrombus associated with the acute lesion is generally dealt with by repeated and prolonged (2–3 min) balloon inflations promoting mechanical lysis. We have resorted to intracoronary thrombolytic agents infrequently and have not been impressed by their benefit. Fortunately, distal embolization of thrombus rarely complicates the procedure and generally responds to guide wire disruption or balloon inflation in the few instances in which it is observed. Rarely, refractory thrombi have been aspirated through guiding catheters carefully inserted adjacent to the infarct lesion with gratifying results (2). If other significant lesions are present in the infarct artery, they are also dilated with appropriately sized balloons. Stenoses in arteries other than the infarct vessel are not dilated regardless of severity so as not to jeopardize multiple circulations in the setting of an acutely injured or stunned ventricle. A very rare exception to this dictum is the patient in cardiogenic shock who continues to have hemodynamic embarrassment following dilation of the infarct vessel and who has other critically narrowed arteries supplying viable myocardium. If transient hypotension occurs during the procedure, we employ intravenous boluses of 0.0625–0.125 mg neosynephrine. Sustained hypotension is managed with continuous dopamine infusion and/or intraaortic balloon pump counterpulsation. Rarely, consideration of emergency referral for emergency coronary bypass surgery is appropriate. The identification of critical proximal three-vessel coronary artery disease or left main disease may be best managed with surgery following reestablishment of antegrade flow in the infarct artery. Alternatively, patients with cardiogenic shock refractory to successful reestablishment of coronary flow or with mechanical complications of myocardial infarction may benefit from immediate surgical referral although the prognosis for recovery is poor. The entire angioplasty procedure generally takes an average of 20–30 min in the uncomplicated patient. Prior to transfer from the catheterization laboratory, a pulmonary artery catheter is often placed for hemodynamic monitoring in patients with large infarctions. Following successful angioplasty, the heparin drip is continued for 48 hr followed by sheath removal and repeat heparinization for an additional 24–48 hr. Partial thromboplastin times are monitored periodically and are adjusted to 2.5 times control values. Aspirin, a calcium channel blocker, and topical nitrates are continued until discharge, although consideration of long-term beta-blocker therapy is reasonable. Prior to discharge, a treadmill exercise test is performed. Spontaneous or inducible ischemia is an indication for restudy of the infarct vessel or consideration of revascularization of other systems by angioplasty or bypass surgery.

Figures 9–1 to 9–8 demonstrate an example of the technique and results of direct infarct angioplasty. The patient was a 54-year-old man presenting with a first anterior myocardial infarction 4 hr after the onset of chest pain. Figures 9–1 and 9–2 show end diastolic and end systolic frames from a left ventriculogram in the right anterior oblique projection obtained at the beginning of the acute procedure. Akinesis of the anterior wall is present. Figure 9–3 demonstrates total occlusion of the proximal left anterior descending artery, with associated narrowing of a diagonal branch.

Figure 9–4 shows the balloon catheter inflated across the total occlusion after passage of a floppy-tipped guide wire. Following several inflations, wide patency of the infarct vessel was achieved (Fig. 9–5). The patient consented to restudy 1 week later. End diastolic and end systolic frames demonstrate dramatic improvement of anterior wall motion, and the global ejection fraction increased from 37 to 67% (Figs. 9–6, 9–7). Repeat arteriography demonstrates sustained patency of the left anterior descending artery (Fig. 9–8).

RATIONALE

Direct infarct angioplasty offers several potential advantages over reperfusion therapy with thrombolytic agents. Virtually all patients admitted through the emergency room with an evolving myocardial infarction can be treated with emergent coronary angiography and balloon angioplasty (1). In contrast, the majority of patients presenting to emergency rooms with acute myocardial infarction are not receiving thrombolytic agents because of contraindications to therapy. In the Western Washington Emergency Room Tissue Plasminogen Activator Study, only 24% of 547 patients admitted with a documented infarct were eligible for therapy, and only 81% of those patients actually received it (3). Similarly, Cragg et al. reported that only 13.5% of 1,206 infarct patients admitted during the first 24 months of the TIMI IIB time frame met criteria for thrombolysis (4). Table 9–1 lists patient-related factors currently contraindicating thrombolytic and angioplasty therapy (5,6).

Current thrombolytic agents, whether used alone or in combination, demonstrate an acute reperfusion ceiling of approximately 75% (7). This continues to hold true even with the combination of thrombolytic agents (8). In patients with infarctions involving the right coronary or circumflex arteries, even lower patency rates are observed (9). Therefore, despite the expense and risk of thrombolytic agents, at least 25% of patients receiving these agents are not benefited. Furthermore, approximately 85% of patients are left with a residual stenosis in the infarct artery. For comparison, the data available for reperfusion with direct infarct angioplasty from multiple centers are summarized in Table 9–2 (1, 10–14). The majority of centers report acute reperfusion rates considerably higher than those achieved with current thrombolytic agents. Unlike thrombolytic therapy, direct angioplasty is equally effective for all three native arteries (1). Furthermore, the efficacy of reperfusion therapy in many

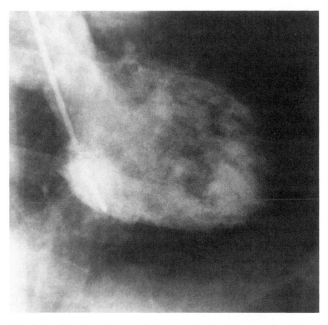

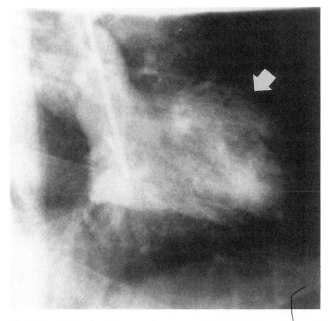

Fig. 9–1. Baseline left ventriculogram in the right anterior oblique projection obtained during acute anterior infarction. The end diastolic frame is displayed.

Fig. 9–2. Akinesis of the anterior myocardial wall is observed at end systole (arrow).

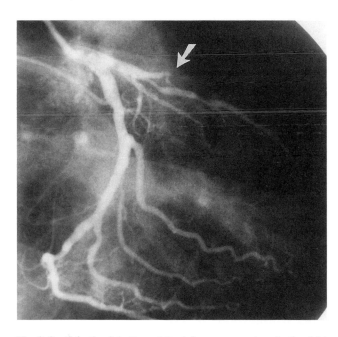

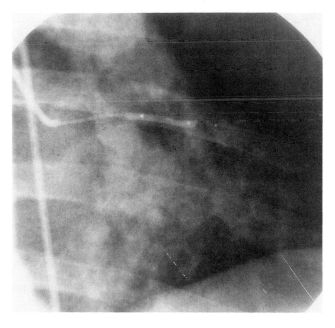

Fig. 9–3. Selective injection of the left coronary artery in the right anterior oblique projection. Total occlusion of the proximal left anterior descending artery is present (arrow).

Fig. 9–4. An over-the-wire balloon catheter is positioned across the site of occlusion, and full balloon expansion is demonstrated.

important and substantial patient subsets is largely unknown with thrombolytic agents. These include patients with prior bypass surgery, patients with cardiogenic shock, and those patients over age 75. Data are available demonstrating the efficacy of direct angio-

plasty in each of these groups as will be discussed below.

A further impetus for direct angioplasty for acute myocardial infarction is the desire to avoid the hemorrhagic complications characteristic of thrombolytic

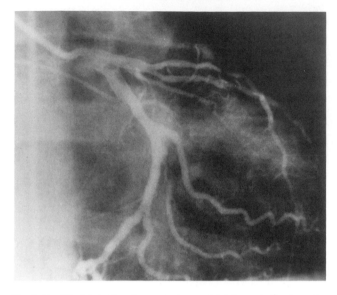

Fig. 9–5. Final injection demonstrates reestablishment of antegrade flow in the left anterior descending artery with minimal residual stenosis. There is improved patency of a large diagonal branch that was also dilated.

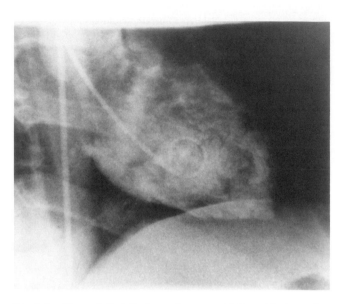

Fig. 9–6. The end diastolic frame from repeat left ventriculography 1 week following direct infarct angioplasty is shown.

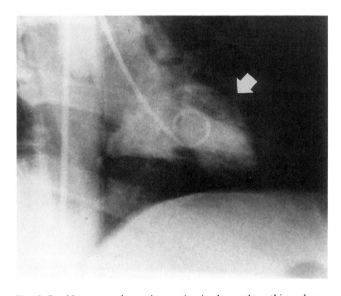

Fig. 9–7. Near-normal anterior motion is observed on this end systolic frame (arrow).

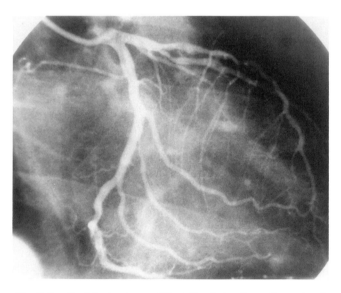

Fig. 9–8. Persistent patency of the left anterior descending artery is demonstrated.

therapy. Rates of serious intracranial hemorrhage as high as 5% following thrombolytic therapy have been reported in community hospitals (15). Hemorrhagic stroke has not been observed following direct infarct angioplasty without antecedent thrombolytic therapy. Conditions that may masquerade as acute myocardial infarction, such as aortic dissection or acute pericarditis, may prove fatal if treated erroneously with thrombolytic agents (16). In contrast, emergent catheterization allows immediate confirmation of the diagnosis before further therapy is offered.

RESULTS

From 1980 through April 1988, 500 consecutive patients were treated with direct infarct angioplasty by five experienced cardiac interventionalists at the

TABLE 9–1. Patient-Related Contraindications to Thrombolytic Therapy or Direct Angioplasty for Acute Myocardial Infarction

Thrombolytic therapy	Direct angioplasty
Active bleeding	Lack of vascular access
Cardiogenic shock	Severe contrast allergy
Age > 76	
History of cerebrovascular disease	
Blood pressure > 180–200 mmHg systolic or 110 mmHg diastolic	
Bleeding disorder	
Surgery within 2 weeks	
Recent prolonged CPR	
Trauma within 6 months	
Prior bypass surgery	
Proliferative retinopathy	

Mid America Heart Institute (1). Clinical criteria for inclusion were chest pain persisting > 30 minures and ≥ 1 mm of ST-segment elevation in ≥ two contiguous electrocardiographic leads. Patients were excluded if they were pretreated with thrombolytic agents or if the index infarction followed PTCA complicated by acute closure. Patients were not excluded for advanced age, shock, prior bypass surgery, hypertension, history of trauma, CPR, stroke, or associated medical diseases. Patient demographics of the group are listed in Table 9–3. Of note, 17% of patients were ≥ 70 years old, 8% presented in cardiogenic shock, 10% had prior bypass surgery, and 82% were treated within 6 hr of symptom onset. Table 9–4 lists the angiographic findings in the 500 patients. Multivessel disease was present in 57% of patients. TIMI grade 0 or 1 flow was present in 82% of vessels. The overall angioplasty success rate, defined as reduction of a stenosis to ≤ 40% without death or urgent surgery, was 94%. Neither the vessel dilated nor the elapsed time from pain onset altered the success rate of angioplasty. Overall, in-hospital mortality was 7.2% with 36 deaths in 500 patients. Table 9–5 lists the variables associated with hospital mortality. Using logistic regression analysis, age ≥ 70 years, cardiogenic shock, three-vessel disease, baseline ejection fraction ≤ 45%, anterior infarction, and failed angioplasty were identified as independently associated with in-hospital mortality. Among patients who were candidates for thrombolytic therapy using the TIMI IIB criteria, but were treated with direct infarct angioplasty, the in-hospital mortality was only 1.8%.

Acute and predischarge left ventriculograms were available in 261 patients. The global ejection fraction increased from 53 to 59% at the time of discharge ($P < .001$). In patients presenting in cardiogenic shock, the mean ejection fraction increased from 28 to 44% ($P < .005$). Regional wall motion, analyzed with the centerline chord method, improved significantly in the infarct segments in 53% of patients with follow-up studies. Independent predictors of regional wall motion improvement included a patent infarct artery at follow-up, reduced baseline ejection fraction, and anterior infarction.

Bleeding complications involving retroperitoneal hemorrhage or vascular trauma requiring surgery or transfusion occurred in 3% of patients. Neither stroke nor myocardial rupture was observed. Ten patients (2%) required urgent coronary bypass surgery. Predischarge antiographic follow-up was available in 307 patients. Reocclusion of the infarct vessel was identified in 47 patients (15%). As this group included all symptomatic patients but only a fraction of asymptomatic patients, this number probably overestimates the true frequency of reocclusion. If the 47 reocclusions are expressed as a percentage of the total number of patients, the reocclusion rate was 9.4%.

All but five hospital survivors were followed for a mean of 33 months. Of hospital survivors, 95% were alive at 1 year and 84% were alive at 5 years (Fig. 9–9). Multivariate analysis identified reduced predis-

TABLE 9–2. In-Hospital Experience With Direct Angioplasty Without Antecedent Thrombolytic Therapy for Acute Myocardial Infarction

Reference	Patients	PTCA success (%)	Urgent CABG (%)	Mortality (%) Overall	Mortality (%) Thrombolytic candidates
O'Keefe et al. (1)	500	94	1.6	7.2	1.8
Brodie et al. (10)	383	91	6.7	9	3.9
Rothbaum et al. (11)	151	87	0	9	NA
Kimura et al. (12)	58	88	NA	NA	NA
Marco et al. (13)	43	95	0	9.3	NA
Ellis et al. (14)	271	73	NA	NA	NA
Blaine[a]	188	96	NA	7%	3

NA, not available.
[a]J.R. Blaine, M.D., Springfield, MO (personal communication).

TABLE 9–3. Demographics for 500 Patients Treated With Direct Angioplasty for Acute Myocardial Infarction

	No.	%
Mean age (years)	59 ± 11	
Age range (years)	27–85	
Sex: M/F	364/16	73/27
Age ≥ 70 years	85	17
MI location		
Anterior	217	43
Inferior	283	57
Ischemic time (min)		
Mean	312 ± 256	
Median	244	
Range	30–1440	
≤ 2 hr	69	14
2–4 hr	225	45
4–6 hr	117	23
> 6 hr	89	18
Cardiogenic shock	39	8
Prior bypass surgery	49	10

From O'Keefe JH et al.: Early and late results of coronary angioplasty without thrombolytic therapy for acute myocardial infarction. Am J Cardiol 64:1221–1230, 1989, with permission.

TABLE 9–4. Baseline Angiographic Characteristics in 500 Patients With Acute Myocardial Infarction

	No.	%
One-vessel disease	215	43
Two-vessel disease	163	33
Three-vessel disease	122	24
Infarct related artery		
Left main	3	1
Left anterior descending	194	39
Left circumflex	65	13
Right	203	40
Bypass graft	35	7
TIMI grade antegrade flow		
0	304	61
1	107	21
2–3	89	18
Ejection fraction ≤ 30%	50	10

From O'Keefe JH et al.: Early and late results of coronary angioplasty without thrombolytic therapy for acute myocardial infarction. Am J Cardiol 64:1221–1230, 1989, with permission.

charge ejection fraction, three-vessel disease, age ≥ 70 years, and the absence of collaterals as independently related to long-term mortality. Survival at 1 year in thrombolytic candidates was 97%. It was concluded that direct infarct angioplasty was highly effective in reestablishing infarct-vessel patency and salvaging ischemic myocardium, resulting in low in-hospital and long-term mortality.

From these 500 patients, Stone et al. analyzed in detail the results of infarct angioplasty in 215 patients with single-vessel disease (17). Wide patency of the infarct-related artery was restored in 212 patients (99%). Complications consisted of one urgent bypass surgery; there were no procedural deaths. Recurrent ischemic events prior to discharge occurred in eight patients (4%). The in-hospital mortality was 1%; five of six patients presenting in cardiogenic shock were alive at discharge. Follow-up data were available in 214 patients at a mean interval of 35 months. The actuarial 3 year cardiac survival was 92%. Similarly, Kahn et al. analyzed in detail the 285 patients with multivessel disease (18). Two-vessel disease was found in 163 patients, and three-vessel disease was present in 122 patients. Cardiogenic shock was present in 33 patients (12%). PTCA of the infarct related artery was successful in 256 patients (90%) and was similar for two-vessel (92%) and three-vessel (88%) disease. Hospital death occurred in 33 patients (12%) including 13 patients with two-vessel disease and 20 with three-vessel disease ($P < .05$). Mortality was only 4% in the subgroup of thrombolytic candidates. The actuarial 1 and 3 year survival was 92 and 87% and was significantly better in two-vessel disease patients. Patients with three-vessel disease and poor left ventricular function had the worst outcome with only a 60% 4 year survival (Fig. 9–10). Thus, direct PTCA in patients with multivessel disease results in high reperfusion rates, good hospital survival, especially in non-shock patients, and favorable long-term outcomes.

An updated series through April 1989 involving 614 patients treated with direct infarct angioplasty identified 72 patients with prior coronary artery bypass surgery. These patients were analyzed in detail by Kahn et al. (19). Anterior myocardial infarction was present in 26 patients and inferior infarction in 46. Eleven patients (15%) presented in cardiogenic shock. Data from the acute angiographic study are presented in Table 9–6. In 48 patients, the infarct vessel was a vein graft, and in 24, it was a native coronary artery. Coronary angioplasty was successful in 65 of 72 patients. PTCA was successful in 41 of 48 (85%) vein grafts and all 24 native arteries. No patient required urgent surgery. There were 65 hospital survivors (90%), including 95% of nonshock patients and 64% of shock patients ($P < .01$). Symptomatic reocclusion occurred in only one patient. Baseline and predischarge ventriculography was available in 26 patients. The mean left ventricular ejection fraction increased from 44 to 51% ($P < .01$). At late follow-up (mean 31 months), actuarial 1 and 3 year survival was 89 and 87%, respectively. The only predictor of better survival was a baseline ejection fraction of ≥ 40%. It was concluded that prior coronary surgery should not preclude reperfusion therapy with direct angioplasty, which can be accomplished with low procedural risk,

TABLE 9–5. In-Hospital Mortality Among 500 Patients With Acute Myocardial Infarction Treated With Direct Angioplasty

	No. patients	Mortality (%)	Univariate odds ratio	Multivariate odds ratio
One-vessel disease	3/215	1.4		
Two-vessel disease	13/163	8.0	5.7	4.1
Three-vessel disease	20/122	16.4	11.7	6.3
Cardiogenic shock	16/39	41.0	9.5	8.6
Nonshock	20.461	4.3		
Age (years) ≥ 70	15/85	17.6	3.5	3.7
Age < 70	21/415	5.1		
Anterior MI	24/216	11.1	2.6	2.1
Inferior MI	12/284	4.2		
Successful angioplasty	25/468	5.3		
Failed angioplasty	11/32	34.3	6.5	5.4
Elapsed time (hr)				
≤ 2	3/69	4.3		
2–4	16/225	7.1		
4–6	7/117	6.0		
≥ 6	10/89	11.2	2.6	—
Prior bypass	5/49	10.2	1.5	—
Thrombolytic candidates	2/222	1.8		
Thrombolytic exclusions	34/278	12.2	6.8	—

From O'Keefe JH et al.: Early and late results of coronary angioplasty without thrombolytic therapy for acute myocardial infarction. Am J Cardiol 64:1221–1230, 1989, with permission.

improvements in ventricular function, and excellent in-hospital and late survival.

Patients presenting in cardiogenic shock were reported in detail by Laramee et al. (20). Through October 1987, 39 patients were treated with direct infarct angioplasty without antecedent thrombolytic therapy. The mean age was 64 years, and 87% had multivessel disease. Intraaortic balloon pump counterpulsation was required in 90% of patients, and cardiopulmonary resuscitation was needed in 33%. PTCA was successful in 86% of 56 lesions. There were 23 hospital survivors (59%). During follow-up, survival at 12 and 24 months was 39 and 32%, respectively.

To provide further information regarding the safety of direct infarct angioplasty, we reviewed the catheterization laboratory records of 250 patients treated in our recent experience. Patients were selected to in-

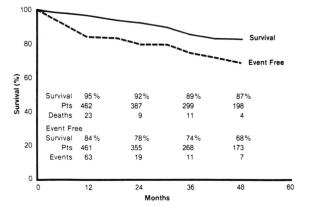

Fig. 9–9. Survival and event-free survival of all patients discharged from the hospital among 500 patients treated with direct infarct angioplasty. Event-free is defined as absence of death, reinfarction, or need for coronary artery bypass surgery. (From O'Keefe JH et al.: Early and late results of coronary angioplasty without thrombolytic therapy for acute myocardial infarction. Am J Cardiol 64:1221–1230, 1989, with permission.)

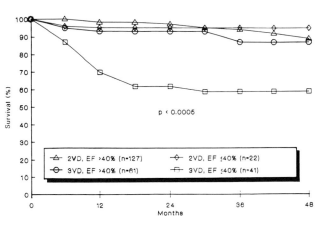

Fig. 9–10. Actuarial survival curves following hospital discharge from an initial cohort of 285 patients with multivessel coronary disease treated with direct infarct angioplasty. Patients with two-vessel disease (2VD) and three-vessel disease (3VD) are separated by a baseline left ventricular ejection fraction (EF) > 40% or ≤ 40%. The numbers in parentheses indicate the patients in each group at discharge.

TABLE 9–6. Initial Angiographic Findings in 72 Patients With Prior Bypass Surgery Treated With Direct Infarct Angioplasty

	No.	%
Infart related coronary artery		
Left anterior descending	2	3
Left circumflex	4	6
Right	17	23
Left main	1	1
Saphenous vein graft to		
Left anterior descending	25	34
Left circumflex	6	9
Right	17	24
Initial antegrade TIMI flow		
0	49	68
1	14	19
2–3	9	13
Infarct location		
Anterior	26	36
Inferior	46	64
Ventricular function		
Mean ejection fraction	46 ± 15%	
Range	20–82%	
Ejection fraction < 40%	47	65

From Kahn JK et al.: Usefulness of coronary angioplasty for acute myocardial infarction in patients with prior coronary artery bypass grafting. Am J Cardiol (in press), with permission.

gery were excluded from this analysis of native vessel infarction. Catheterization lab events were divided into major events (death, cardiopulmonary resuscitation, ventricular tachycardia/fibrillation requiring cardioversion, sustained hypotension requiring dopamine and/or intraaortic balloon pump counterpulsation) and minor events (transient hypotension responding to intravenous bolus neosynephrine, bradycardia responding to atropine or transvenous pacing). The results are summarized in Table 9–7. A total of 61 patients (24%) had events including 22 patients (9%) with major events and 39 with minor events only (15%). Major in-lab events occurred in 16 of 16 shock patients and in only six of 234 nonshock patients ($P < .001$). The majority of events in shock patients were supportive measures to maintain adequate perfusion due to preexisting hypotension. Minor events were more frequent in patients with reperfused right coronary arteries. Overall, successful PTCA was achieved in 239 of 250 patients (96%), and hospital survival was observed in 94% of patients. Predischarge arterial patency was documented in 139 of 153 patients (91%) consenting to restudy. It was concluded that anticipation and careful management of catheterization lab events during infarct angioplasty can lead to excellent procedural and hospital outcomes.

To analyze the impact of direct infarct angioplasty on the mechanism of death following myocardial infarction, hospital and late causes of death were determined for the 614 patients treated through April 1989 (Table 9–8). Overall, 49 patients died in-hospital. Twenty-two patients presented in cardiogenic shock

clude 100 consecutive patients with infarction involving the left anterior descending (LAD) artery, 100 consecutive patients with infarction involving the right coronary artery (RCA), and 50 consecutive patients with infarction involving the left circumflex (LCX) artery. Patients with prior coronary bypass sur-

TABLE 9–7. Catheterization Lab Events During Direct Infarct Angioplasty in 250 Consecutive Patients

	LAD infarct (n = 100 patients)	RCA infarct (n = 100 patients)	LCX infarct (n = 50 patients)	P value
Major events				
Total (%)	10	8	8	NS
Death (%)	1	0	0	
Urgent surgery (%)	1	0	4	
Intraaortic pump (%)	10	4	8	
Cardioversion (%)	1	5	2	
Dopamine infusion (%)	3	3	2	
Total-nonshock patients (%)	2	4	0	
Minor events				
Total (%)	6	27	12	<0.001
Bolus neosynephrine (%)	4	13	4	0.02
Atropine (%)	2	19	6	<0.001
Temporary pacemaker (%)	2	13	8	0.01
Total events	16	35	20	0.01
PTCA success (%)	96	98	90	NS
Hospital survival (%)	93	96	94	NS

TABLE 9–8. Mechanism of In-Hospital and Late Death
Following Direct Infarct Angioplasty in 614 Patients

Mechanism	No.
Cardiogenic shock	22
Abrupt vessel closure	6
Sudden	
Ventricular arrhythmia	5
Myocardial rupture	2
Cardiac tamponade	1
Postcoronary bypass	
Elective	6
Urgent	2
Line sepsis	2
Peritonitis	1
Respiratory failure	1
Pneumothorax	1
Late death	
Cardiac deaths	36
Arrhythmic	
Witnessed	8
Nonwitnessed	12
Sleep	3
Deaths in circulatory failure	
Congestive heart failure	6
Recurrent infarction	7
Noncardiac deaths	18

and died of low-output failure. An additional five patients died after acute reclosure of the infarct vessel, including two patients still in the catheterization laboratory. Eight deaths were sudden. Five of these were due to documented arrhythmias. Two others were determined to be due to myocardial rupture; both patients had failed infarct angioplasty. Death followed coronary bypass surgery in eight patients. Following hospital discharge, 55 patients died during a mean follow-up of 32 months. The cause of death was cardiac in 36 patients. An arrhythmic death occurred in 23 patients. Circulatory failure was the cause of death in 13 other patients. It was concluded that successful direct infarct angioplasty may prevent in-hospital myocardial rupture. Further inroads in mortality must focus on patients with cardiogenic shock and late on reducing arrhythmic deaths. More frequent use of beta-blockers at discharge occurred later in the study, but benefit from this adjuvant therapy following direct infarct angioplasty remains to be determined.

CONCLUSIONS

The author's experience with direct infarct angioplasty at the Mid America Heart Institute indicates that this therapy is the most effective method of restoring infarct vessel patency. Other advantages over alternative reperfusion therapies include the applicability and demonstrated efficacy in virtually all patient groups, objective definition of left ventricular function and coronary anatomy, identification of anatomic high-risk patient subsets, unequivocal demonstration of arterial patency following reperfusion, and facilitation of adjunctive invasive therapies including intraaortic balloon pump insertion and coronary artery bypass grafting. Direct infarct angioplasty is not associated with intracranial hemorrhage and can usually be performed with few procedural complications. A comparative trial of direct infarct angioplasty and tissue plasminogen activator is in planning stages, and the results of that trial will provide further insight into the range of reperfusion strategies. Until that time, there is sufficient experience with direct infarct angioplasty to suggest it as the therapy of choice for evolving myocardial infarction in centers with angioplasty availability and expertise willing to expeditiously transport patients to the catheterization laboratory.

10. Recurrence Following Successful PTCA

As indicated in previous chapters in this book, the indications for coronary angioplasty in the treatment of coronary artery disease have expanded greatly in the 1980s. This is due to technologic improvements in guiding catheters, guide wires, and balloon catheter systems as well as to improve techniques and greatly increased operator experience. When discussing the alternative of angioplasty with the patient and the patient's family, one can confidently predict that the patient has a 95% chance of initial success with angioplasty, and only a 3% chance of going to emergency bypass surgery at experienced centers and with experienced operators performing the procedure. However, recurrence (restenosis) after coronary angioplasty continues to be the main negative aspect of the procedure. Since the publication of the first edition of this book in 1987, there has been really very little improvement in the treatment of restenosis or has there been a dramatic decrease in the amount of restenosis. The understanding of restenosis continues to be a subject that obsesses many investigators, and once it is solved, as I would confidently predict that it will be within the next 5 years, the procedure of angioplasty will be even more palatable as an alternative to bypass graft surgery.

In the following discussion of recurrence, much of the development and interpretation of the data base used occurred in conjunction with my colleagues at the San Francisco Heart Institute in the mid-1980s.

PROBLEMS AND DEFINITIONS

To understand recurrence and discuss it, one must first define it. There have been many major definitions of restenosis that have been presented in the literature, but there are three major criteria on which most investigators agree. They are 1) residual stenosis of more than 50% at follow-up angiography; 2) loss of 50% of the luminal diameter gained at the time of the initial angioplasty; and 3) an increase of greater than 30% in the immediate percent diameter stenosis following angioplasty. The interpretation of reports regarding restenosis must be viewed with the clear understanding of what the author means by restenosis. Variations in results obtained when a variety of definitions are applied to the same sample of cases have been reported. In an analysis of different definitions, Leimgruber and his colleagues show that there was a significant overlap in classifying their follow-up sample of nearly 1,000 patients with angiographic restudy (249 of the 998 patients were classified as having recurrence by all three definitions listed above). However, the number of patients classified differently ranged from five to 36, depending on which definition or combination of definitions was used.

A concise definition of recurrence would be helpful to compare various reports in the literature, but it is not clear how the different definitions correlate with actual myocardial ischemia in restenotic vessels. It would be hoped that the presence of a severe stenosis with demonstrable reversible myocardial ischemia would be the basis for performing a repeat angioplasty on a recurrent lesion, just as it is in selecting the patients for angioplasty in the first place. There have been several studies done which show that it is difficult to determine a relationship between major luminal diameter and actual coronary flow. For example, Gould and his associates found that in order to achieve a significant decrease in the coronary flow in the canine model, more than an 80% luminal diameter reduction was necessary at rest and over 60% with hyperemic stimuli. In that same series in some stenoses of 80% in the left circumflex coronary artery, flow distribution at rest was normal. These anatomic-physiologic inconsistencies were not only characteristic of severe stenoses. Thallium studies in man have shown that abnormalities can exist with lesions as minimal as 20–40% diameter stenosis. Given this assumption that a given luminal diameter does not necessarily correlate with myocardial ischemia in these studies or in other studies reported, it is obvious that caution must be exercised in assessing angiographic recurrence and that angiographic studies, although necessary to demonstrate a recurrent lesion, should not be used alone but rather in combination with physiologic assessment of the myocardial blood flow with thallium exercise studies. If these thallium studies can be obtained prior to the initial PTCA, shortly after the PTCA as a baseline "normal," and then at 6 months postprocedure or at a time of suspected recurrence, the validity of the test will be greatly enhanced.

Since 1983, there have been hundreds of abstracts and articles published in journals using a variety of statistical analyses systems to identify and try to relate factors to recurrence. A lot of problems exist with these studies since they are not all coordinated and certainly do not all agree in a variety of definitions or groupings.

In attempting to assess factors relating to recurrence, they can generally be categorized in the following categories: 1) clinical; 2) morphological; 3) technical or procedural; and 4) pharmacologic. Clinical factors include diabetes and smoking and would be factors in the patient's habits or environment that might exert an influence on recurrence. The morphologic factors are defined as characteristics that describe the severity, location, and/or composition of a specific lesion. Technical factors relate to the procedure itself and aspects of the performance of angioplasty. Pharmacologic factors reflect various medications given to angioplasty patients prior to, during, and following the procedure. This seems to be a logical organization of study for factors relating to recurrence, and the reference material presented in the Bibliography referring to this section would allow the reader to delve more deeply into the statistical analysis of factors presented. This chapter, however, will deal more with the practical aspects of, particularly, the morphologic and technical factors relating to recurrence. A complete review of the clinical and pharmacologic factors is discussed in Jang et al. (1982).

In addition to general categories, morphologic subgroups may exist that represent characteristics of the disease process that may be meaningful in comparing patients who recur with those who do not. Morphologic characteristics of the disease itself include the extent of the disease (e.g., single vs. multiple vessel), lesion severity (e.g., subtotal vs. total occlusion), lesion location (e.g., bifurcation stenoses, origin stenoses, obstructions on tortuous segments of arteries, etc.), and vessel type (e.g., native vs. vein graft). These various subgroups have been examined to see if any more or less favorable morphologic features can be found.

A recurring theme throughout this book, when discussing restenosis, has been that the true extent of restenosis cannot be determined without having 100% angiographic follow-up. This relates to the observation that some patients will develop pain at a variety of intervals following angioplasty, and when restudied, in fact, the target vessel for angioplasty is widely patent with good flow and no obvious restenosis. On the other hand, a number of patients who have remained asymptomatic have come to restudy, and there have been cases of "silent" restenosis that have not been predicted either by the patient's symptoms or by thallium treadmill testing. These discrepancies make it difficult to assess on clinical or noninvasive grounds the presence or absence of restenosis and certainly do not allow one to assess the severity of a recurrent lesion.

In our current medical system, both for financial and traditional reasons, 100% angiographic follow-up is simply unrealistic. We therefore must be somewhat vague in discussing restenosis with patients and their families, but it should be emphasized to them that there is a significant amount of restenosis, that it is probably in the 30% range, and that it is very important for the patient to have follow-up thallium treadmill testing to both provide a baseline study shortly after angioplasty and another study at the end of the recurrent 6 month time.

It is also obvious from following a large number of patients that the vast majority of recurrences do become clinically obvious within 6 months. There are rare recurrences that surface between 6 and 12 months postangioplasty and beyond 12 months postangioplasty if the patient returns with a recurrent symptom or has a change in thallium treadmill testing. It is almost always another lesion rather than the original lesion treated with angioplasty. In considering and accepting these statements, it should be obvious that the timing of recurrence must be considered to be when the patient began to feel repeat anginal symptoms, not when the patient finally got around to going to the physician to report these symptoms. The same is true for the timing of the thallium exercise testing.

MORPHOLOGIC FACTORS AFFECTING RECURRENCE

Morphologic factors that consistently are associated with restenosis in a number of reports include lesions with greater than 90% diameter stenosis before PTCA and residual percent diameter stenosis of less than 30% after PTCA. In the earlier days of angioplasty when transstenotic pressure gradients were commonly measured, only one study (10) reported that high transstenotic pressure gradients before angioplasty were significant as being a predictor of recurrence. Numerous studies, however, reported that significantly high gradients after angioplasty had some significance as a recurrence predictor. In general, the data suggest that lesions that are initially more severe are more likely to recur, but that working hard at these lesions to try to achieve the best post angioplasty result possible may somehow alter the incidence of recurrence.

Whether restenosis occurs more frequently in different arteries or at different areas of these various coronary arteries has been the subject of several studies. Studies from two centers agree that the left anterior descending coronary artery has a higher chance for recurrent stenosis; however, these centers disagree as to which of the other two major vessels (the left circumflex or right coronary artery) are the next most likely to recur. In addition, other reports have noted findings about the location of the lesion related to higher rates of recurrence. One early study reported that lesions at or near the origin of the left anterior descending coronary artery developed restenosis more frequently than elsewhere in the LAD. Other studies have not confirmed this, and it is certainly possible that recurrence in lesions at the origin of the LAD are more frequent because of the tenderness with which the angioplasty physician treats these areas. By definition, inflating a balloon to cover the area of stenosis at the origin of the LAD must involve inflation of the balloon in the left main coronary artery. Operators tend to undersize balloons in this situation in order to prevent damage to the left main trunk and to lessen the chance of completely obstructing flow in the distribution of the left main trunk during the balloon inflation. The amount of pressure exerted on the stenosis at that site may also be less than thought, since dissipation of the pressure in the left main trunk or toward the circumflex branch may, in fact, provide less pressure exerted on more tightly stenotic segment, i.e., the origin of the LAD.

Another area that has a higher recurrence rate is the ostium of the right coronary artery or the aortic anastomosis of a bypass graft. It has long been thought that these areas are not representative of pure coronary or graft lesions but also involve some degree of disease of the aorta itself. Obviously, dilating these areas not only dilates the origin of the vessel but also the wall of the aorta adjacent to its origin. Pressure forces in the balloon are also dissipated somewhat in the larger aorta since the balloon must be partially in the vessel and in the aorta. One way to try to decrease this phenomenon is to have as small an amount of balloon in the aorta as possible during balloon inflations.

Another area of apparent increased restenosis involves bifurcation lesions. This was reported in one study but not confirmed by numerous other studies. It is certainly likely that in the early days of kissing balloon angioplasty that the balloons were somewhat undersized for the individual vessel lesion so that simultaneous inflations could be carried out and not be too large an additive diameter for the proximal artery. If sequential inflations are used and appropriate-sized balloons are chosen for each vessel, the recurrence with bifurcation lesions should not be higher than in other subgroups.

Earlier reports of the NHLBI Institute Registry suggested that vein grafts were more likely to exhibit recurrence than were native coronary arteries. Other studies suggested that this finding was not necessarily true. Some studies of vein graft angioplasty reported that the proximal and middle portions of the graft were more likely to recur than was the distal portion of the body of the graft. These initial findings, however, were based on extremely small follow-up samples, and more recent studies found no significant difference in the risk of recurrence for various segments within the vein grafts.

The morphology of lesions has also been assessed in reference to association with higher risk of recurrence. Most notably, diffuseness of disease and length of lesion diameter greater than 15 mm have been reported as predictors of recurrence. The Montreal group reported other anatomic characteristics, such as eccentricity, calcification, and poor distal runoff associated with recurrence, although these factors have not been included in other studies of recurrence. Certainly, the inflation of a balloon several times in a long segment of disease in an overlapping manner would at least theoretically make one believe that recurrence at some area along that length of disease might recur. This should be discussed fully with the patients and their family prior to their acceptance of angioplasty as the treatment of choice, but since repeat angioplasty is so successful in most cases, even in anatomic situations where it is believed that the risk of restenosis is greater than usual, this should not be a strong factor in turning down a patient for angioplasty. When one considers that the alternative to angioplasty is coronary bypass surgery, in most patients it is less traumatic to perform one or two angioplasties to solve the problem without open-chest surgery than to reject the patient for angioplasty on the theoretical chance of recurrence.

TECHNICAL FACTORS PREDICTING RECURRENCE

Intraprocedural technical factors have been dissected to try to pick out features during the procedure that might positively or negatively influence recurrence. One factor that seemed to be quite consistent is the use of higher dilatation balloon catheter inflation pressures. Although this technique might have been used during the procedure to try to effect a larger balloon diameter, it could also reflect difficulty during the procedure with a "hard" lesion and total occlusion or represent a situation in which repeated dilatations were performed because of a dissection or other unsatisfactory result observed intraprocedurally. For whatever underlying reason, higher balloon inflation pressures have been found to be related to a greater risk of recurrence. Tandem or multiple lesions dilated in a vessel was found in one study to be a predictor of recurrence, but this has not been found in other studies.

One finding that has seemed consistent over several studies and potentially has an impact on the performance of angioplasty is the balloon-to-vessel ratio. This refers to the ratio between the meausred size of the balloon diameter at maximum inflation at the site of the lesion divided by the measured vessel diameter. Several studies have demonstrated that lower balloon-to-vessel (or graft) ratios are associated with higher risk of recurrence. The ideal balloon-to-vessel ratio for optimal success of PTCA and reduction of restenosis appears to be about 1.1:1.0. This is obviously a very close call and requires precise measurement, but the finding does suggest that balloons should be as large as the presumed normal adjacent native vessel to achieve the best immediate and long-term results. This again may be one reason that proximal LAD lesions appear to have recurred more frequently than lesions in other areas if, in fact, undersizing the balloon has occurred in these proximal LAD lesions because of concern about the left main trunk. It should be emphasized, however, that oversizing of balloons may result in higher rates of immediate complications, particularly dissection, which is a high price to pay in attempting to reduce the recurrence rate.

The absence of an uncomplicated "intimal dissection" has been reported to be associated with restenosis. However, the wide variety of definition of "intimal dissection" (ranging from a simple tear that probably occurs in most angioplasties to extravasation of contrast outside the lumen) suggests that the term needs to be defined more carefully and incidence of recurrence may need to be assessed separately for each angiographic "dissection" pattern. Insufficient revascularization has also been related to higher rates of recurrence.

Review of the current literature implicating morphologic and technical factors that may affect recurrence suggests that the physicians performing angioplasty may be able to positively affect recurrence rates by careful choice of balloon size, overinflating PVC balloons if they have been undersized, and by attempting to reduce residual percent diameter stenosis to the lowest possible levels. It appears clear that earlier studies reporting higher incidences of recurrence in branch lesions and vein grafts are not supported by the majority of studies. The effect of the site of dilatation on restenosis is unclear, although it is probable that long areas of disease and multiple lesions in vessels with diffuse disease have higher incidences of recurrence. These considerations need to be factored into the initial evaluation of the patient who is a candidate for angioplasty. The possibility of recurrence, however, should not eliminate patients from being offered the procedure since the alternative is much more traumatic and costly and certainly no one can absolutely predict that an individual lesion will recur.

TREATMENT OF RECURRENCE

Since recurrence or restenosis remains a significant fact of life in the field of angioplasty, the treatment of recurrence will be necessary in approximately 20% of patients who undergo an initially successful procedure. The exact recurrence rate cannot be known without 100% angiographic follow-up of patients with initial success, as it has been stated earlier in this book that ultimate goal is needed to define the recurrence problem and is most likely not attainable.

Theoretically, one would expect that each position in which a balloon is inflated in an artery is a potential site for recurrence. This possibility should be kept in mind in several situations. If a "moderate" lesion is present in an artery, e.g., a 50–60% lesion, the chance of recurrence following balloon inflation in that area ultimately may worsen the overall situation. If a 50–60% lesion recurs as a 90% restenosis, and a second angioplasty is not successful, the patient may need to have bypass surgery for a lesion that, if left alone, could probably have been treated medically. The warning in this situation is that lesions should be documented to be both angiographically and hemodynamically significant before balloon inflations are carried out. It is important that only hemodynamically significant lesions be dilated, and this should be proved by documentation of ischemia prior to selection of the patient for angioplasty and also documentation of a significant pressure gradient across the lesion prior to balloon inflations if any questions still exist. The use of the Pinkerton balloon with a 0.014 wire to obtain excellent pressure gradient measurements has been discussed elsewhere, and I use this technique not infrequently to become convinced that a lesion is one that should be dilated for hemodynamic reasons. Particularly in multiple-vessel disease, in the case of a lesion that seems to be of borderline angiographic anatomic significance, if a significant pressure gradient is not demonstrated, then balloon inflations should not be carried out because of the potential for recurrence.

In the case of left main coronary artery disease, the concern about recurrence is one of the main reasons for not accepting patients wtih unprotected left main lesions for angioplasty. Although left main lesions are generally technically straightforward as far as being able to reach and cross the lesion and dilate the stenosis, if recurrence does occur in the left main position, the reappearance of a significant stenosis in that area could be catastrophic. Intraprocedurally, the left main trunk could be handled quite nicely using full cardiopulmonary support equipment, but the concern about restenosis still exists. Therefore, because of this concern, unprotected left main disease should still be treated with bypass surgery.

In multiple-vessel disease, theoretically, each stenosis dilated has an independent chance of recurrence. In fact, as is discussed elsewhere in this chapter and in the chapter on multiple-vessel disease, the probable multifactorial etiology of restenosis speaks against this theory expressing itself as fact. Certainly, the "host" factors would skew a patient with multiple dilations toward having recurrence at all sites. The "lesion" factors would tend to act independently at each dilatation site. This consideration would also seem to be of theoretical importance in tandem disease or long segmental stenoses. All of these possibilities should be kept in mind when discussing the probable incidence of recurrence with the patient and the patient's family.

Since the treatment of recurrence must be faced by any practitioner of angioplasty, some general philosophies must be kept in mind when faced with a patient with recurrence. The documentation of recurrence should be angiographic restudy. This should correlate with the patient's symptoms and noninvasive thallium treadmill testing, and as has been stated before, the mere appearance of a restenotic narrowing does not necessarily prove a hemodynamically significant recurrence. The suspicion of recurrence can come from the return of clinical symptoms and/or the return of ischemic response on EKG or thallium treadmill testing. This method of early suspicion and detection points out the importance of both close clinical follow-up after an initial successful angioplasty and also the importance of a baseline stress EKG as soon after the angioplasty as possible to document the exercise response at a time when the dilated artery or arteries are presumably open. Follow-up stress electrocardiography should then be performed either at the time of return of anginal symptoms or on a routine basis at 4–5 months postangioplasty to watch for recurrence within the well-documented 6 month window following successful dilatation. As has been documented elsewhere, there are both false positive and false negative signs of recurrence clinically and by stress electrocardiography; therefore, the proper documentation

of recurrence is by correlating these features with a follow-up angiogram.

Once recurrence has been documented by angiographic follow-up, the practitioner is faced with the decision of how to treat the recurrent stenosis. The obvious three treatment modalities would be to maintain the patient on medical therapy, perform a repeat angioplasty, or refer the patient for coronary bypass graft surgery.

The maintenance of the patient on medical therapy is usually the least attractive of these treatment modalities. The patient was first selected for angioplasty because of significant angina not responsive to medical therapy, and if the symptoms return, it is likely that medical therapy will again be unsuccessful. Some patients may wish to consider this potential course of therapy, however, and it should be given to them as an option just as it was prior to the initial decision for angioplasty. If multiple-vessel angioplasty has been performed, recurrence of one of several lesions may, in fact, be proven, but the patient may be clinically enough better than maintenance on medical therapy can then be carried out.

Repeat angioplasty has been shown to be very effective in the treatment of restenosis. There is no greater risk of a significant cardiac complication with repeat angioplasty than with a first procedure, and, in fact, many times repeat angioplasty is technically somewhat easier than is the first angioplasty because the equipment has been tried and chosen and the selection of optimal equipment can be made quite definitively based on the first experience. The incidence of emergency bypass surgery or myocardial infarction is not higher during a repeat angioplasty attempt. It has been estimated, and our series statistics would tend to substantiate, that repeat angioplasty is successful in the long term in about 80–85% of cases, so the recommendation of a second angioplasty to a patient is certainly a worthwhile treatment alternative in recurrence.

Coronary bypass surgery, obviously, is a potential treatment of recurrence that should be discussed with the patient and the patient's family. In certain cases, the recurrence may assume an anatomical configuration that does not appear as well suited to angioplasty as does the original lesion, and such an anatomic appearance may be a strong indicator that bypass surgery should be recommended rather than a second angioplasty. Conversely, a recurrence may be more favorable than the original lesion and a more optimistic picture may be painted in presenting the patient with the various treatment alternatives. For example, if a patient's original lesion was in the proximal third of the left anterior descending coronary artery and the restenosis involves not only that area but also the entire proximal third of that vessel leading to its origin from the left main coronary artery, which would necessitate balloon inflation in the left main segment, the practitioner may feel more comfortable in referring the patient for surgery rather than performing repeat angioplasty. It may also be true that the "failure" of angioplasty as manifest by a recurrence will sway the patient's preference toward surgery, and as is true with the initial procedure, angioplasty should not be "sold" to any patient or the patient's family as the only means of treatment for arterial stenosis. In spite of this statistical success of repeat angioplasty, some patients will feel more comfortable with a different procedure, and since they view the recurrence as a failure of angioplasty in their case, they may choose this course.

The role of other nonsurgical technical means of treating recurrences is discussed in detail in Chapter 13 (New Technologies for the Treatment of Obstructive Arterial Disease). Certainly, one of the hopes of the development of new mechanical devices, such as atherectomy catheters, lasers, and stents, was that obstructive lesions relieved by these devices would have less recurrence than would balloon angioplasty. In fact, in most series, all of these new instruments have had a higher recurrence rate than the recurrence rate reported with a balloon angioplasty. Certainly, the patients treated with any of these mechanisms represent a skewed sample in that a number of the patients have already recurred several times and the other factors affecting recurrence may adversely affect whatever type of mechanism is used. The presentation of atherectomy, laser, or stent as a treatment alternative in a patient who has recurred should be considered, but, at least at the present time, none of these procedures seem to have any substantial value over a repeat angioplasty attempt using the standard balloon angioplasty catheters.

In treating restenosis with repeat balloon angioplasty, usually the same guiding catheter that worked the first time will be acceptable for the second attempt as well. If the stenosis is more severe or if a longer segment of stenosis has appeared with the recurrence, more back-up from the guide may be needed and this should be considered when selecting the guiding catheter. Generally, the wire used can be the same wire as was used the first time. If the anatomic appearance of the restenosis is different, then selection of the guide wire will necessarily be different as well.

In terms of selection of the dilatation catheter in the case of restenosis, it is generally important to try to select a balloon size that will achieve as large a lumen as possible to approximate an undiseased segment of the artery. In many cases, this results in the selection of a slightly larger balloon than used with the initial angioplasty. There certainly should be no downsizing of balloon during treatment of recurrence. Perhaps at the time of initial dilatation, a smaller-than-ideal balloon had to be used because of the tightness of the stenosis or difficulty in crossing the lesion with the "ideal" dilatation catheter system. It is also true that since the advertised balloon sizes are measured in water, the actual measured diameter of the balloon during the first angioplasty may have been smaller than that expected, and if a resultant 30 or 40% stenosis was angiographically present following the first angioplasty, then perhaps a slightly larger balloon or higher-pressure balloon should be used the second time to try to achieve a more ideal and larger lumen. The amount of pressure used to inflate the balloon with a repeat angioplasty is often higher than was used the first time and also generally that used in order to try to achieve a slightly larger balloon diameter with the PVC balloons or to exert a little more force in an attempt to compact the area of stenosis more completely. Longer balloon inflations may also be considered, and the use of the Stack perfusion balloon catheter is helpful in this technical management of restenosis.

In general, then, with repeat angioplasty, the old term of "longer and stronger" is advisable in that the goal is to achieve ideal lumen size and to compact the material as completely as possible. In my series of patients treated for restenosis, I usually use a slightly larger balloon catheter (with quarter sizes now available this is somewhat easier) and inflate the balloon to higher pressures. Longer balloon inflations are made for as long a time as tolerable, and hopefully at least 1 min of significant balloon inflation can be achieved if the patient's symptoms and objective demonstration of ischemia do not preclude this length of time. The use of the Stack perfusion balloon catheter can be considered if this is a problem.

The question of how many repeat angioplasties it is reasonable to perform will inevitably arise in cases of repetitive restenosis. Certainly, the second angioplasty is an acceptable and advisable modality for the treatment of recurrence, but if a third angioplasty is contemplated, in general, the length of time between recurrences should have increased and some indication that the third angioplasty would be successful should be present. If the length of time between recurrences actually decreases, then in most cases we would recommend bypass surgery or the use of another mechanical device as the treatment of choice. For example, if the patient has had a recurrence at 4 months following the initial successful angioplasty and then has another recurrence at 6 or 7 months following the second procedure, this would seem to be favorable for trying angioplasty the third time. If the initial recurrence occurs at 4 months, and the repeat recurrence occurs at 3 months, the time interval between recurrences is decreasing, and one must face the fact that the lesion is most likely not going to respond well in the long term to balloon angioplasty. A case demonstrating angioplasty persistence and a good long-term result is seen in Figure 10–1.

The patient's clinical situation, particularly regarding age and concurrent disease of a noncardiac nature, may lead one to perform repeated angioplasties rather than to subject the patient to a bypass surgical procedure. Certainly, one should not make a career of redilating recurrent stenoses in any given patient, but each patient must be evaluated individually as to the advisability of treatment with repeat angioplasty and the likelihood of success of sequential procedures.

The treatment of restenosis by repeat angioplasty, therefore, statistically, is a viable treatment modality. In general, I try to do something different the second time, namely, to use a slightly larger balloon, inflate the balloon to slightly higher pressures, and/or hold the pressures for longer periods of time. As long as restenosis remains a significant factor in the field of angioplasty, the practitioner of angioplasty must understand the possibility of recurrence and be able to accept it not as a defeat of the procedure but as an inherent fact of the procedure that must be dealt with in an intelligent and competent manner, always keeping in mind that the safety and health of the patient are of primary importance in selecting the treatment modality for recurrence.

Some interesting additional modalities for the treatment of recurrence have been tried. It had been demonstrated using an angioscope that a "shaggy" appearance of a dilated segment exists following angiographically successful angioplasty. It was hoped that attempts to "glaze" that area and smooth its surface with a thermal laser probe following balloon angioplasty would leave a lining more resistant to restenosis. The use of permanently implantable stents in an area of stenosis that has recurred may someday provide the support needed to prevent restenosis in elastic lesions. These techniques and others currently under active investigation are documented in Chapter 13 (New Technologies for the Treatment of Obstructive Arterial Disease), and I am sure that their value will become clarified in the near future.

PREVENTION OF RESTENOSIS

One of the most commonly asked questions when patients present with restenosis is, "Why?" Most of the time the patient wants to know what he/she could have done to prevent this recurrence from happening. Hopefully, the initial explanation of angioplasty included a thorough airing of restenosis possibilities, and this explanation had some impact on the patient so that it is not an entirely unexpected happening.

Numerous medical manipulations have been tried to aggressively lower the restenosis rate. A number of reports have suggested that aggressive management in lipid lowering could decrease the restenosis rate. Diet and a variety of medications have been used, and in one series, the restenosis rate dropped to only 12.5%, compared to 38% for the control. Again, this series did not have adequate angiographic follow-up in the control group, and the results of the study may well have been biased toward suggesting that aggressive lipid lowering can change the restenosis rate. Certainly, lowering the lipids in patients postangioplasty should be part of the medical regiment, but at this time, it would appear that the true efficacy of aggressive lipid lowering remains unknown.

The use of steroids in various dosages and regimens have been tried to affect the recurrence rate. Most of these studies have shown that there is no significant difference between patients treated aggressively or minimally with steroids and those not treated with steroids at all.

The effect of short-time prostacyclin (PGI_2) on the incidence of restenosis was studied, and an excellent angiographic follow-up rate of 93% was obtained in this Canadian study. The conclusion of this study was that the short-term administration of prostacyclin did not significantly lower the risk of restenosis after coronary angioplasty.

Preliminary reports from centers trying long-term, low-dose heparin postangioplasty have indicated that in some cases of chronic recurrence there seems to be a salutary effect to administering subcutaneous heparin over a 30-day postangioplasty period. The dosage used is 5,000 units b.i.d. subcutaneously, and this is very similar to the regimen used following bypass surgery in the early days of that procedure. Numbers of patients included in the studies are almost anecdotal, and no conclusion has been made regarding the efficacy of this addition to the postangioplasty treatment regimen.

The use of high-dose fish oil has been reported by several authors. It would appear that the best regimen must be started at least 1 week to 10 days prior to a repeat angioplasty in the case of restenosis and continued for about 3 months afterward. The high-dose fish oil preparations are costly, but if the conclusion of these several trials continue to show that there is a reduction in the restenosis rate, it may well

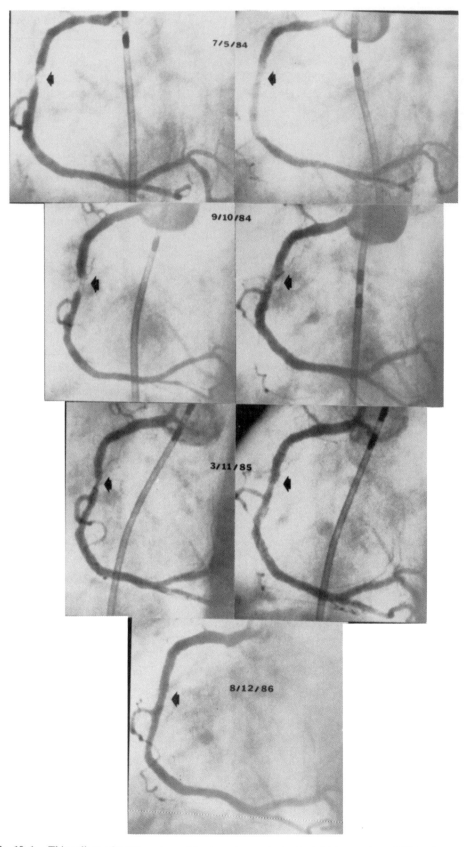

Fig. 10–1. This collage of LAO angiographic views demonstrates the initial stenosis and PTCA (7/5/84) as well as the recurrences and repeat angioplasties (9/10/84 and 3/11/84) with eventual excellent long-term result (8/12/86).

prove to be an efficacious addition to the medical regimen.

Platelet inhibitors, including aspirin, dipyridamole, and sulfinpyrazone have been widely used in patients following successful initial angioplasty. These agents, alone or in combination, have been reported in many trials, and their influence on restenosis in human beings remains unproven. The use of Coumadin has likewise not shown to decrease the incidence of restenosis.

Most patients undergoing angioplasty are placed on calcium blockers for several months following the procedure. It is hoped that since patients with documented spasm have a high incidence of restenosis that reducing coronary rates and vasospasm would have a positive effect on the restenosis. Recent studies in animals and humans have shown that neither nifedipine nor diltiazem has had any significant effect.

In conclusion, it can be safely stated that the etiology of restenosis is currently unknown and that probably until restenosis is better characterized from a pathophysiologic standpoint the treatment for it will remain not entirely satisfactory. I would certainly anticipate that the incidence of restenosis will fall as the understanding of recurrence increases, and it is most likely that some pharmacologic method of treating restenosis or preventing restenosis will emerge. Even at the current rate of restenosis (25–30%) in patients, it should be remembered that it is effectively treated by repeat angioplasty in most of these patients.

11. Complications of Coronary Angioplasty

The complications of PTCA usually involve injury done to the coronary artery during an angioplasty attempt. The term "dissection" has been liberally used in the literature and perhaps wrongly so. The pathologic term dissection means disruption of the media of the artery, and in most cases, the "dissection" that occurs during angioplasty involves the disruption of the intima rather than extension into the media.

It is obvious from the 3% risk of emergency bypass surgery and the 2.8% risk of significant myocardial infarction as a result of the procedure that serious complications of angioplasty still continue to occur in spite of the increased safety of the equipment and increased operator experience. The extension of the procedure into more difficult and complicated lesions has also contributed to holding the complication rate at a steady level. The most serious complication, of course, is death of the patient, and perhaps the greatest precaution that can be taken to avoid this complication is the presence of formal cardiac surgery standby in each and every case of angioplasty. Although one can theoretically identify patients at higher risk for complications during the procedure by study of the preangioplasty anatomy of the arteries (i.e., tortuous vessels, lesions on bends in arteries, etc.) or patients who are at higher risk for death because of significant left ventricular dysfunction, there is still no certain way to identify a risk-free patient. Even in patients with total occlusions and good collateral supply to the totally occluded vessel, whom one might expect would have very little chance of having to go to emergency bypass surgery, a 2.3% emergency surgery rate continues.

Significant damage to the coronary artery at the time of the procedure can be caused by the guiding catheter, the guide wire, or the balloon catheter itself. The guiding catheter has a greater potential of inducing arterial trauma than do routine diagnostic catheters because the tip of the guiding catheter is often seated more deeply in the proximal vessel. The tips of the early guiding catheters were stiffer and somewhat larger than were the diagnostic catheters, but over the past several years, the catheter companies have made a great effort to soften the material used in the tip of the guiding catheter, thereby reducing the likelihood of guiding catheter-induced trauma. At times during the angioplasty procedure, the guiding catheter may be advanced far into the coronary arteries, either on

purpose or inadvertently, and disruption of the intima can be caused by the tip of the guiding catheter. Guiding catheter trauma also provides a nidus for the later development of atherosclerotic lesions stimulated by the damage to the artery by the guiding catheter. The time when deep seating is of particular concern during the procedure is that following balloon inflations, when the balloon catheter is being withdrawn back into the guiding catheter so that injections of contrast can be made to assess angiographic progress. This maneuver often causes the tip of the guiding catheter to dive far into the target artery, and if at all possible, this should be avoided by a push-pull technique involving two experienced operators. As the balloon catheter is withdrawn into the guiding catheter, the guiding catheter must also be slightly withdrawn and the guide wire advanced forward so that the entire system does not fling out of the target vessel when the "suction" pressure of the withdrawal motion of the balloon catheter is released once the balloon enters the guide.

At times, the guiding catheter is advanced on purpose farther into the vessel than the ostium in order to achieve a better back-up system to force the balloon across the tight stenosis. The presence of the balloon catheter in the artery as a stent during this maneuver somewhat reduces the chance of arterial trauma, but certainly great care must be taken during these manipulations to avoid trauma induced by the guiding catheter.

A particularly dangerous area for guiding catheter trauma is the origin of the internal mammary artery if that artery must be cannulated in order to achieve dilatation either of the internal mammary artery itself or of the coronary artery supplied by that bypass conduit. It has long been recognized that the internal mammary artery is a fragile artery, and great care must be taken in the positioning of the guiding catheter at the origin of the internal mammary artery in order to avoid trauma to that vessel. The tips of various internal mammary guiding catheters vary from company to company, and the angulation of origin should be assessed angiographically and then the most coaxial tip design selected as the guide for the internal mammary artery.

Currently available guide wires that are 0.014 inches in diameter or smaller with flexible and non-coated tips have very limited capabilities of damage to the traversed artery in experienced hands. There are many wire-tip configurations available, and the trade-off for flexibility and safety is sometimes the inability to achieve pushability of the wire at the lesion. This can be overcome by advancing the balloon catheter over the wire to stiffen the tip at the level of the lesion or by removing the flexible-tipped wire necessary to safely reach the lesion once the balloon has been passed over this wire to the area just proximal to the lesion and then replacing it with a stiffer wire to cross the stenosis. A "feel" must be developed for the manipulation of the guide wire, however, since even these inherently safe guide wire systems can travel under a plaque and cause disruption and dislodgment of the offending material. During advancement of the guide wire, constant maneuvering of the tip should be done to assure that the tip is free and torqueable. If the tip is not free and easily removable by torquing the system, one should be concerned that the tip of the wire is either in the side branch or under a plaque, and the wire should be withdrawn slightly until the tip is free and only then advanced in the usual manner. The advancement of the guide wire should not be hurried, and great care should be taken in traversing the vessel both proximal and distal to the lesion since the wire inevitably will be followed by a larger profile system, namely, the balloon catheter. If a plaque or arterial wall is dissected by the initial passage of the wire, then a larger tract will certainly be made in a false lumen when the balloon catheter is passed and even when balloon inflations occur. This is a common cause for dissection of the vessel.

If stiffer wires such as 0.016 inch guide wires or 0.018 inch guide wires are to be used, the chance of trauma increases somewhat, and extreme care must be used in advancing the guide wire down the artery. Compared with standard wires, however, the high-torque floppy 0.018 inch system from ACS, although larger in diameter, is a very safe wire, and the tip has the soft flexible characteristics of the smaller 0.014 inch wires.

Inflation of a balloon in an artery can and does cause some degree of trauma to the artery every time. The goal of angioplasty is to achieve a controlled injury to the artery, but in some cases, a significant "dissection" or disruption of the intima occurs. This can usually be identified during the procedure by injection of contrast through the guiding catheter and subsequent identification of an irregular or disrupted lumen. If contrasts "hangs up" in the area of balloon inflation during the guiding catheter injections, then concern for significant damage to the artery must be entertained.

Spasm can and does occur during angioplasty, both secondary to guide wire passage and irritation of the vessel and also secondary to balloon catheter inflation. This generally has a smoother appearance than does a dissection and is reversed by the administration of intracoronary nitroglycerin and/or sublingual or intracoronary calcium blockers. The discussion in Chapter 6 (Complex PTCA II: Total Occlusions) dealing with totally occluded coronary arteries details the downstream spasm that often occurs following the successful angioplasty of totally occluded vessels with reestablished antegrade flow. This can also occur in a nontotally occluded artery that has slow flow distally. When the artery is opened and increased pressure in the distal vessel occurs, reflex spasm can be seen. This again can be identified by its angiographic appearance and proof that it is spasm rather than dissection, or downstream fixed stenoses can be demonstrated by the administration of intracoronary nitroglycerin through guiding catheter injections.

The presence of thrombus in the coronary artery to be dilated certainly increases the risk of intraprocedural complications and abrupt reclosures in the early postangioplasty period. Thrombotic material generally has a rather typical appearance that is different from that of a dissection and, when identified, should be treated appropriately, and attempts to resolve the situation in the catheterization laboratory should be made. Sending a patient back to the heart unit with thrombus present in the artery constitutes a situation that certainly has a high risk for an abrupt reclosure. In some cases, prolonged heparinization will "clean up" areas of thrombus, but, in general, it is better if this is taken care of in the laboratory.

Distal emboli can occur in any angioplasty, but is most likely to be a complication in patients with totally occluded coronary arteries, thrombus in the coronary artery at the time of the angioplasty, or in saphenous vein bypass graft angioplasty. When distal embolization occurs, the patient commonly has chest pain and ischemic changes in EKG that do not resolve with time, nitroglycerin, or other medical intervention. The emboli have most likely lodged in small distal vessels, and the best way to identify this phenomenon is to either see pruning or squaring of the distal arteries. Sometimes, if the emboli embed in vessels too small to clearly identify, another feature consistent with distal embolization is slow flow of contrast through the vessel because of the increased resistance and plugging of the distal arteries with decreased runoff.

Abrupt reclosure occurs in 3–6% of cases of angioplasty. This is generally defined as a reocclusion of the artery anywhere from minutes after the procedure is concluded to 24–48 hr later. The mechanism of abrupt reclosure varies, but can be from dissection of the artery at the time of the procedure, which progresses over time to a total closure of the vessel. It may also be due to the accumulation and propagation of thrombus in the artery at the site of the distal lesion or thrombogenesis in conjunction with dissection or spasm of the vessel. It is interesting that abrupt reclosures have not been seen in patients treated with atherectomy (see Chapter 13, New Technologies for the Treatment of Obstructive Arterial Disease), and therefore removal rather than compression of the plaque seems to preclude this complication phenomenon. If abrupt reclosure occurs and is identified, the patient should be returned to the catheterization laboratory immediately to identify fully the anatomic situation. It is usually heralded by chest pain and EKG changes consistent with ischemia, and a rapid return to the laboratory is of utmost importance. The catheterization laboratory crew should be on call full-time while patients are still in the early postangioplasty period, and the goal should be to be able to return the patient to the catheterization laboratory within 45 min. Diagnostic angiography should be quickly carried out, and if the artery is totally occluded, an attempt to cross the area of total occlusion with a flexible-tipped wire should be carried out while the cardiac surgery team is attaining full readiness to transport the patient to surgery very quickly. If the wire can be passed across the total occlusion, an appropriately sized balloon catheter should be inflated a few times to try to reestablish antegrade flow in the vessel. One must be aware of the likelihood of reperfusion arrhythmias, and lidocaine or other antiarrhythmic agents may be given prophylactically in this setting. Once antegrade flow is reestablished, attempts to achieve a good angioplasty result can be made within an appropriate time-frame. Case 12 in Appendix I demonstrates one such case where surgery was avoided and a good long-term result achieved. If, however, the result from angioplasty following an abrupt reclosure does not angiographically appear to be of the quality that can be trusted, the physician must make the difficult decision to send the patient to surgery, even with a patent artery. If an artery has abruptly reclosed once and a near-perfect result is not achieved with repeat angioplasty, that artery should not be trusted and the patient should have bypass surgery so that the repeated abrupt reclosures do not jeopardize the patient's life or myocardium.

Other complications of the procedure with angioplasty pertain to the procedure of angiography as well.

Entry-site complications, either thrombosis or hemorrhage of the brachial or femoral artery entry sites, can certainly occur and should be treated in an appropriate manner consistent with one's treatment of diagnostic angiographic complications. In the early series of patients, there were some protamine reactions, and this drug is no longer generally used following angioplasty, both to preclude the occurrence of allergic reactions and also to lessen the chance of thrombotic abrupt reclosure. Reaction to contrast media can and does occur with angioplasty, and if the patient has a history of dye reaction or intolerance to shellfish, then appropriate preprocedural and intraprocedural means should be carried out to decrease the likelihood of a contrast reaction. One protocol for contrast reaction treatment is listed in Appendix II–B.

TREATMENT OF COMPLICATIONS DURING ANGIOPLASTY

If trauma is induced by the guiding catheter as described above, an attempt to "tack back" the damaged lining of the artery can be made by balloon angioplasty. If damage can be identified angiographically, then a balloon catheter can be inserted and positioned at the site of trauma and inflated to adequate pressures for as long as possible to try to reattach the area of intimal disruption. A modest oversizing of the balloon catheter in these instances is often helpful, and when this is done, the larger balloon catheter can be held at a lower pressure for longer periods of time in order to achieve a reattachment of the damaged arterial lining. Since this may occur in proximal vessels, the amount of myocardium held ischemic during balloon catheter inflations is sometimes considerable. If this is true, then the use of a flow-through perfusion balloon catheter system (STACK) will generally allow one to achieve the longer inflations necessary to tack back flaps of intima. The liberal use of intraaortic balloon pumps and even cardiopulmonary support in these cases is encouraged, and with appropriate care and planning, even in cases of significant damage to the artery by the guiding catheter, the situation can be resolved by angioplasty and bypass surgery avoided.

If damage is done by the passage of the guide wire and can be identified as an area of narrowing, presumably by the raising of a flap in that area, careful manipulation of the wire past that area in the true lumen of the vessel and placement of a balloon catheter at the site of dissection to reattach the flap to the wall of the artery can be attempted. It is clear that in cases of severe stenosis, the moment at which the wire crosses the lesion is often the moment of truth as far as the success or failure of the angioplasty is concerned. If the wire crosses the true lumen and subsequent balloon inflations are carried out, a good result could be anticipated. If the wire crosses beneath the plaque or through a false channel, then balloon inflations carried out at that site will produce an even larger false channel, and it is often these cases that show significant dissection or are candidates for abrupt reclosure, as described elsewhere in this chapter. As with guiding catheter-induced trauma, dissections caused by the wire should be tacked back by balloon inflations at the site of the dissection. Prolonged inflations are often helpful, and the use of a perfusion balloon catheter will often be the salvaging decision. It should also be recognized that dissection of an artery in this manner increases the chance of abrupt reclosure, and the patient should be kept on heparin for at least 24 hr following the procedure and then carefully watched once the heparin is stopped. In some cases, heparin can be restarted after removal of the sheaths, and the patient kept on heparin for a few days. It is not unreasonable to return patients with either guiding catheter trauma or dissections caused by the wire to the laboratory before discharge and to perform an angiogram to see just how well that area has healed. This is certainly a safety feature and more reliable than the patient's symptoms or thallium treadmill testing.

If excessive trauma occurs during the balloon inflation, a decision must be made at that time as to the most likely etiology of the problem. Disruption of the intima or raising of a flap can be treated by prolonged balloon inflations, as described above, to try to reattach the offending material to the wall of the artery. Again, slight oversizing of the balloon may be helpful in such cases. The use of an extended or exchange wire to put in a larger balloon is important, and repeat crossing of such an area, while commonly done by some practitioners, is better avoided in these situations.

Spasm following balloon inflations or wire manipulations can occur, and this may be difficult to identify during the procedure. Differentiation between spasm and the presence of significant arterial tearing can be difficult. The appearance is somewhat different, with a smoother appearance of spasm and a more ragged appearance when dissection has occurred, and the liberal use of intracoronary nitroglycerin infused directly into the target artery can sometimes relieve the spasm and thereby identify the source of the problem. If spasm does occur, it is a good idea to leave the wire across the area of balloon inflation for a longer than usual period of time to make sure that the spasm is not a recurrent problem. Sublingual nifedipine can be very helpful in instances of equipment-induced spasm. Pa-

tients should be watched for as long as necessary to assure that the spasm has been controlled, and on some occasions, patients will need to be sent to surgery because of the inability to obliterate the spasm process. The use of intracoronary verapamil and other efforts to break the spastic circle should be made, but if these are not successful, then the transport of the patient to bypass surgery, in the manner described below, is necessary and appropriate.

SAFE TRANSPORT OF THE PATIENT TO EMERGENCY BYPASS SURGERY

As stated in other chapters of this book, the prime consideration in the acceptance of a patient for angioplasty should be the development, in the operator's mind, of a worst-case scenario in which the patient would have to be taken to emergency bypass surgery. Each patient must be individually analyzed as to the anatomy of the target lesions, the amount of myocardium supplied by the vessels to be dilated, and the quality of the coronary supply to and the functioning of the myocardium that is not jeopardized and will not be directly affected by the angioplasty attempt. The operator should be convinced that, should the target vessel or vessels become irreversibly occluded, safe transport to emergency bypass surgery can be carried out. As described elsewhere in this book, the use of the intraaortic balloon pump in patients with significantly compromised left ventricular function is encouraged either on a standby or an operative basis during the procedure. The use of full cardiopulmonary support with a heart-lung bypass machine in place and functioning has extended the procedure of angioplasty to some very high risk patients who, without this precaution, could not be safely and quickly transported to the operating room. The use of the intraaortic balloon pump or cardiopulmonary support system provides a margin of safety that can often make the difference between being able to present the surgeon with a stable patient for emergency bypass or transporting a patient to surgery who is undergoing cardiopulmonary resuscitative efforts. The more stable a patient can be presented to the surgeon in the operating room, the more likely that the patient will survive and have a good result from the revascularization surgery.

If an artery closes during the procedure by trauma induced by the guiding catheter, the guide wire, or the balloon catheter, an attempt should be made to continue flow through the artery while the patient is transported to surgery. Often, simply maintaining the presence of the guide wire across the lesion and in the distal vessel will keep the artery patent with adequate flow, and transfer to the surgical suite can be accomplished with this hardware in place. The use of multihole perfusion catheters in this situation is also very helpful. These catheters have several holes, positioned both proximal and distal to the area of closure, and can provide distal flow in much the same manner as side-hole guiding catheters do. These multihole perfusion catheters should be immediately accessible during all procedures. The maintenance of flow during transport to surgery will not only preserve myocardium, but will also allow the surgery to take place in a more calm and orderly setting and increase the chances of success of the surgery. The previous placement of a right heart catheter with a central lumen and pacing capability provides the ability not only to measure pulmonary pressures to monitor the situation, but also provides a large central line to infuse fluids or medication through the large lumen system. The immediate availability of pacing capabilities is often important, particularly in the case of procedures performed on the right coronary arteries. During transport to the operating suite, the catheter systems that are left in place should be sewn in position so that inadvertent dislodgment does not occur. If the patient is transferred to the surgical suite with a wire or a multihole perfusion catheter across the area of closure, care should be taken to withdraw the guiding catheter from the ostium of the main artery, particularly in the case of the left coronary artery, so that prolonged ischemia or trauma to the main ostium does not occur during transport. Leaving the guiding catheter in place during such transport also presents the potential for reduction of flow not only in the target artery, but also in other branches of the left coronary system.

The question of surgical back-up during cases of angioplasty has been debated at length at various institutions. The quality and availability of surgical back-up varies from institution to institution, but some generalities can be made. All cases of angioplasty should have some level of immediate access to the surgical suite in order to assure that the procedure is safe for the patient. In some institutions, attempts have been made to identify higher-risk vs. lower-risk patients and different levels of back-up support instituted. Although it may be possible to identify higher-risk patients than usual, i.e., patients with lesions on a bend in the artery or patients with diffuse and long segmental disease, it is not possible to identify a patient who is at no risk to go to bypass surgery. This includes patients with total occlusions, a phenomenon that has been discussed elsewhere in which patients with previously totally occluded arteries have them opened, and then with either a dissection or

abrupt reclosure, the situation develops into a full-blown myocardial infarction event. This presumably is due to the dislodgment of material and distal embolization that cuts off the collaterals that were present prior to the angioplasty attempt. It is up to the individual operator to assess the patient preangioplasty and to assure him- or herself and the patient that the safety of the procedure is preserved by the availability of appropriate surgical back-up. whether an anesthesiologist need to be present in the catheterization laboratory or whether the surgeon needs to be in the room or only immediately available is a situation that will vary from institution to institution. The prime factor in all cases, however, should be that no case should be done without some form of surgical back-up available and that surgical back-up should be appropriate so that if a catastrophic event occurs, i.e., dissection of the left main coronary artery with the guiding catheter, the patient can be transported in an expeditious manner to receive bypass surgery. The main safety feature in angioplasty is the ability to get out of trouble if it occurs, and this mandates that excellent bypass surgery coverage be available for all cases.

ABRUPT RECLOSURE

Abrupt reclosure can occur within minutes of removing the balloon and wire system until up to 48 hr, or even longer in rare cases. This event is usually heralded by the onset of pain and/or EKG changes.

If, during the procedure, a suspicion of spasm, dissection, or thrombus has been raised or if, on the postangioplasty angiogram, a significant intimal disruption is present, it is wise to leave the sheaths in place if the femoral approach has been used and maintain the patient on heparin and IV nitroglycerin for at least 24 hr after the procedure. This precautionary measure not only allows continued anticoagulation during the early healing process, but also provides rapid reaccess to the arterial and venous systems if a return to the catheterization laboratory is necessary.

If there is clinical evidence of abrupt reclosure, the patient should first be stabilized with medications as much as possible, including antiarrhythmic medications, and then quickly returned to the catheterization laboratory. The exact anatomic problem should be delineated both to determine if anything can be done further from an angioplasty standpoint to correct the situation and also to identify the exact problem for the surgeons if the patient is transferred immediately for surgery. In cases of abrupt reclosure, an attempt to reopen the vessel by angioplasty is usually undertaken. This is appropriate to occur while the operating room is being prepared for the patient, but if recrossing the area of abrupt reclosure with the guide wire is difficult or time-consuming, the operator should be ready to make the decision to transfer the patient quickly to surgery so that prolonged damage to the myocardium by ischemia does not occur. In general, the same-style guiding catheter, guide wire, and balloon catheter used initially can be used for this repeat attempt, and a gentle attempt to recross the area of abrupt reclosure should be carried out. A very flexible wire should be utilized in this type of case. If it is possible to recross the area of abrupt reclosure with wiring of the distal vessel, then balloon inflations carried out at the site of closure can often salvage the situation and prevent having to send the patient to surgery. If, however, recrossing the area is not accomplished easily and with rapidity, the decision to transfer the patient to surgery should be made quickly so that undue ischemic time of the myocardium supplied by the target vessel is avoided.

If a vessel is reopened after an abrupt reclosure, it is wise to leave the wire across the area of reclosure for a prolonged period of time (30 min to 1 hr) and observe the situation in the angiographic suite to be certain that a repeat abrupt reclosure does not occur. During that time, of course, the surgical back-up must be kept at ready, and continual consultations with the surgical team carried out so that they are aware of the progress or lack thereof in the situation.

If there is any question concerning the adequacy of the results after an abrupt reclosure has been reopened, it is wise to leave either the wire or a multihole perfusion catheter across the area of closure and transfer the patient to the surgical suite in a stable situation rather than returning the patient to the coronary care unit and having another abrupt reclosure occur. If the repeat angioplasty of the segment appears to be excellent, then a return to the coronary care unit for further close observation is appropriate.

When patients are returned to the laboratory for an abrupt reclosure, a subsequent inflation with a larger balloon is sometimes helpful in achieving a better "tacking back" of the offending flap in the case of a dissection. If a thrombus is implicated in the abrupt reclosure, the administration of a thrombolytic agent can be considered. Urokinase is particularly helpful, and the doses used to dissolve identifiable thrombus are small enough that the option of a safe trip to surgery is still within the realm of reality. The administration of thrombolytic agents in this setting must be undertaken with the caution that the amount of time necessary to administer thrombolysis should be carried out in the setting of an artery in which flow is maintained so that an extra 20–30 mi of myocardial ischemia does not occur.

OTHER COMPLICATIONS OF ANGIOPLASTY

Other complications of the angioplasty procedure include local trauma to the site of entry, contrast medium reaction, and neurological complications. The danger of trauma at the site of entry is the same as that with routine angiography and should be dealt with expeditiously. If thrombosis of a brachial artery occurs, this should be treated by thrombectomy and/or resection of the brachial artery by a vascular surgeon. If a tear of the femoral artery occurs, vascular surgery should be undertaken in an expeditious fashion. The prolonged anticoagulation sometimes necessary after angioplasty will often be in direct conflict with the need to stop a hematoma formation and appropriate judgments must be made to try not to cause a thrombotic closure of an angioplasty segment, but also to preclude the occurrence of a serious peripheral complication. The possibility of a retroperitoneal hematoma must be kept in mind, particularly in patients on prolonged heparinization.

If the patient has a history of allergy to previous contrast administration or to iodine or shellfish, then the patient should be pretreated for contrast reaction. An appropriate protocol is listed in Appendix II–B.

Neurologic complications of angioplasty are rare. One possible source of emboli that is more likely with angioplasty than with routine angiography involves the use of the long sheath from the femoral approach. This long sheath is a potential source of emboli even with full heparinization (10,000 units before the angioplasty equipment is inserted and additional heparinization at hourly intervals if the procedure is prolonged). A flush system should be attached to the side arm of the long sheath and continuously flushed if catheter changes are necessary. Leaving a guide wire in the system and exchanging guiding catheters over the guide wire rather than preloading the guide wire system is also advisable. Wiggling of the guide wire between catheter changes and allowing back-bleeding through the sheath can reduce the threat of thrombus introduced by passing the guiding catheter through the sheath and into the ascending aorta.

Complications when attempting angioplasty of saphenous vein bypass grafts or of native vessels through the grafts involve the irregular grumatous material that often lines these bypass conduits. The passage of the wire down the bypass graft can function as a mixer blade and raise flaps in its trip through the bypass. The use of a "U"-shaped wire and other ways to handle this situation are discussed in Chapter 8 (Complex PTCA IV: Bypass Grafts). Inflation of the balloon catheter in the graft can also fragment the material lining the graft and send showers of emboli distally. These complications, of course, could be avoided by not attempting angioplasty of bypass grafts, but in cases where repeat surgical procedure is necessary, it is acceptable to attempt angioplasty of grafts, particularly if they are 5 years old or younger. Great care should be taken in attempting angioplasty of grafts older than 5 years, and the patient and family should be so informed of the increased risk of complication during the procedure. If a dissection in a graft does occur, then prolonged inflations, perhaps with a larger balloon, can be attempted to try to tack back the material raised by either the guide wire or the balloon catheter. If distal embolization occurs in a diffuse manner, the resultant ischemia often has to be accepted and some amount of myocardial damage will occur. The use of streptokinase in these situations is usually not helpful because the material in the grafts that is embolized is usually not thrombus but simply a toothpastelike lining in the graft.

12. Patient Care Aspects of PTCA

Delivery of safe and effective care to the PTCA patient requires a diligent health care team. The PTCA team is composed of physicians who are responsible for the highly technical aspects of angioplasty and nurses who are required to lend their expertise both before, during, and after the procedure. Preprocedure nursing responsibilities include evaluation, planning, and teaching. Treatment plans are made taking into account both the patient's physical and emotional needs. Instruction is provided that is tailored to the patient's level of understanding. Steps in patient care before, during, and after the procedure will be outlined below.

Most angioplasty patients are admitted to the cardiac unit or outpatient department on the day of their procedure. Therefore, time is of the essence for the nursing staff who must work expeditiously to thoroughly prepare the patient for PTCA. The first nursing step undertaken is conducting the patient interview.

PATIENT INTERVIEW

History

Information regarding the patient's medical history and current functional status must be obtained directly from the patient. The interview process reveals the patient's understanding of his/her limitations as a result of coronary artery disease and the result they expect to achieve with angioplasty.

History of allergic reaction must be carefully noted. Some contrast agents used for arteriography during PTCA are iodine-based and can cause a localized reaction such as rash or itching or anaphylaxis. Intravenous corticosteroids or antihistamines may be ordered prior to the procedure depending on the potential for reaction and severity of any previous reaction.

Information regarding the patient's sensitivity to anesthetics is valuable in the event the patient should require emergency surgery. Local anesthesia is given at the catheter insertion site. The administration of intravenous sedatives is not uncommon.

Medications

All medications taken by the patient should be reviewed, and any medication taken the day or morn-
ing of the procedure documented. Also, it is important to note medications that might be taken normally but were held the day of the procedure. Patients taking anticoagulation medications are instructed to discontinue this medication 2 days prior to the procedure. The nurse should inquire as to when the last dose was taken to ensure that the patient will have adequate coagulation. Diabetic patients requiring insulin or oral hypoglycemic agents will most likely require adjustments in dosage prior to the procedure.

PATIENT EDUCATION

The educational needs will vary among patients. It is recommended that the patient's family be included in the teaching session so they too will gain an understanding of both the procedure, the expected outcome, and the subsequent hospital course.

The following areas should be discussed: coronary anatomy, physiology, the pathophysiology of coronary artery disease and its associated risk factors, and treatment options (i.e., bypass surgery, medical management, angioplasty). Teaching will also cover the procedural steps, risks, and potential complications of PTCA and coronary artery bypass surgery. In addition, a discussion should occur that focuses on the prolonged hospital stay should an emergency surgery or complication occur. The teaching process can be enhanced by the use of aids such as a balloon catheter demonstration, illustrated brochures, and audiovisual equipment.

The simplicity of the procedure, relative to coronary bypass surgery, can contribute to the patient's misconception of the potential risk and long-term consequences related to the disease. It must be stressed that coronary artery disease (CAD) is a progressive, chronic disease. A realistic appreciation of the inherent risks of the disease will encourage compliance with the necessary medical regimen and lifestyle adjustments. Having the patient's family included in these discussions can help them support the patient in their long-term health management.

Following instruction, the patient should be encouraged to express his/her concerns, and in return, the nurse should provide comprehensive information that addresses the issues raised.

101

PREPARATION FOR PTCA

The nurse must ensure that the appropriate steps are taken to prepare the patient for angioplasty. It is important to have recordings of current height, weight, blood pressure, pulse, and temperature and documentation of the presence and quality of peripheral pulses. This will provide a baseline for use in evaluating changes or monitoring trends throughout the hospitalization. Patients are instructed to take nothing by mouth, other than their medications, after midnight on the night prior to the procedure. The NPO status will be maintained until after the procedure is completed.

Placement of a peripheral intravenous catheter can facilitate adequate fluid hydration prior to the procedure. The peripheral IV also provides access for administering emergency medications or may be used for the infusion of heparin postprocedure.

Routine preprocedure laboratory tests may include serum electrolytes, renal panel, hemogram, and partial thromboplastin time (PTT). Electrocardiogram and chest X-ray may also be performed. Results of previous studies (e.g., thallium stress test) should be available and incorporated into the permanent record.

In preparation for catheter insertion, both groins and/or right anticubital areas should be cleansed and shaved. The catheter insertion site will be determined by the physician based on the anatomical location of the obstructive coronary lesion.

Obtaining informed consent is ethically and legally imperative. The consent must include details of the procedure to be performed and the potential risks or complications. The physician will discuss with the patient the risks as well as the expected outcome. All necessary consent forms should be completed prior to transferring the patient to the catheterization laboratory.

Upon arrival in the catheterization laboratory, the patient will be introduced to the staff of highly trained nurses and technicians who will assist in the PTCA procedure. It is the staffs' responsibility to orient the patient to the laboratory setting and explain procedural steps. They will assist in meeting the patient's physical needs as well as provide emotional support. Thorough documentation of the procedure and patient's condition upon PTCA completion is critical to providing optimal postprocedure care.

IMMEDIATE POSTPROCEDURE MANAGEMENT

The incidence of complications after angioplasty is low. However, when required, the nurse must be readily available to critically assess the patient and be capable of directing immediate intervention. For this reason, the postprocedure patient is placed in a designated monitored area or a special care unit for those patients at higher risk for complications or hemodynamic decompensation. An immediate assessment of the patient is critical in establishing a baseline for decision making thereafter. The initial assessment should focus on indications of 1) acute occlusion of the dilated vessel, 2) bleeding at the cannulation site, and 3) compromised perfusion to the extremity distal to the access site. Thereafter, the nursing care should provide patient comfort, sheath removal management, and discharge education.

CORONARY ARTERY OCCLUSION

The incidence of acute occlusion within the first 24 hr ranges from 2 to 11% (Popma and Dehmer, 1989). Of that group, 84% occlude within the first 6 hr postprocedure. The ischemic episode experienced by the patient will be demonstrated by chest pain, EKG changes, and possible dysrhythmia. Without intervention, ischemia will advance to myocardial infarction. Therefore, it is essential that the nurse is able to assess the presence of all subtle changes during the initial postprocedure period.

The patient should be assessed for chest pain upon arrival to the unit and instructed to notify the nurse of any occurrence of chest pain. In the presence of chest pain, the nurse must assess the duration, severity, precipitating factors, and its similarity to the patient's typical angina. Prior to the administration of nitrates, a 12-lead EKG should be obtained during the chest pain and then compared to the pre- and postangioplasty EKG. The health team must be notified of any EKG changes such as ST elevation or depression, T wave changes, and Q wave development. Coronary artery spasm from vessel manipulation is common after angioplasty. If the administration of nitroglycerin rapidly relieves the ischemic pain, it is likely to be related to spasm (Popma and Dehmer, 1989). Other patients may complain of mild chest discomfort up to 4 hr after PTCA; this is likely to be caused by the stretching of the coronary artery during balloon inflation (Clark, 1987). Often, this pain is distinguished from ischemic pain because it is atypical of the patient's characteristic angina.

HYPOTENSION

Hypotension unrelated to hypovolemia warrants frequent vital sign assessment because it could represent ischemia. When hemodynamic monitoring is available, the nurse should alert the physician of a nonvolume-related rise in PCWP,PA, and RA pressures associated with a decrease in cardiac output or cardiac index and an increased systemic vascular resistance (SVR). Any of these changes may be indicative of cardiac failure or myocardial ischemia.

Ischemia is usually treated with nitroglycerin, sublingual or intravenous. If IV nitroglycerin is used, it can be titrated to relieve chest pain while maintaining an adequate systolic blood pressure. Calcium channel blockers are utilized for the treatment of coronary artery spasm. Beta-blockers may also be initiated to decrease myocardial oxygen demands and increase oxygen supply through an increased diastolic filling time.

Heparin is conventionally used postprocedure to prevent thrombosis at the site of the dilatation, although there is conflicting evidence in opposition of this practice (Ellis et al., 1989). With heparin administration, it is essential to monitor the partial thromboplastin time to maximize the anticoagulation effect. To assure accuracy, the blood sample for a PTT should be obtained from a venipuncture site or through the arterial sheath (Rudisill, 1989). Diligent monitoring of the PTT values in accordance with heparin administration may be crucial in preventing reclosure of the vessel (Gabliani et al., 1988).

BLEEDING MANAGEMENT

The increased risk of bleeding postangioplasty is due to the use of anticoagulation during and after the procedure. In most cases, the venous and arterial catheter introducer sheaths are not removed in an anticoagulated state to avoid excess bleeding. Therefore, the access site with sheaths intact requires frequent observation to assure bleeding management.

When the patient arrives in the unit, the nurse should thoroughly inspect the access site for latent bleeding, oozing, hematoma formation, and patency of introducer sheaths. Should dressing of the access site be necessary, it should allow for clear observation of the area. If latent bleeding is present, direct pressure should be applied above the puncture site. Sand bags should be discouraged in the management of bleeding because the pressure exerted by the bag is insufficient in controlling the bleed and prevents visual assessment of the site. When present, the perimeter of a hematoma should be clearly delineated to assure identification of increasing size. Oozing around the sheaths is not uncommon, but as with all the above situations, the health team should be notified of the initial assessment and any changes thereafter.

Patients need to be instructed to avoid sneezing, coughing, and lifting their head because of the increased pressure at the insertion site. The head of the patient's bed should be maintained at 30° or less, and the nurse must assist the patient in keeping the affected extremity straight to minimize shearing of the sheaths at the insertion site. These combined efforts should reduce the likelihood of bleeding at the insertion site.

COMPROMISED CIRCULATION

The extremity distal to the access site is at risk, especially when the indwelling sheaths are present. The extremity needs to be frequently assessed for motion, sensation, temperature, color, and the presence and quality of peripheral pulses. The preangioplasty assessment should be reviewed to provide a basis for comparison. Any change should be followed and reported to the medical team.

PATIENT COMFORT

Postprocedure patients are required to lie in bed with their affected extremity virtually immobile. The nurse must make every effort to provide the patient with comfort measures during this period of bed rest. Although the extremity of the insertion site needs to remain straight, the patient should be turned off of their back while maintaining leg immobility. Nurses should offer back massages and analgesics to increase relaxation and comfort. The active involvement of family members in providing patient comfort measures generally aids in the anxiety reduction of the patient and their family.

SHEATH REMOVAL

Sheath removal is typically uneventful, but can elicit a vasovagal response associated with bradychardia and hypotension. To adequately prepare for this situation, the patient should be monitored at the bedside and have patent peripheral IV access for fluid management, if emergently required. In addition, during sheath removal, atropine and supplies necessary for sheath removal should be on hand. Heparin infusion should be discontinued to allow the partial thromboplastin time to return to near normal. After removal, the physician and/or nurse must be prepare to apply direct pressure to the puncture site manually or with a C-clamp until hemostasis is achieved. To provide a safe sheath removal, the nurse must be avail-

able for continuous assessment and must be prepared
to respond immediately to the situation. The patient
is required to lie flat for 4–6 hr post-sheath removal
to ensure hemostasis. Following this, the patient can
be mobilized.

DISCHARGE INSTRUCTION

Prior to discharge, the patient should be instructed
on the administration, dosage, action, and potential
side effects of medications with emphasis on those
newly prescribed. An individualized discharged activity prescription will be based on the patient's previous
activity level and extent of disease. Upon discharge,
the patient should be instructed to report any unusual
drainage from the catheter insertion site. There may
be some discoloration of this area and a small lump
may be noted. Any change in sensation of the extremity distal to the catheterization site should be reported. If the anticubital space was cannulated, the
patient may need instruction regarding an appoint-
ment for suture removal.

The plans for follow-up examination or diagnostic
studies should be scheduled and reviewed with the
patient prior to discharge. Because of the short hospitalization, the teaching on risk factor modification is
minimal. However, the patient does learn that there
are certain risk factors contributing to coronary artery
disease that he/she cannot control, i.e., age, sex, and
family history. It is encouraging, however, for them to
discover that other risk factors such as blood pressure,
smoking, cholesterol, weight, diabetes, and stress *can*
be modified. Therefore, the patient should be provided
with risk factor modification teaching materials and
referred to modification programs in the area.

13. New Technologies for the Treatment of Obstructive Arterial Disease

INTRODUCTION

Despite the effective and widely practiced application of balloon angioplasty for the treatment of atherosclerotic peripheral and coronary artery disease, all practitioners in this field are well aware of the limitations inherent in balloon dilatation. The widespread acceptance of PTCA combined with this awareness of the limitations of balloon angioplasty has provided the impetus for the development of a veritable explosion of new technologies intended to improve both the short- and long-term results of catheter-based revascularization. A summary of the major limitations of balloon angioplasty and the associated rationale for the development of new technologies (e.g., laser catheters, atherectomy devices, intravascular stents, etc.) is outlined in Table 13–1.

Most notable among the current limitations of balloon angioplasty are the problems of abrupt vessel closure and restenosis (1–4). Improvements in balloon catheter and guide wire technology during recent years has improved primary success rates of PTCA but has had little impact on the incidence of abrupt vessel closure or restenosis (5).

Even in the most experienced hands, abrupt closure following balloon angioplasty occurs in approximately 3–5% of PTCAs, probably as the result of intimal dissection, thrombus formation, and/or coronary vasospasm (6–9). When repeat balloon dilatation proves ineffective in restoring luminal patency after abrupt coronary closure, the patient faces the prospect of emergent coronary artery bypass grafting surgery with relatively high morbidity and mortality (2, 10). Although there are certain clinical and angiographic predictors of increased risk for abrupt vessel closure after PTCA (9, 11, 12), this adverse outcome is essentially unpredictable, adding to the anxiety of performing PTCA, particularly in patients with multivessel disease and/or anatomically unfavorable lesions. One of the major rationales for the development of many of the new technologic approaches to revascularization is to provide a means to treat arterial obstruction in a predictable fashion such that the risk of abrupt vessel closure is minimized.

Although abrupt vessel closure is possibly the most dreaded complication of balloon angioplasty, restenosis remains the most frequently encountered problem limiting the long-term efficacy of PTCA (3,4). Clinically evident restenosis occurs in approximately 25–40% of cases after successful PTCA and is most frequently observed between 3 and 6 months after the procedure (3,4,13–15). The angiographic incidence of restenosis appears to be significantly greater than the clinical recurrence rate (16). To date, no pharmacologic intervention or variation in the technical approach to balloon dilatation (e.g., prolonged balloon inflation or increased balloon sizing) has been convincingly demonstrated to alter the incidence of restenosis (17–25) after PTCA. Pathologically, restenosis is caused by a rapid proliferation of intimal and medial smooth muscle cells and/or fibroblasts with an associated extracellular matrix of fibrous tissue (3). Balloon-induced vessel wall trauma, with transient stretching of the media, exposure of plaque elements with platelet adhesion and aggregation, and eventually an inflammatory response to the injury, appears to provide the major stimuli for smooth muscle cell growth and proliferation after PTCA (3,26). Although it may be unrealistic to expect nonballoon technologies to completely eliminate this response to injury scenario, there is still some rationale for developing revascularization devices that debulk plaque, create a smooth lumen to minimize turbulence and platelet aggregation, and minimally injure the normally quiescent smooth muscle cells of the media. There are some data to suggest that debulking of plaque with either laser or mechanical systems may reduce the incidence of restenosis (27–30). Alternatively, intravascular stents may provide a means for decreasing the clinical occurrence of restenosis. This will be discussed later in the chapter.

Several other limitations of balloon angioplasty that may be overcome by some of the newer catheter-based technologies include the difficulties in treating chronic total occlusions (31–33), diffuse disease (5), ostial lesions, and lesions associated with intraluminal thrombus (9).

As mentioned above, there has been a rapid proliferation of technologies (see Table 13–2) aimed at dealing with these limitations of balloon angioplasty. Although it is beyond the scope of this textbook to review in detail every new device that has been devel-

105

TABLE 13–1. Rationale for Development of New Approaches to Recanalization

Based on current limitations of balloon angioplasty:

1. **Restenosis:** unresolved problem, 25–40% of cases, with higher rates for long lesions, LAD, Prinzemetals, etc.

   Rationale: Plaque *removal,* rather than just remodeling, may lower restenosis rates

2. **Total** (old subtotal) **occlusions:** > 3 months' old occlusions — > very poor success rates (10–15%), limits potential for "complete revascularization"

   Rationale: New technology (mechanical, hot tip, laser) may allow high success rates, with or without adjunctive balloon angioplasty

3. **Thrombus removal:** High occlusion rates in lesions with visible thrombus (up to 73%) and particularly in setting of acute MI

   Rationale: Difficult to compress thrombus; why not try to remove it?

4. **Abrupt closure:** Because of intimal dissection, thrombus and/or spasm occurs in 3–8% — > 40% MI rate, 3% mortality with emergent bypass surgery. Unpredictable

   Rationale: Mechanical systems and/or laser plaque removal may be predictable and safer

5. **Other:** Certain anatomic situations difficult to treat; e.g., diffuse disease, ostial lesions, etc., may be more effectively treated with newer technologies

TABLE 13–2. New Devices for the Treatment of Obstructive Arterial Disease

Direct application of laser energy
- GV Medical, balloon centering, argon
- USCI multiple-fiber circumferential array, pulsed argon
- MCM (pulsed dye laser), with spectral fingerprinting, "smart laser"
- AIS, Excimer (pulsed) laser systems
- Other: Spectronetics excimer, Eclipse (pulsed), ACS, MIT (argon)

Indirect application of laser energy
- Trimedyne LaserProbe ("hot tip")
- Nd:YAG sapphire tip "hot tip"
- USCI/Spears, laser-assisted balloon angioplasty, Nd:YAG, (welding)

Mechanical systems (atherectomy or atheroabrasion)
- DVI/Simpson, directional atherectomy catheter (Atherocath®)
- Cordis/Kensey, high-speed rotational atherectomy (abrasion)
- Biophysics International/Auth, Rotablator® (abrasion)
- Transluminal extraction catheter (TEC)
- MedInnovations/Fischell, pullback atherectomy catheter (PAC)
- Other: Bard atherectomy, ultrasonic plaque ablation (Siegel), etc.

Intravascular stents
- Johnson & Johnson/Palmaz-Schatz, woven wire stent, over balloon
- Medinvent/Sigwart, self-expanding stent
- Cook/Gianturco-Roubin, balloon expandable stent
- Other: biodegradable stent, Medtronics stent, Cordis stent

Other devices
- Radio-frequency "hot tip"
- Magnum wire for total occlusions
- Slow rotational probe for total occlusions

oped in the last several years, this chapter will attempt to provide an overview of this rapidly moving field, highlighting the status of specific devices in each of the following categories: 1) direct application of laser energy 2) indirect application of laser energy, 3) mechanical systems for plaque ablation or removal, and 4) intravascular stents.

LASER ANGIOPLASTY

Overview

Ever since the early 1960s when the first lasers were developed, physicians and the lay public have been intrigued with the notion of harnessing this energy to treat a variety of medical conditions. The first use of a laser to ablate human atheroma was reported by McGuff et al. in 1963, when they used a ruby laser to irradiate a segment of atheromatous aorta obtained at autopsy (34). However, the clinical application of laser technology to treat obstructive arterial disease did not evolve until the 1980s when the success of balloon angioplasty combined with the refinement of

fiber optics to transmit the energy along the length of a catheter kindled an intense interest in the promise of "laser angioplasty." Early studies by Abela and co-workers demonstrated the feasibility of continuous wave laser energy transmission (Nd:YAG and argon lasers) via flexible fiber optics to ablate atheromatous plaque (35–37). The histopathology from these in vitro studies demonstrated a zone of ablation surrounded by areas of thermal injury, raising concerns regarding the focality of laser energy delivery (35–38). Severe thermal injury to the arterial wall associated with continuous wave laser application has been demonstrated to induce smooth muscle cell proliferation and collagen formation, leading to restenosis and limiting the long-term efficacy of continuous wave laser angioplasty (39). Subsequent studies have suggested that the use of pulsed delivery of laser energy at various wavelengths helps to minimize this thermal effect (40–42) and has provided the rationale the increased interest in pulsed lasers for clinical application.

Despite the promise and hype of laser angioplasty, this technology has had a number of limitations that have been difficult to overcome. The most important problem limiting the safe application of laser energy to atherosclerotic coronary artery disease has been the unacceptably high incidence of arterial perforation (35,37,43). Historically, this complication has resulted from both mechanical perforation due to the stiffness of bare fiber optics and from laser-induced perforation due to dispersion of laser energy to the more "normal" portion of the vessel wall (43–46). A variety of innovative approaches have been developed to try to overcome the problem of vessel perforation during laser angioplasty. These include the encapsulation of the fiber optic within an elliptical cap ("hot tip" laser), the use of pulsed laser delivery with multiple fibers delivered coaxially over a central guide wire (e.g., the AIS excimer laser), the use of fluorescence (spectral feedback) guided laser delivery (i.e., "smart laser"), the coaxial delivery of a divergent laser beam using a balloon catheter for centering the laser beam, and others. The ability to use angioscopy to "guide" the delivery of laser energy has proven impractical because of the need for continuous intracoronary flushing of saline, the large size of the catheters, and the poor ability to estimate lumen size secondary to pincushion distortion. Although other new technologies, such as catheter-based ultrasonic imaging, may eventually prove useful in guiding the delivery of laser energy, the feasibility of incorporating this type of diagnostic device in a laser catheter remains to be demonstrated.

The other current limitations of laser angioplasty include 1) the relatively small channel size created by laser catheters, often necessitating the use of adjunctive balloon angioplasty; 2) the potential for thermal injury (primarily with continuous wave lasers); 3) increased vessel wall thrombogenicity (e.g., excimer lasers) and potential for reocclusion (47); 4) arterial spasm (particularly with thermal injury, cw) (48–51); 5) the potential for embolic debris that appears to be more pronounced with pulse laser systems, and 6) the substantial cost of purchasing and maintaining complex laser systems; and 6) the substantial cost of purchasing and maintaining complex laser hardware (52,53). Despite these limitations, the newest generation of laser angioplasty catheters, as described below, are beginning to show some clinical promise. It will likely be many years, however, before the exact role of laser angioplasty in the treatment of atherosclerotic coronary artery disease is reasonably defined.

Direct Application of Laser Energy: Specific Devices

Balloon centered argon laser (GV Medical, LAS-TAC®). This balloon-centered continuous wave argon laser system represents one of the first direct laser devices developed to seriously address the problem of laser-induced vessel perforation. The device incorporates a single fiber optic passed through a central lumen of a relatively conventional coronary balloon angioplasty catheter. The initial device utilized a bare optical fiber, but more recently has incorporated a lens assembly at the distal fiber tip that is used to create a 40° divergence of the laser beam. The divergence of the laser beam is intended to rapidly decrease the energy delivered to the vessel as one moves radially or axially away from the fiber tip (54,55). Theoretically, this should decrease the risk of perforation. Balloon inflation is used to coaxially align the centrally located optical fiber and lens assembly (Fig. 13–1).

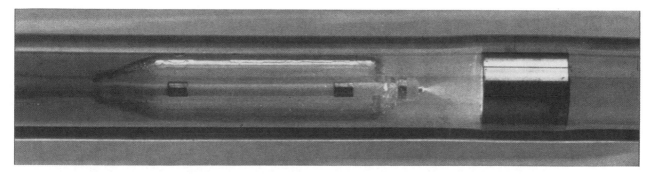

Fig. 13–1. Picture of LASTAC® continuous wave argon laser catheter for the treatment of total coronary artery occlusions (simulated use in plastic tubing). The divergent laser beam is aligned coaxially by a balloon-centering mechanism.

This particular device is designed to be used adjunctively with standard balloon angioplasty in cases of total or subtotal occlusion when conventional guide wires (or balloon catheters) are unable to cross a lesion. Since conventional balloon angioplasty is performed after the creation of a very small (laser-created) luminal channel, it is unlikely that this approach will have any significant impact on the incidence of abrupt vessel closure or restenosis.

Although this device has been used in clinical trials in both peripheral vascular disease and in the coronary arteries, there is relatively little published data summarizing the results. Nordstrom and Dorros have reported the preliminary results using this device in the treatment of peripheral vascular disease (56). In this series, 34 iliac or superficial femoral artery lesions were treated (20 total occlusions) using the laser system followed by balloon angioplasty. The laser (argon, continuous wave, 2–10 sec, 8–10 W energy) was successful in crossing 32/34 lesions (94%). It is not clear how many of these lesions could have been crossed using conventional techniques. Complications of the procedure included three emboli (9%), one perforation (3%), and two early closures (6%). There was inadequate long-term follow-up data to evaluate the incidence of restenosis. Foschi and colleagues have described the preliminary results using this device in the treatment of high-grade and total occlusions in both native human coronary arteries and aortocoronary saphenous vein bypass grafts (57). In this series, 67 lesions were treated in 67 patients. Fourteen of the 67 cases were in saphenous vein grafts, and in 55 of 67 cases the laser system was used to treat total occlusions. Three-quarters of the total occlusions were believed to have been present for 2 months or longer. Using repeated 1–2 sec exposures the laser allowed the operators to cross 51/67 lesions (76%). The laser treatment, when successful, was followed in each case by conventional balloon angioplasty, with most lesions reduced to less than 50% stenosis. There was one mechanical perforation, two abrupt closures necessitating emergency bypass surgery, and one distal embolus causing myocardial infarction. Long-term follow-up data was limited but suggested restenosis rates comparable to PTCA alone. Although these results are somewhat preliminary in nature, they suggest that the GV Medical balloon-centered argon laser may be one of the tools available to successfully expand the ability to treat chronic total occlusions. Obviously, more experience with the device is necessary before its role in treating coronary artery disease, and its effects on long-term vessel patency, if any, are better defined.

Direct excimer laser system. Recent developments in excimer laser technology have led to increased optimism regarding the ability to safely deliver laser energy in the coronary arteries. The term "excimer" stands for excited dimer. This type of laser energy is created by high-voltage electrical discharge in a mixture of an inert gas (e.g., helium, argon, xenon) in the presence of a highly dilute halogen compound (e.g., chlorine, fluorine, etc.). The laser energy emitted is within the ultraviolet portion of the spectrum (i.e., 193–351 nm wavelength) and contains a very high energy content. The application of this type of laser system to plaque ablation in human coronary arteries was initially limited by technical problems relating to radio-frequency interference generated by high-voltage electrical discharge, the need to dampen discharge-related acoustical effects, noxious properties of the halogen component of the gas mixture, and difficulties in coupling the laser output to fiber optics.

One of the appealing characteristics of pulsed excimer lasers is the ability to ablate atherosclerotic tissue with minimal thermal effect (42,58) and reasonably precise control of tissue ablation (59). Unlike some of the continuous wave lasers that may create peak tissue temperatures of 160°C during brief exposures, the peak tissue temperatures during pulsed excimer laser energy delivery typically does not exceed 65°C (42,58). The dose-response characteristics of the excimer laser also provide a desirable linear relationship between the depth of tissue ablation and the number of pulses applied. The relatively clean tissue cuts, without evidence of significant thermal effects, observed with excimer laser ablation have led some investigators to postulate that the tissue ablation with this device is due to a "photochemical desorption" (60). However, recent observations that there is minimal thermal effect with nonexcimer pulsed laser energy (e.g., argon or Nd:YAG lasers) suggest that the excimer laser ablates tissue via a localized thermal effect with heat being dissipated rapidly so that little thermal injury to surrounding tissue is observed (60,-61). Part of the tissue ablation observed with pulsed laser energy may also be the result of a photoacoustic effect, which may also explain the increased embolic potential of pulsed laser delivery.

Animal experiments have demonstrated that excimer laser energy can be applied in a controlled fashion in vivo with little evidence of thermal injury to surrounding vascular tissue (62). In addition, there are data suggesting that excimer-induced vascular injury heals more rapidly and completely than does injury induced by continuous wave lasers (62).

Although the potential of excimer laser angioplasty has been appreciated for some time, it has taken many years to improve the understanding of laser energy delivery and fiber-optic design to allow excimer lasers to be applied in the clinical arena. Several excimer laser devices have been developed and are in various phases of clinical evaluation. To date, none has been approved by the FDA for commercial sale to treat coronary artery disease.

The largest clinical experience with the excimer laser has been obtained using a system manufactured by Advanced Interventional Systems (AIS). This system uses a XeCl gas mixture and emits laser light with a wavelength of 308 nm, with energies of up to 350 mJ per 200–300 nanosecond pulse. The initial device developed by AIS consisted of a single laser fiber optic with a balloon catheter for coaxial alignment of the 400 μM fiber, similar to the design of the GV Medical device (see above). This device has been used in the treatment of peripheral artery disease (63). In these cases, the excimer laser (1.2 mm catheter) was used adjunctively with conventional balloon angioplasty, achieving an overall acute success in 24 of 31 cases (77%) of femoropopliteal stenoses and occlusions (63). Recanalization was accomplished in 17 of 22 total occlusions (77%), with improved success in later cases due to introduction of balloon-centering for coaxial alignment. There was one case of clinically significant embolization (3%) to the popliteal artery, one case of acute femoral artery thrombosis (3%), and

one case of late (12 hr) thrombosis (3%) treated with intraarterial urokinase. At a mean follow-up of 9.1 $\pm$ 3.5 months, seven patients (28%) had developed clinical evidence of restenosis.

The first successful intracoronary application of the 308 nm XeCl excimer laser was reported in 1989 (64). The device used in the majority of cases in the recently reported multicenter coronary trials is a 1.6 mm diameter catheter containing a circumferential array of twelve 200 micron optical fibers, surrounding an 0.018 inch central guide wire lumen (65) (Fig. 13–2). The laser energy delivery is such that plaque ablation occurs only when the catheter tip actually comes into contact with the plaque (i.e., contract ablation). More recently, a 2.0 mm device with 50 micron fibers has been introduced. The investigators have also described plans to study a 2.4 mm diameter device.

The results of the initial 110 cases of percutaneous excimer laser coronary angioplasty have recently been reported (65). In this series, a total of 134 lesions (40 LAD, 18 LCX, 41 RCA, 10 saphenous vein grafts) were treated either with excimer laser alone ("stand alone," 31%) or with adjunctive balloon angioplasty (n = 76, 69%). An average of 1202 $\pm$ 1131 laser pulses were used in each case. Acute angiographic

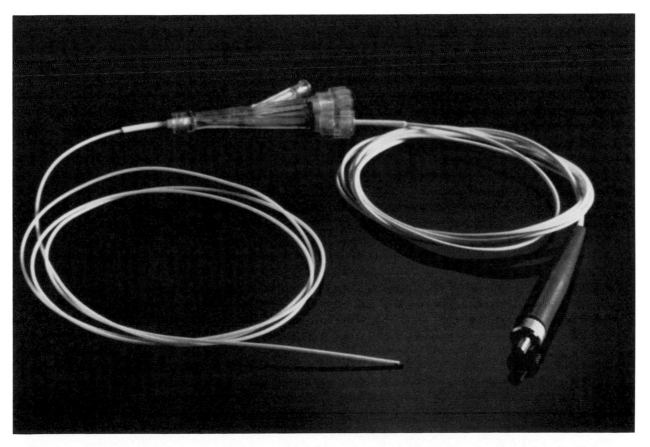

Fig. 13–2. Photograph of the 1.6 mm (4.8 French) multifiber AIS excimer laser catheter, shown introduced through a Y-adaptor.

success was achieved in 94 of 110 patients (85%), with a reduction in the mean stenosis severity from 89 ± 11% (preprocedure) to 48 ± 25% (after laser alone) to 24 ± 16% (after balloon). There were no deaths or clinically detected perforations. However, approximately 15% of cases were associated with clinically significant complications, including emergency bypass surgery (n = 3, 3%), myocardial infarction (n = 2, 2%), embolic events (n = 2, 2%), transient vessel closure (n = 3, 3%), and spasm (n = 5, 5%). An additional eight patients (7%) had angiographic dissection. More recently, the principal investigators have reported a 1% perforation rate with this device. In a separate report describing the use of the excimer laser in treating totally occluded coronary arteries after a guide wire had crossed the lesion, three of 18 lesions (17%) had reoccluded within 24 hr (66). Despite the encouraging lack of perforation with this device, the overall success rate and incidence of complications appear comparable to balloon angioplasty alone. Ultimately, it may be desirable to use larger diameter laser catheters to increase the ability to perform "stand alone" laser angioplasty. However, it is not certain that the safety profile (i.e., no perforations) of the 2.0 or 2.4 mm diameter devices will be comparable to those observed with the 1.6 mm diameter system. No detailed long-term follow-up data have been presented, but preliminary communications suggest that restenosis rates after either "stand alone" excimer laser angioplasty or excimer laser angioplasty combined with balloon angioplasty yields restenosis rates similar to those observed with PTCA alone (i.e., ~30%). The data presented from the coronary trials to date suggest that the excimer laser does not improve the predictability of the outcome, decrease acute complications, or alter restenosis rates compared to plain old balloon angioplasty (POBA). Thus, based on the results from these early trials of the excimer laser angioplasty, the exact role of this expensive new technology in the interventionalist's armamentarium remains uncertain. It is also uncertain whether the pulsed excimer laser offers any significant advantage(s) over other less costly pulsed laser systems (e.g., pulsed midinfrared laser). It is possible that the single fiber coaxially aligned device may ultimately prove useful in treating chronic total occlusions. The multifiber guide wire-following device may have advantages over balloon angioplasty in the treatment of diffuse disease, heavily calcified lesions, and coronary stenoses that are crossed with a guide wire but cannot be crossed with low-profile balloon catheters.

Direct laser with spectral feedback (fluorescence-guided, "smart laser"). One of the more in-

triguing approaches to improving the safety and tissue selectivity of applying laser energy in tortuous, beating human coronary arteries has been the concept of using spectral feedback to distinguish normal from diseased portions of the arterial wall and then using this information to guide the laser ablation process. Ideally, such a system would be capable of performing definitive (stand alone) plaque ablation with an acceptably low risk of coronary perforation.

The fluorescence-guided, "smart laser" approach is based on the ability to use the technique of fluorescence emission spectroscopy to differentiate normal from atherosclerotic vascular tissue (67,68). Extensive in vitro testing of this type of system utilizing a low-energy helium cadmium (325 nm) laser to produce laser-excited fluorescence indicated that this technique could differentiate atherosclerotic plaque from normal vascular tissue (69,70). This low-level "diagnostic" laser was then interfaced with an ablative pulsed dye (480 nm, "treatment") laser to create an integrated prototype dual-laser system (MCM Laboratories, Mountain View, CA). The system is controlled by a computer that integrates the diagnostic and treatment lasers designed to turn off the firing of the treatment laser when the characteristic fluorescence spectra indicating normal media is identified (71,72) (Fig. 13–3). Preliminary clinical studies suggested that this spectral feedback laser system could be used to identify plaque in vivo via a flexible fiber-optic catheter delivery system (73,74). The system has been designed to allow transmission of both the low-level diagnostic laser energy and the high-energy abla-

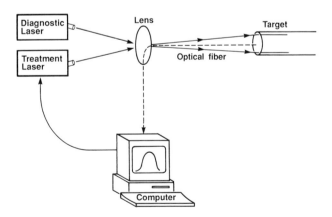

Fig. 13–3. Schematic showing the configuration of fluorescence guided ("smart") laser catheter system. The tissue fluorescence characteristics of the target tissue are assessed by the diagnostic laser, which is transmitted by the same optical fiber(s) used to transmit the therapeutic (ablative/treatment) laser energy. The computer is used to analyze the fluorescence spectra of the target tissue and, ideally, will determine when to fire the treatment laser (i.e., when the fiber optic is aligned with atherosclerotic tissue rather than to normal medial tissue).

tive ("treatment") laser over a common fiber optic. The computer-based plaque discrimination algorithm parameters have been designed to provide high sensitivity for normal tissue recognition (72,73) to improve safety and decrease the risk of perforation.

This system, initially utilizing a single 200 or 500 μM fused silica optical fiber, was used in an adjunctive role with balloon angioplasty to treat patients with obstructive peripheral vascular disease (75). The fluorescence-guided laser system successfully recanalized 47 of 55 (85%) total femoropopliteal occlusions that could not be crossed using standard guide wire technology. In eight cases, most often in lesions with heavy calcification, the laser was not able to open a channel. Balloon angioplasty was performed in all 47 patients in whom the laser was passed successfully, with an acceptable angiographic result in 42 patients (76%). Plaque ablation with the treatment laser did not appear to affect the ability of the diagnostic laser to identify plaque. Although the system was reasonably successful in recanalizing these occlusions, the process is somewhat time-consuming, requiring repeated realignment of the fiber optic to steer away from the normal wall. The more striking limitation of

the technique was related to a high incidence of mechanical (n = 15, 27%) and laser-induced (n = 2, 4%) vessel perforations. Vessel dissection was also frequent (n = 12, 22%) because of the passage of guide wires and balloon catheters through the laser-created neolumen. Subacute vessel closure (< 24 hr) occurred in four cases (7%), and long-term follow-up suggested a restenosis rate of > 30% at 3–6 months after the procedure (75). More recent reports have described a limited experience using an improved multifiber design in five patients with peripheral vascular disease and have mentioned "encouraging" early clinical results using a flexible 5 French multifiber (14 × 150 microns) laser catheter in coronary arteries (Fig. 13–4) (76).

The future success of fluorescence-guided laser angioplasty, like that of the excimer laser and the balloon-centered argon laser, will ultimately depend on a convincing demonstration that this complex and expensive new technology improves the safety, expands the applicability, and/or decreases the incidence of restenosis of catheter-based revascularization compared to balloon angioplasty. The very low incidence of coronary perforation using coaxial, guide

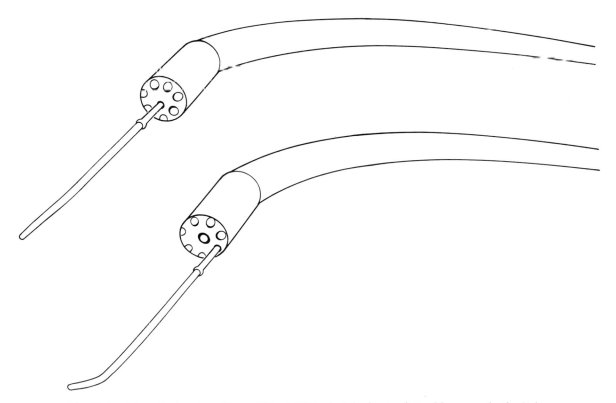

Fig. 13–4. Schematic drawing of the multifiber MCM pulsed dye laser catheter. More recently, the device has incorporated up to 14 optical fibers. The upper drawing shows a device with the guide wire in a central lumen. The lower figure shows the device with an eccentrically placed guide wire, which could theoretically be used to treat eccentric lesions.

wire-directed delivery of the pulsed excimer laser suggests that one does not need the sophisticated dual-laser computer-based guidance system of the "smart laser" to prevent laser-induced vessel perforation. Although it is possible that further refinements of the "smart-laser" will improve the safety and/or the efficacy of this approach, it appears unlikely that this technique will compete effectively with simpler and less expensive mechanical systems currently being tested to definitively treat obstructive arterial disease.

Indirect Application of Laser Energy: Specific Devices

LaserProbe ("hot tip laser"). The LaserProbe consists of an argon laser coupled to a fiber-optic catheter with a rounded metallic cap (see Fig. 13–5). The device is powered by a 12 watt argon laser. It is coupled to a 300 micron diameter fiber-optic catheter that delivers laser energy to a 1.5–2.0 mm metallic cap at the tip of the catheter.

The LaserProbe has been evaluated in the cholesterol-fed rabbit model of iliac atherosclerosis. In initial experiments, it was compared to a first generation direct laser fiber-optic catheter (77). Laser recanalization of the iliac vessel was achieved in two of 12 animals randomized to treatment with the direct laser fiber-optic system. Eight of 12 iliac artery segments treated with the LaserProbe were improved. The occurrence of perforation was significantly less in animals treated with the LaserProbe (9%) compared to those treated with the bare fiber-optic catheter (75%). Histologic examination of iliac arteries treated with the bare laser fiber-optic catheter demonstrated a relatively small defect along one side of the treated vessel that was associated with charring and thrombus formation. Vessels treated with the LaserProbe proto-

type catheter showed evidence of circumferential thermal injury with minimal charring and less thrombus formation. In a comparison to balloon angioplasty in the same model, Sanborn et al. reported less restenosis following LaserProbe angioplasty compared to conventional balloon angioplasty. Histology at 2–4 weeks following LaserProbe treatment demonstrated reendothelialization and the formation of only a thin fibrocellular intimal layer (77–79).

Significant experience using the LaserProbe in peripheral arterial disease in humans has been obtained. Typically, a peripheral arterial procedure using the LaserProbe is performed through an 8–9 French sheath introduced into the superficial femoral artery in the anterograde direction. Patients routinely receive heparin. Following baseline angiography, the LaserProbe is inserted through the sheath and advanced under fluoroscopic guidance to the proximal end of the lesion. Laser angioplasty is then performed using 5 or 10 sec pulses of 8–13 watts of argon laser energy as the probe is advanced through the lesion with continuous motion. The procedure is monitored fluoroscopically. In virtually all cases, conventional balloon angioplasty is necessary following initial laser therapy to achieve an adequate lumen in the peripheral arteries. Following angioplasty treatment, patients are commonly treated with heparin for 24 hr and most patients receive antiplatelet therapy in addition (78).

The majority of reported clinical experience with the LaserProbe is in peripheral arterial atherosclerosis. Sanborn et al. reported a 93% angiographic success rate in a total of 42 peripheral arterial vessels treated with the LaserProbe (80). This series included 28 total occlusions. There were no laser-related perforations; however, there were two cases of detachment of the metallic tip from the fiber-optic catheter. This resulted in a modification of the catheter system that

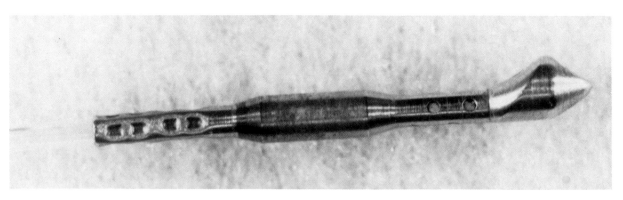

Fig. 13–5. Photograph of the distal tip of a 1.6 mm LaserProbe catheter.

prevented any further such episodes. Follow-up at a mean of 11 months following procedure in 45 patients with femoropopliteal lesions demonstrated a cumulative patency rate of 70% (81).

Recently, a multicenter experience using the Laser-Probe catheter has been reported (82). A total of 219 peripheral arterial lesions were attempted in 208 patients. Angiographic and clinical success was achieved in 155 (71%) of the attempted lesions. Perforation occurred in 4.1% of attempted lesions. Although probe tip detachment occurred early in the overall clinical experience, this complication was prevented when a 0.014 inch safety (anchor) wire was incorporated into the device. Balloon angioplasty was performed following initial successful treatment in all cases. No posthospitalization follow-up data were reported.

The LaserProbe has proven to be more difficult to use in the coronary arteries. The initial report of LaserProbe coronary angioplasty was from two hospitals involving a total of 11 patients (79,84). Eight of the 11 patients were described as having successful procedures. Vessel tortuosity prevented successful application of the technique in three patients. Although no perforations resulted, myocardial infarction occurred in three of eight patients who were described as successfully treated. A larger series of patients were treated by the LaserProbe in a report by Linnemeier et al. (84). Twenty-two vessels (15 saphenous vein grafts and seven native vessels with restenosis lesions) were attempted, and 21 (95%) were successfully crossed with the LaserProbe; all successfully crossed lesions underwent subsequent balloon angioplasty that was necessary because of the small lumen created by the LaserProbe. Furthermore, despite use of aspirin, dipyridamole, calcium, antagonists, nitroglycerin, heparin, and dextran, there was still a 14% incidence of significant thrombosis or spasm. A new prototype LaserProbe with a 1.9 mm diameter tip has been developed. This device has been used in two patients to successfully treat coronary stenosis. In each case, no adjunctive balloon angioplasty was necessary (85). Despite the development of this larger-diameter LaserProbe, the lumen that is achieved using this device still may not be adequate in many coronary arteries. Adjunctive balloon angioplasty will continue to be necessary in many instances after successful Laser-Probe coronary angioplasty. A different tact in the use of the LaserProbe concept is its application to a guide wire. A 0.018 inch laser guide wire is being developed with the anticipation that it will assist in recanalizing totally occluded coronary arteries. This device can be used in conventional balloon angioplasty catheters

that allow passage of a 0.018 inch guide wire. Whether this laser guide wire will be adequately steerable to allow its safe use in coronary arteries remains to be seen.

The LaserProbe has been approved by the Federal Drug Administration for peripheral angioplasty. In virtually all instances, the LaserProbe is used to achieve initial recanalization and then is followed by conventional balloon angioplasty." This mode of use has resulted in the term "laser-assisted balloon angioplasty." The long-term efficacy of LaserProbe angioplasty remains to be defined. It is clear that application of the peripheral LaserProbe technology to the coronary arteries is fraught with difficulty. Problems with tortuosity limit trackability of the LaserProbe. Even when the LaserProbe can be successfully applied to coronary lesions, the maximal tip diameter of 1.9 mm is likely to yield a definitive result in only a portion of treated lesions; adjunctive balloon (or other type of) angioplasty is likely to be necessary. The potential applicability of this technology in human coronary arteries therefore remains in doubt. For this technology to be successfully applied in the coronary arterial tree, significant modifications of the current device will be necessary.

Laser balloon angioplasty. A second approach for the indirect application for laser energy during the course of angioplasty has been developed by Richard Spears and is termed "laser balloon angioplasty" (86). This initial device was adapted from a standard balloon angioplasty catheter such that it contained a heating element that was 1.5 cm long and was centered in the balloon portion of the catheter. Neodymium:YAG laser energy is transmitted via a fiber-optic catheter to the heating element. Activation of the laser creates a cylindrical pattern of heat radiation over the 1.5 cm heating element. Heat is generated by conversion of the laser energy in the adjacent arterial wall tissue (87). The concept of laser balloon angioplasty evolved as the mechanism of standard balloon dilatation became better understood. Inflation of a balloon in an atherosclerotic lesion creates one or several splits in the intimal layer of the vessel (88,89). Often, these intimal splits extend into the media and occasionally into the adventitia. These splits are responsible to a variable degree for the improvement in lumen that results in improved coronary blood flow. However, the intimal splits can also serve as a nidus for platelet deposition leading to thrombus formation. In addition, deposition platelet in intimal splits may lead to the initial stages of the cellular proliferation process that results in restenosis in a significant number of patients undergoing balloon angioplasty. Laser balloon angioplasty has been developed in an attempt to minimize the luminal "roughness" present following conventional balloon angioplasty. Spears suggested that the laser balloon angioplasty device can "thermally coagulate" tissue layers adjacent to the luminal surface of freshly dilated lesions (90). The thermally coagulated (or "sealed") surface is thought to reduce the probability of thrombus formation at the sites of intimal splits and also to prevent the development of dissecting intramural hematomas within the wall of the arterial vessel. These effects should reduce the risk of acute complications of angioplasty. In addition, it is hypothesized that reduction in platelet deposition following the "sealing" process should result in a decreased release of platelet-mediated growth factors that may play a role in the cell proliferation process culminating in restenosis.

The Laser Balloon Angioplasty Catheter System has been developed by USCI, Incorporated. It consists of a triple lumen catheter: One lumen allows passage of a standard PTCA guide wire; the second lumen allows inflation and deflation of the balloon portion of the catheter; and the third lumen carries the fiber-optic fiber for transmission of the laser energy. The catheter system is coupled with an Nd:YAG laser. The Nd:YAG laser can generate radiation at two wavelengths: 1.064 microns and 1.319 microns. The laser energy is transmitted via the fiber-optic cable to a terminal diffusing tip. The energy is emitted from the diffusing tip in a circumferential pattern such that temperatures of 80–150°C are achieved at a radius of 1.5–2.5 mm from the diffusing tip (86). In recent months, the laser balloon angioplasty catheter has undergone significant modification. The heating element has been lengthened to correspond with the entire balloon length. To prevent laser energy from diffusing out the ends of the balloon catheter, gold leaf deflecting shields have been attached to the ends of the balloon portion of the catheter (Fig. 13–6). These modifications allow a larger portion of the vessel to receive laser energy treatment yet minimize the chance of thrombus formation from heat generation at the ends of the balloon catheter.

Laser balloon angioplasty is typically performed following conventional balloon angioplasty (86). The initial laser balloon angioplasty catheter system was limited to a 3.0 mm balloon size. When conventional balloon dilatation is completed, the laser balloon angioplasty catheter system is placed over the lesion using an exchange technique. A final dilatation at moderate pressure (4 atm) over 15–20 sec is performed. Laser energy is delivered in a decremental manner with the peak energy in the first 5 sec of the inflation and lower energies subsequently. In vitro studies indicated that an initial laser dose of 35 watts provided optimal rapid heating (91); however, a peak laser energy level of 25 watts has been adopted in human trials (92). The issue of optimal laser energy dose format is being further evaluated in randomized clinical studies (92,93), and it is uncertain at this time what the optimal energy dosing format will be. Following the 15–20 sec exposure to the decremental laser energy dose, the balloon remains inflated for an additional 15–30 sec to allow cooling of the treated vessel wall; this may prevent "thermal contraction" of the vessel after treatment (91). Immediately before balloon inflation and initiation of laser energy, the treated vessel is filled with saline injected through the guiding catheter. This causes "hemodilution" in the treated vessel and may decrease the risk of thermal coagulation of blood in and around the balloon during heating. The guide wire is left in place through the guide wire lumen of the catheter during laser treatment; to prevent excessive heating of this wire, the guide wire lumen is constantly flushed with a saline solution during laser treatment.

Extensive in vitro and in vivo research has been performed evaluating laser energy levels, duration of exposure to laser energy, and potential mechanisms of effect with laser balloon angioplasty (91,94–98). For instance, a comparison of laser balloon angioplasty and conventional angioplasty was carried out in normal rabbit iliac arteries (97). One month following initial treatment, vessels subjected to moderate-dose laser balloon angioplasty demonstrated better patency than did vessels treated with conventional balloon an-

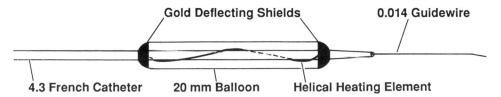

Fig. 13–6. Diagram of a laser balloon angioplasty catheter. The helical heating element that traverses the length of the balloon is indicated. In addition, gold deflecting shields are present at the ends of the balloon to prevent laser irradiation of the contents of the lumen.

gioplasty. Additional observations have been made in the atherosclerotic cholesterol-fed rabbit model using laser balloon angioplasty (98). Laser balloon angioplasty was performed in one iliac artery, while conventional balloon angioplasty was performed in the other in a series of ten animals who had developed atherosclerosis following intimal denudation. Use of laser balloon angioplasty was associated with the maximal improvement stenosis lumen diameter. Surprisingly, platelet deposition (studied using an indium labeling technique) was greater in iliac vessels following laser balloon angioplasty than it was following conventional balloon angioplasty. Furthermore, the authors reported no histologic evidence of "sealing" in the majority of treated vessels. The authors postulated that improvement in lumen diameter following laser balloon angioplasty must be due to some process other than "sealing" and suggested that loss of elastic recoil of the vessel may be important.

Laser balloon angioplasty has been tested primarily in the human coronary arteries and not in the peripheral vessels. Based on perceptions developed during the early stages of device development, it was theorized that laser balloon angioplasty would be helpful in settings of acute closure, in opening total occlusions, and possibly to prevent restenosis. The device is being evaluated in each of these clinical settings. Sinclair et al. reported the results of using the laser balloon angioplasty device in nine patients suffering acute closure following conventional balloon angioplasty (99). Acute closure was defined as a $\geq 75\%$ diameter stenosis reduction with progressive reduction in flow to TIMI grade 1 or 0 despite multiple balloon inflations. Patients meeting these criteria were treated with laser balloon angioplasty (peak laser dose = 25 watts, 1–13 doses). Eight of the nine patients were recanalized successfully using the laser balloon technique; one patient required nonurgent coronary bypass graft surgery because of recurrent luminal obstruction. In the setting of chronic total occlusions, laser balloon angioplasty has been used in a series of 13 patients (100). Ten of the 13 patients were successfully recanalized. Recanalization persisted for 48 hr in all patients; however, restenosis occurred in four of the six patients at 4 months following initial treatment.

Spears and colleagues have been performing a multicenter randomized trial evaluating the effects of laser balloon angioplasty on restenosis rates (92,93). The trial is designated to evaluate restenosis rates following initial treatment with laser balloon angioplasty at three different energy levels and to compare these results to initial treatment with conventional balloon angioplasty. In the first 61 patients treated in this protocol, laser balloon angioplasty has been associated with a better improvement in stenosis lumen diameter compared to conventional balloon angioplasty. Three months following initial therapy, however, the stenosis lumen diameter has decreased substantially in both laser balloon-treated and conventionally balloon-treated patients. Although there are interim report on the status of this trial frequently presented at national meetings, patient recruitment is not complete and follow-up is too short at this time to allow definite conclusions about the efficacy of laser balloon angioplasty for prevention of restenosis.

Laser balloon angioplasty represents a significant improvement over the first generation of direct laser devices. It is a reasonably trackable device that retains the safety of the "over-the-wire" balloon angioplasty systems. It appears to be efficacious in a growing series of patients treated for acute closure syndromes (99,-101). Any beneficial effect on long-term restenosis rates remains to be determined. Furthermore, the mechanisms of action of laser balloon angioplasty are possibly quite different from those mechanisms initially postulated. At least in an animal model, laser balloon angioplasty has been associated with increased deposition of platelets following treatment compared to conventional balloon angioplasty (98). It has been difficult to demonstrate the phenomenon of "sealing" in vivo. Thus, further investigation is necessary to understand both the basic mechanisms of interaction of laser balloon angioplasty with the arterial wall and the potential long-term effects of the device in the clinical setting. A comparative summary of direct and indirect laser catheter systems are shown in Tables 13–3 and 13–4, respectively.

MECHANICAL SYSTEMS: ATHERECTOMY AND ATHEROABLATION CATHETERS

Overview

A number of mechanical systems have been developed during the last 4–5 years to treat obstructive peripheral and coronary artery disease (102). The impetus for the development of these mechanical-based catheter systems has been outlined above. Compared to laser angioplasty systems, mechanical devices have the potential advantages of greater predictability and decreased cost and complexity.

Semantically, it is important to distinguish between *atherectomy* devices (e.g., Simpson AtheroCath ® and pullback atherectomy catheter), which cut and remove obstructing atheromatous material, and *atheroablation* devices, such as the Rotablator ®, which grind the atheroma into small particles, allowing them to embolize distally. The relative advantages

TABLE 13–3. Comparison of Direct Laser Angioplasty Devices (Coronary Application)

Device	Balloon-centered argon	AIS excimer laser	Fluorescence-guided laser
Treatment laser type	Continuous wave argon	Pulsed excimer (XeCl, uv)	Pulsed dye
Number of fibers	1	12	14
Luminal alignment	Balloon centered	Guide wire[a]	Guide wire[a]
Catheter size(s)	?	1.6, 2.0 mm	1.7 mm
Cost vs. balloon angioplasty	↑↑	↑↑	↑↑↑
Flexibility/trackability	+++	+++	+++
Simplicity of use	++	+++	+
Thermal injury	Yes	No	?
Create lumen larger than device	No	No	No
Treatment of total occlusions	Yes	No	No
Risk of dissection	++	+	?
Risk of perforation	++	+[b]	?
Risk of embolization vs. PTCA	↑	↑	Probably ↑
Overall acute complications vs. PTCA	↑↑	↑	?
Need for adjunctive PTCA	100%	40–70%	?
Restenosis (compared to PTCA)	=	=	=

Flexibility, simplicity, etc., are ranked on a + to ++++ scale.
[a]Used as lone fiber to treat total occlusion in peripheral arteries.
[b]Perforation risk may be increased with larger sizes (2.0 and 2.4 mm), data not available.

TABLE 13–4. Characteristics of Indirect Laser Devices

Characteristic	LaserProbe	Laser balloon angioplasty
Common names	Laser thermal angioplasty Laser-assisted angioplasty "Hot-tip"	"LBA"
Catheter sizes	1.6–1.9 mm	2.5 mm, 3.0 mm, 3.5 mm
Cost vs. balloon angioplasty	2× or more	2× or more
Flexibility/trackability	+	+++
Simplicity of use	++++	++
Thermal injury	+	+
Create lumen longer than device	No	Yes[a]
Treatment of total occlusions	Yes	Yes[b]
Risk of dissection vs. balloon	↑	=
Risk of perforation vs. balloon	↑↑↑	=
Risk of embolization vs. balloon	↑	=
Need for adjunctive PTCA	~ 100%	~ 100%
Restenosis	No data	=[c]

Flexibility/trackability and simplicity are ranked on a + to ++++ scale.
[a]Creates lumen longer than associated with conventional balloon PTCA.
[b]Only if occlusion can be crossed with guide wire
[c]Based on verbal presentation of preliminary data.

or disadvantages of these two approaches have not been compared in any controlled fashion, but will be commented on in the following discussion of specific mechanical devices. The idealized mechanical system should 1) efficiently (i.e., rapidly) debulk atheromatous lesions, including segments with diffuse disease; 2) be flexible and trackable to allow device delivery to both proximal and distal coronary vessels; 3) be compatible with standard balloon angioplasty techniques and equipment (i.e., not require specialized guide wires or guiding catheters); 4) minimize dissections, perforations, and early and late abrupt closure (i.e., provide a predictable result); 5) be capable of treating eccentric stenoses; 6) minimize injury to the media and adventitial layers in order to decrease the incidence of restenosis (3,103,104); 7) create a smooth, cylindrical lumen to allow laminar blood flow thus minimizing turbulence and shear-related platelet aggregation (105); 8) minimize embolic debris and remove tissue for histopathologic examination; 9) be capable of treating lesions that are anatomically unfavorable for PTCA; and 10) be capable of creating a luminal channel larger than the outer diameter of the atherectomy/atheroablation device. Like laser angioplasty catheters, the mechanical approaches to atheroma removal are in an early stage of development, and all of these currently available devices have certain limitations. Although none of these mechanical systems meet these criteria for an idealized device, future generations of atherectomy catheters may eventually come closer to achieving these goals.

Mechanical Systems: Specific Devices

Directional atherectomy (Simpson Athero-Cath®). The directional atherectomy catheter (AtheroCath®, Devices for Vascular Intervention, Inc., Redwood City, CA) developed by Dr. John B. Simpson was the first mechanical system developed for the treatment of obstructive arterial disease. The device was first tested in cadaver arteries and atherosclerotic rabbit vessels in 1985 (106). Since that time it has undergone a number of design changes, with significant modifications made to allow the safe application of the device in coronary arteries. The device consists of a cylindrical ("cup-shaped") steel cutting blade that is housed in a rigid cylinder/capsule at the distal end of the device. The distal cylinder has a 10 mm-long longitudinal window encompassing approximately 25% of the circumference of the cylinder and a balloon on the opposite side. The coronary device has a tapered and relatively flexible nose cone that functions as a specimen collection chamber. The cutting blade is connected to a hand-held disposable motor drive unit via a cable that extends for the length of the catheter. Depressing a switch on the hand-held driver activates the motor and spins the cutter at approximately 2000 rpm. During atherectomy, the cutter is manually advanced by the movement of a trigger/level on the hand-held driver. The balloon, which is used to force the atheroma into the cutting window prior to activation of the blade, is inflated via a standard balloon inflation device. The coronary device has been manufactured in 5, 6, and 7 French versions and can be advanced over movable coronary guide wires. Currently, because of the size and stiffness of the coronary device, the use of a specially designed 11 French guiding catheter (9 French internal diameter) is required. A photograph of the coronary catheter is shown in Figure 13–7.

The procedure used to perform atherectomy with this device is somewhat complex and more time-consuming than is conventional PTCA. After cannulation of the coronary ostium with the 11 French guiding catheter, the lesion is crossed with an 0.014 inch guide wire. The AtheroCath® is then advanced across the lesion using a gentle torquing motion. The roughness of the open cutting window may occasionally make passage of the catheter difficult, particularly in nonrestenotic native coronary lesions. If the device cannot be passed, an exchange is performed for a lower profile device or predilatation is performed with a 2.0 mm balloon catheter. After the atherectomy catheter is advanced into the lesion, the proper orientation of the cutting window is performed manually by torquing the catheter. Some expertise is required to correctly orient the cutting window. After retracting the cutting blade, the balloon is inflated to relatively low pressure ($\sim$ 20 psi) in order to force the plaque into the cutting chamber. The motor drive unit is activated and the cutting blade advanced forward, thus cutting the plaque within the chamber and pushing it into the nose cone collection area. The balloon is deflated and the entire catheter rotated into the next quadrant where the inflation, cut, deflation, rotate sequence is repeated. After three to six cuts, the device is removed to clean the collection chamber. The compaction of the atheroma in the nose cone, against the guide wire, necessitates the removal of the guide wire when the catheter is removed (i.e., guide wire is entrapped within the nose cone). This may add to the complexity of the procedure if further cuts or adjuvant balloon angioplasty is required. Higher balloon inflation pressures (up to 50 psi) may be required to treat calcified lesions or vessels in which there is a residual stenosis of > 30%. The initial procedural approach with this device was to aggressively try to debulk coronary lesions, given early experience in peripheral arteries, suggesting that this strategy might reduce restenosis. However, recent data from coronary atherectomy with this device demonstrating an increased risk of restenosis with deep cuts into the media or adventitia has resulted in a less aggressive debulking strategy.

During the last 2–3 years, this device has been used in more than 1,000 coronary cases at multiple centers. A substantial experience has now been reported with data describing the acute and long-term results and complications of directional atherectomy (107–111). As significant learning curve has been observed with this technology, as one would predict, with improved results at large centers with the greatest experience with the device. In a recently reported experience from the most experienced center (Sequoia Hospital, Redwood City, CA), 260 patients underwent directional atherectomy of 308 lesions, with an acute success rate of 91% (success defined as < 50% residual stenosis and > 20% improvement in luminal stenosis) (112). Lesion severity was reduced from 76 $\pm$

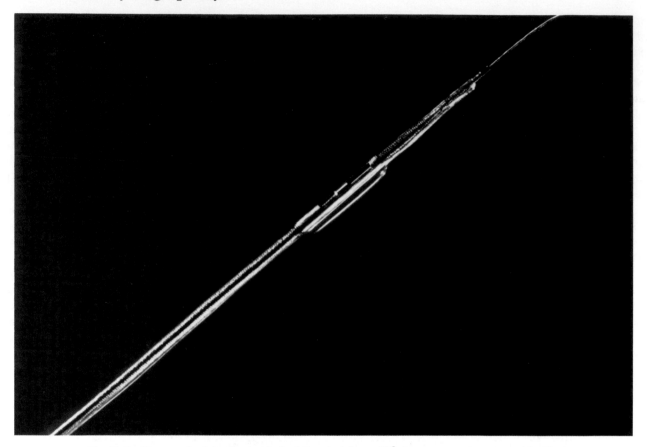

Fig. 13–7. Photograph of the distal end of a 6 French Atherocath ® for coronary atherectomy. The distal tapered end of the device provides the collection chamber for specimens cut by the cylindrical cutting blade shown in the center of the cutting window. The balloon is inflated on the outer surface of the cutting capsule opposite the cutting window. The device tracks over a 0.014 inch guide wire.

14% to 13 ± 22%. There were no deaths, but procedural complications included need for emergency CABG surgery in nine patients (3.5%), Q wave myocardial infarction in four patients (1.5%), and perforation in three patients (1.2%). Abrupt vessel closure was seen in an additional two patients. The experience from a multicenter trial of directional coronary atherectomy (n = 534 lesions) reported an overall complication rate of 18% with an emergency bypass surgery rate of 4.4%, a 4.8% incidence of myocardial infarction, a 2.3% incidence of embolization, and a 0.6% (n = 3) mortality rate (107).

In the Sequoia Hospital experience, the procedure was more likely to be successful in restenotic lesions and in lesions of the LAD or saphenous vein grafts. The device was much less successful in treating lesions with calcification (96% success without calcium, 66% success if calcified). Calcification was also associated with a higher acute complication rate (113). These differences in success rates are probably accounted for by the observation that it is easier to cross lesions that are softer (i.e., restenosis, vein graft lesions) in larger vessels with nontortuous access with the relatively bulky AtheroCath ®.

Despite the reasonably encouraging acute results obtained with this device in carefully selected patients at experienced centers, the long-term restenosis rates in the coronary arteries have been somewhat disappointing (114–117). The overall restenosis rate following directional coronary atherectomy is approximately 40–50% at 6 months following the procedure (114,117). Primary treatment of focal native lesions may yield restenosis rates as low as 23% (116). Higher restenosis rates have been observed after treatment of long (> 1 cm) lesions (~ 60%), in patients with a history of two or more prior PTCAs (50%), in vessels < 3.25 mm diameter (53%), and after atherectomy of saphenous vein grafts (up to 75%) (115–117).

Given our current understanding of the mechanism(s) leading to fibrointimal hyperplasia after arterial injury, and the likely mechanism of luminal improvement following directional atherectomy, it is not too surprising that directional atherectomy has been associated with relatively high restenosis rates (3,26,103,117,118). It has become increasingly clear that the primary stimuli for smooth muscle cell proliferation (intimal hyperplasia) after any form of catheter-based revascularization are 1) injury to the medial smooth muscle cells (stretching, thermal, and/or mechanical), 2) deep injury to the media leading to greater platelet deposition with the release of platelet-deposition with the release of platelet-derived growth factors (119), and 3) irregular residual luminal geometry leading to nonlaminar flow patterns, increased shear rates, and enhanced platelet deposition (3,103,-105). Baim and colleagues have recently analyzed the possible mechanism(s) of directional atherectomy and have proposed that tissue removal accounts for a minority of the acute luminal improvement observed after this procedure (118). The remainder of the luminal improvement may be caused by a Dotter effect and marked stretching of the media and adventitia by bal-

loon dilatation of the vessel after it is weakened by deep atherectomy cuts (i.e., "facilitated angioplasty"). The excellent acute angiographic results following directional atherectomy may be related to this "facilitated angioplasty" effect with aneurysmal dilatation of the weakened arterial wall following even low-pressure balloon inflations after the initial cut(s). The observation that 51–64% of atherectomy samples contain medial tissue and 23–30% have adventitial tissue suggests that directional atherectomy makes frequent deep cuts into the arterial wall (109,118). The investigators' proposal that the resultant luminal contour has a scalloped appearance has been confirmed in some cases by intravascular ultrasonic imaging. Thus, it appears likely that directional atherectomy often causes severe, deep injury to the arterial wall due to a Dottering effect, deep cutting, and "facilitated angioplasty." Despite the excellent acute angiographic results seen after this procedure (Fig. 13–8), it is likely that the residual luminal contour is irregular with scalloping. All of these factors

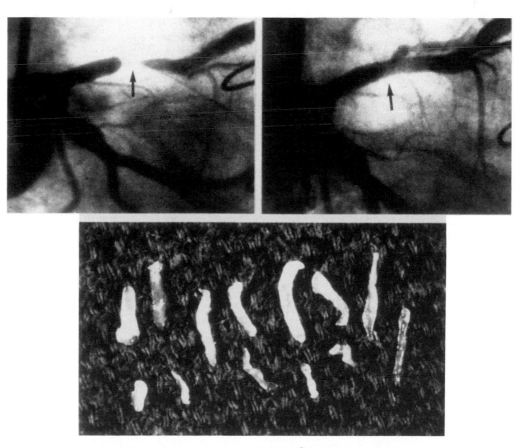

Fig. 13–8.   Results of coronary atherectomy using Atherocath® in high-grade LAD stenosis. Panel in upper left shows a high-grade lesion in the proximal portion of the LAD. The photograph in the upper right panel shows the final excellent angiographic result after atherectomy. The lower panel shows the atheromatous material removed from the lesion.

may contribute to the relatively high restenosis rates observed following directional atherectomy. Recent procedural changes, including lower-pressure balloon inflations, less aggressive tissue removal, and changes in catheter design to use a "dumbbell" balloon on the outside of the cutting capsule or ultrasonic guidance of cutting (120) may help to minimize this deep injury problem. It is too early to tell whether these changes will impact either the short- or long-term success rates.

In summary, directional atherectomy is a promising new technique that is capable of achieving excellent acute results in the treatment of coronary artery disease. Although the procedure of directional atherectomy is relatively complex and more time-consuming than is balloon angioplasty, it may have a role in the treatment of proximal coronary lesions that appear morphologically unfavorable for PTCA. The acute complication rates appear to be similar to those observed with PTCA. Restenosis rates following directional atherectomy are similar to those seen after balloon angioplasty in native lesions that have not been previously dilated, but may be higher than PTCA in long lesions, in saphenous vein grafts, and in patients with recurrent restenosis. Further refinements in the device and in procedural approaches may ultimately decrease the incidence of deep arterial trauma and improve the long-term results.

Rotational angioplasty (Atheroablation, Auth Rotablator ®). The Rotablator ® is a high-speed atheroablation catheter that has been used investigationally for the treatment of coronary artery disease since 1988 (121,122). The device consists of a distal abrasive metal burr (1.0, 1.25, 1.50, 1.75, and 2.0 mm diameters for coronary application) welded to a long flexible drive shaft that tracks over a flexible 0.009 inch guide wire (see Fig. 13–9). The distal one-half of the burr is coated with tiny diamond chips (30–40

μm) that are embedded into the metal. The metal drive shaft is sheathed within a 4 French Teflon catheter and is driven at rotational speeds of approximately 150,000 rpm by an air-driven turbine. The high-speed rotation of the roughened distal burr is designed to grind the atheroma into embolic particles that are small enough to pass freely through the coronary capillary bed without obstructing blood flow. The flexible 0.009 inch guide wire used with the device does not spin during plaque abrasion.

Hansen et al. initially demonstrated the feasibility of rotational angioplasty using the Rotablator ® in ablating plaque in atherosclerotic rabbit iliac arteries (121). The device was also successfully used to debulk calcified and/or fibrous plaque from atherosclerotic human arteries (122). The microparticles so generated were generally smaller than 5μm and caused no significant embolic sequelae after peripheral injection into dogs (122). In other experiments described by Fourrier, approximately 25% of the debris generated by the device was > 15μm, with even larger particle sizes seen with large burrs (e.g., 4.5 mm) (123–125). Histologically, the Rotablator ® appears to leave a relatively smooth lumen without deep cutting into the media (126).

The device was used successfully in treating six patients with femoropopliteal stenosis (123). Shortly thereafter, Hansen and co-workers demonstrated the feasibility of delivering the device in canine coronary arteries (127). In 1988, Fourrier et al. reported the first use of the device in human coronary arteries 9122). The coronary procedure is carried out similarly to PTCA. In general, patients are medicated with orally administered calcium channel blocking agents and aspirin and intravenous heparin. Some operators have routinely administered intracoronary nitroglycerin to try to lessen the coronary artery spasm that may be seen after rotational angioplasty (128,129).

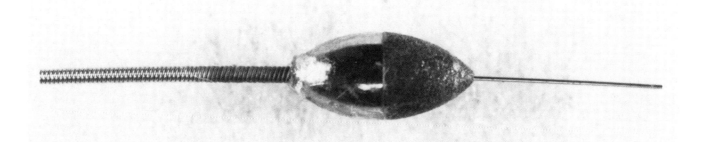

Fig. 13–9. Close-up photograph of the distal abrasive tip of the Rotablator ®. The distal one-half of the oblong burr is coated with tiny diamond particles, used for high-speed rotational abrasion of atheromatous plaque. A 0.009 inch guide wire exits the distal tip of the burr.

The coronary ostium is typically cannulated with a high-flow 9 French guiding catheter. When possible, the lesion is crossed with the 0.009 inch Rotablator® guide wire. However, this guide wire is not as steerable as are standard PTCA guide wires, often necessitating the use of a floppy 0.014 inch guide wire with a low-profile balloon catheter, followed by an exchange procedure to replace the standard guide wire with the 0.009 inch Rotablator® wire. Once the lesion is crossed with the 0.009 inch guide wire, the abrasive burr of the Rotablator® is advanced to the lesion. The air-driven turbine is activated, and when the burr speed reaches 150–175,000 rpm, the burr is advanced over the guide wire through the lesion. Several passes are typically required to abrade the lesion. Passes are performed until there is no longer a tactile sensation of mechanical resistance as the burr is advanced and retracted. If the angiographic appearance seems adequate, the Rotablator® and guide wire are withdrawn. Because of this burr-size limitation, adjunctive angioplasty may be necessary in cases in which the residual narrowing is greater than percent after the largest Rotablator® burr has been passed.

To date, the Rotablator® has been used in approximately 100 cases to treat coronary artery disease. There has been no comprehensive multicenter reporting of the data from these coronary trials, so one must examine the reports from individual centers in order to assess the safety and efficacy of this procedure. In general the operators in the reported clinical trials were limited to using burrs no larger than 1.75–2.0 mm due to the choice of 9 French guiding catheters with internal diameters ranging from 0.078–0.088 inch. Preliminary experience with the device suggests that one can only expect to achieve a final luminal diameter equal to 80–90% of the final burr size (e.g., 1.4–1.6 mm lumen with 1.75 mm burr, 1.6–1.8 mm lumen with 2.0 mm burr) (124). This luminal opening may prove adequate in smaller distal vessels but tends to leave significant (> 50%) residual narrowing in larger, proximal sites. In one series that reported quantitative angiographic results, the Rotablator® improved the luminal diameters from 0.54 $\pm$ 0.32 mm to only 1.37 $\pm$ 0.31 mm (124). It is difficult to determine the "stand-alone" success rate using the Rotablator®, but it appears to be approximately 65–80% in most series (122,124,128). In approximately 10–35% of cases, adjunctive PTCA has been used to improve the final luminal dimensions. The rate of adjuvant PTCA will likely decrease with the use of larger burr sizes (up to 2.5 mm). There is little data describing the functional results (i.e., noninvasive testing) following coronary Rotablator® therapy.

Although the Rotablator® has proven successful in recanalizing coronary lesions with minimal or no risk of perforation (with currently used burr sizes), the use of this device has been associated with a relatively high complication rate (124,128,129). In the largest reported single series of coronary cases (n = 40), Tierstein and colleagues described the following complications: angina after Rotablation 17/40 (43%), ST-segment shifts 12/40 (30%), transient impairment in coronary blood flow 6/40 (15%), and non-Q wave MI in 8/40 patients (20%) (129). Five of these eight patients with myocardial infarction demonstrated impaired LV contractility with good return of LV contractility at follow-up. There was one death (2.5%) at Stanford University Hospital attributable to Rotablator®-induced thrombotic vessel closure and myocardial infarction. The patient died after emergency coronary artery bypass surgery. In a separate series, Fourrier et al. reported that 3/29 (10%) suffered either early (n = 2) or late (n = 1) thrombotic vessel closure and 2/29 (7%) suffered a non-Q wave MI (122). An additional 6/29 (20%) had transient AV-block, which was believed to be due to ischemia of the AV node secondary to embolic debris. Severe coronary artery spasm in the vascular bed distal to the lesion is frequently seen after Rotablator® therapy despite vasodilator therapy. This spasm may be related to platelet activation by the fine embolic particles and typically improves spontaneously within minutes to hours after the procedure.

There is relatively little data regarding the long-term follow-up with the Rotablator®. In the most recently reported series of 22 patients, 50% (11/22) had > 50% restenosis at a 6 month angiographic follow-up (130). The restenosis rate was not influenced by the use of adjunctive PTCA (i.e., the same rate with "stand alone" Rotablator® vs. Rotablator® plus balloon angioplasty). Although it has not been proven, it is possible that the relatively high restenosis rate after rotational angioplasty is due to thermal injury to the media during Rotablation (due to friction at very high rotational speed) or is merely a function of the significant residual luminal narrowing often present after Rotablator® therapy with the current burr sizes. Despite the complications attributable to embolic debris and the relatively high restenosis rates, most of the investigators testing this device remain cautiously optimistic about its role in treating a variety of lesions that are poorly suited for PTCA (e.g., diffuse disease, heavily calcified lesions, small vessels). Further clinical experience with this device, including better long-term follow-up data, will be required before its role in the therapy of coronary artery disease can be assessed.

Retrograde atherectomy (Fischell pullback atherectomy catheter).   The pullback atherectomy catheter (PAC) is one of the most recently developed approaches to atherectomy and has the potential to overcome some of the limitations of other mechanical devices. The device consists of a flexible outer "closing" catheter with an inner moveable "cut-collect" catheter used to transmit rotational energy ($\sim$ 2000 rpm) from a hand-held, battery-powered "Rotator." Contrast and saline injections can be made via a lumen between the closing and cut-collect catheters. The flexible distal tapered tip of the catheter (attached to the cut-collect catheter) contains a hollow collecting chamber (to collect plaque and/or thrombus) and a sharp, cylindrical (stainless-steel) cutting blade proximally (see Fig. 13–10). The current device, intended for peripheral use, is manufactured with blade sizes of 2.5, 3.0, and 3.5 mm diameter (Arrow/MedInnovations, Inc., Reading, PA). The device is freely moveable over an 0.018 inch guide wire and has lubricity coating on its distal aspect. Plaque can be removed from the collection chamber by flushing through the distal (guide wire) lumen after the device is removed from the body.

The device is in an early phase of development with clinical trials now underway for the treatment of peripheral vascular disease. The PAC has shown promising efficacy in preclinical trials in 13 severely diseased cadaveric superficial femoral arteries. In these experiments, the mean preatherectomy stenosis (all specimens) was 95 $\pm$ 3%, with a final mean posttherectomy stenosis of 21 $\pm$ 5%. Adjuvant balloon angioplasty was not required. The PAC system was very successful in removing atheromatous material (13/13 experiments, 48/49 passes). More pieces of atheroma were removed per pass by the 3.0 and 3.5 mm devices than by the 2.5 mm device. In at least five of the nine ex vivo experiments in totally occluded segments, the guide wire was inadvertently passed in a subintimal plane, thus simulating a "worst case" for cutting in an eccentric lesion. Despite this, only one perforation occurred in an early experiment when

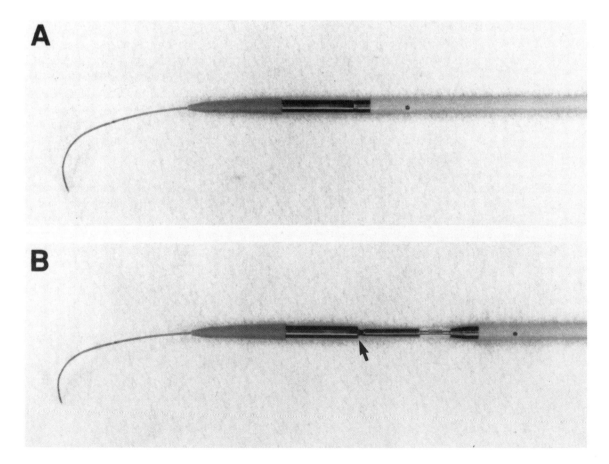

Fig. 13–10.   Photograph of the distal end of a 3.0 mm (9 French) pullback atherectomy catheter (PAC) for the treatment of peripheral vascular disease, shown in its closed (**panel A**) and open (**panel B**) configuration. A sharp cylindrical cutting blade (arrow) is revealed on the proximal end of the collection chamber when the device is in the open configuration. An 0.014 inch guide wire exits from the distal lumen of the catheter.

multiple passes were made with the 3.5 mm device in an improperly mounted segment without interval angiography. The device was very effective in cutting calcified plaque. A representative histologic result (postatherectomy) from an initially totally occluded femoral artery is shown in Figure 13–11, demonstrating a cylindrical (smooth) lumen with the cut limited to the intima.

The pullback atherectomy catheter has several potential advantages over other currently used atherectomy and/or abrasional catheters. Like the Atherocath®, the plaque can be removed from the PAC collection chamber for histopathologic study at the end of the procedure. In contrast to the relatively bulky Atherocath®, the PAC can be made to be extremely flexible and trackable over small guide wires (0.014–0.018 inch) with coronary devices now being developed with cutting blades of 1.7 mm or smaller. In addition, the PAC is capable of cutting a lumen equal to the outer diameter of the cutting blade in a single pass rather than requiring multiple passes in two or more quadrants as is required with the Atherocath®. Unlike the high-speed rotational/abrasional devices, the plaque is collected and removed from the body, which should result in a very low risk of embolization, particularly with the collection

chamber downstream (distal to) the cutting blade. One potential advantage of the PAC compared to the anterograde cutting transluminal extraction catheter (TEC) is the feature that only the distal tip/blades spins with the PAC compared to the entire catheter with the TEC (132). Additionally, the lack of need for aspiration of plaque material during cutting (with PAC vs. TEC) avoids the potential for significant blood loss. Although it remains to be proven in clinical practice, theoretically the PAC should maintain a better coaxial alignment during cutting than anterograde atherectomy devices because of the mechanics of pulling rather than pushing over a flexible guide wire. Finally, compared to anterograde atherectomy, the PAC may also be less likely to "catch" acute angles at bifurcations or occlude side branches. Pullback atherectomy may be well suited to treat ostial stenoses, saphenous vein graft stenoses, intimal dissections after balloon angioplasty, and/or thrombotic occlusions.

The device does have the potential disadvantages, in its current configuration, of requiring staged cutting (e.g., 2.5 mm followed sequentially by larger sizes) and the requirement to gently "Dotter" the tapered tip of the device through the lesion prior to cutting. An expandable version of the device is under

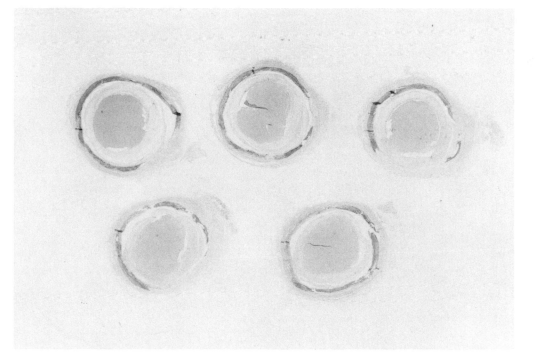

Fig. 13–11. Histopathologic results after pullback atherectomy in a totally occluded cadaver superficial femoral artery. Multiple cross sections (1 mm intervals, hematoxylin and eosin, magnification ×3) are shown following sequential single passes (cuts) using a 2.5, 3.0, and then 3.5 mm-diameter PAC. The dark material filling the lumen is a barium gelatin mixture used to pressure fix the specimen at the end of the experiment. Note the relatively smooth luminal contour after atherectomy.

development. Despite the promising potential of retrograde atherectomy, very little can be said about the clinical utility of such a device at this early stage.

Other mechanical devices. Several other mechanical systems have been developed in the last several years to try to expand or improve upon PTCA. The ultrasonic ablation catheter developed by Dr. Robert Siegel in collaboration with Baxter Healthcare Corp. is one of the more promising devices recently tested for the treatment of total occlusions (132,133). This flexible ultrasound probe can be delivered percutaneously, ensheathed in a 7 French catheter (Fig. 13–12). It transmits ultrasonic energy with a frequency of 19–22 kHz and with a power output of 20–25 watts/cm^2 (133). The advantages of this approach is that the ultrasonic ablation probe has reasonably good tissue selectivity, ablating hard or calcified plaque, and causing little injury to viscoelastic tissue of the normal media and adventitia. The device has been used successfully to recanalize severe femoral and popliteal artery lesions in eight patients (four total occlusions, four severe lesions) (133).

Three of four of the total occlusions and all four stenoses were successfully recanalized in less than 120 sec without emboli, dissection, spasm, or perforation (133) (see Fig. 13–13). Although there was improvement in luminal opening after ultrasonic ablation, adjuvant balloon angioplasty was required in all cases. This device may ultimately prove to be a safe and cost-effective tool for recanalization of total or subtotal occlusions. The risk of distal embolization may limit the application of this device for definitive atheroablation. Further engineering refinements will be required before the ultrasonic ablation probe can be safely tested in the coronary circulation.

The transluminal extraction catheter (TEC) is an anterograde atherograde atherectomy device developed by InterVentional Technologies, San Diego, CA. This device consists of a hollow flexible torquing catheter with a distal conical cutting blade (see Fig. 13–14). The catheter moves freely over a guide wire. The entire catheter is rotated at approximately 750 rpm by a hand-held motor-driven unit. The blades are advanced through the lesion, with suction applied to

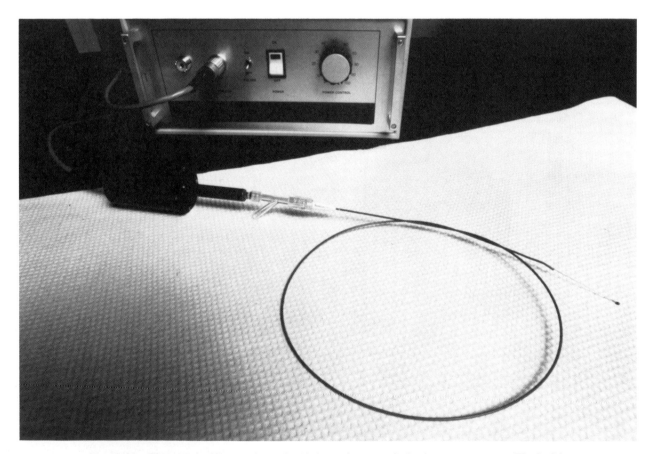

Fig. 13–12.   Photograph of Baxter ultrasonic ablation catheter attached to its power generator. The flexible ultrasonic ablation probe is enclosed in a plastic sheath. There is a small steel burr at the distal tip of the catheter.

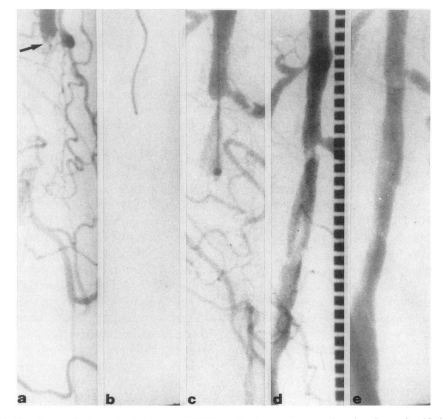

Fig. 13–13. Recanalization of a total superficial femoral artery occlusion using the ultrasonic ablation catheter. **Panel a** shows a long total occlusion (originating at arrow). In **panel b,** a guide wire is advanced into the lesion but is unable to cross the occlusion. **Panels c** and **d** show the recanalization of the lumen using the ultrasonic ablation catheter. Finally, **panel e** demonstrates the final luminal appearance after adjunctive balloon angioplasty.

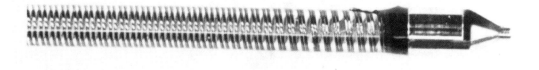

Fig. 13–14. Close-up photograph of the distal tip of the transluminal extraction catheter. The flexible hollow torque tube (catheter) is connected to a distal tip that has two cutting blades. A 0.014 inch guide wire can be passed through the distal-most tip of the catheter.

extract the cut plaque during periods of cutter activation. Material extracted from the artery is collected in a glass collection container. The device has shown some promise in the treatment of peripheral vascular disease. Several hundred peripheral artery procedures have been performed, with initial results suggesting a high primary success rate (92%) and a lessened restenosis rate (14%) when atherectomy was performed without adjunctive balloon angioplasty (134). There

were relatively few acute complications. The device has now been used in the coronary circulation with reasonable success (135). In the most recently reported series, 66 patients were treated with this device (135). The TEC device was used alone, without adjunctive balloon angioplasty, in 45 of the 66 patients. The procedural success rate was 92% (61/66 patients). There were no cases of clinically evident distal embolization. However, there were five patients

(7.5%) who underwent emergency coronary artery bypass graft surgery, two cases (3%) of subacute coronary artery closure requiring PTCA (n = 1) or bypass surgery (n = 1), and one death (1.5%) (135). There have been reports of at least two cases of coronary artery perforation with the device in the early trials that were not reported in this multicenter trial. No significant long-term follow-up data have been reported following the coronary application of the TEC device. Although it is possible that the TEC device will offer some advantages(s) over PTCA, the data reported in this early trial suggest that the device may have a significantly higher acute complication rate than does conventional PTCA. Further comparative studies will be required to adequately assess the clinical utility of this device.

Several other mechanical devices including the Kensey high speed rotational abrasion device (136) and a slow-speed rotational device to recanalize total occlusions (137) have been described but will not be reviewed in detail in this chapter. A comparative summary of several of the mechanical catheter systems now available for the treatment of obstructive arterial disease is shown in Table 13–5.

INTRAVASCULAR STENTS

Overview

The concept of intravascular stenting appeared in the earliest days of transluminal angioplasty. In the late-1960s, Charles Dotter tested plastic tube and metallic coiled stents in canine iliofemoral arteries (138).

Although all the plastic stented segments thrombosed within several hours, Dotter found that the metallic coil stented segments remained free of thrombosis for months. The problems with developing an adequate catheter delivery device and the general limitations of angioplasty (its inability to significantly improve most lumen diameters in diseased arterial segments) prevented further investigation of stenting techniques for a decade. In the late-1970s, a nickel-titanium alloy (nitinol) was discovered that had thermal-shape memory (139). Nitinol undergoes a phase change at specific temperatures. Stents consisting of nitinol wire with expanded diameters of 5–11 mm were formed at high temperature (> 500° C). The nitinol coil could then be straightened in a bath of sterile ice water. The straight nitinol wire was then introduced into the vascular system during a constant cold saline flush through the delivery catheter. Once the wire was in place, the warmer body temperature of the recipient animal reversed the phase change and the wire returned to its coil configuration, thus serving as a stent. Dotter et al. (140) and Cragg et al. (141) tested these heat-sensitive metal alloy stents in animal models. Although the early reports of these stenting devices were optimistic, the large temperature change that was necessary to produce the phase change that resulted in the nitinol converting from the straight wire to the coil wire configuration prevented the clinical application of these devices. By the mid-1980s though, a number of investigators were exploring the concept of endovascular stenting using metallic prostheses (142–144). Again, the daunting problems of thrombogenicity, prediction for precipitating vascular stenosis, and the difficulty of designing adequate deliv-

TABLE 13–5. Comparison of Atherectomy and Atheroablation Devices

Device	Atherocath®	Rotablator®	PAC	TEC
Flexibility/trackability	+	+ + + +	+ + +	+ + +
Simplicity of use	+	+ +	+ + +	+ +
Compatible with PTCA equipment	+ +	+ +	+ + + +	+ + + +
Remove tissue	Yes	No	Yes	Yes
Create lumen larger than device	Yes	Smaller	No[a]	No
Treat eccentric lesions	Yes	+/−	Yes	+/−
Leave smooth cylindrical lumen	No	Yes	Yes	Yes
Risk of deep vessel injury	+ + + +	+	+	+ +
Risk of dissection	+ +	+	+	+ +
Risk of perforation	+ +	+	+	+ + +
Risk of embolization vs. PTCA	↑	↑↑↑	?	↑
Overall acute complications (vs. PTCA)	= or ↑	↑	?	↑
Need for adjunctive PTCA	< 10%	30–50%	?	20–50%
Restenosis (compared to PTCA)	= or ↑	= or ↑	?	=

Trackability, simplicity, etc., are ranked on a + to + + + + scale.
[a]Expandable version can create lumen larger than outer diameter of device.

ery devices combined to keep the increasing interest in endovascular stenting from reaching the clinical arena.

A number of investigators have commented on the characteristics that are desirable for endovascular stents (145–148). In human coronary arteries, intravascular stents must meet a significant number of exacting specifications. The prosthetic device must be strong enough to oppose the "residual circumferential elasticity" of the arterial wall (145) such that the structural integrity of the lumen is maintained. It must be flexible enough to allow its deployment in a tortuous vascular system. The device must have a favorable "expansion ratio" (146) such that it can be tightly compressed on the delivery catheter; the higher the expansion ratio, the larger the diameter of the device following deployment. It should either be inert and very durable or inert and readily degradable. Its deployment must result in very favorable flow dynamics through the "stented" arterial segment, and the device should result in little or no activation of thrombotic pathways.

The practicalities of material science and current design capabilities have yielded a first generation of intracoronary stenting devices that fall short of the above-specified "ideal" criteria for intravascular stents. Nonetheless, a growing number of prosthetic stent devices are becoming available for use in intracoronary therapy. Stent devices have been proposed for treatment of the following conditions: 1) threatened acute closure of coronary artery segments

following conventional balloon dilatation, 2) improvement and "buttressing" of the arterial segment following opening of chronic total occlusions, 3) improvement of the initial luminal result of balloon PTCA, and 4) prevention of restenosis by maintenance of vascular integrity through the "buttressing" of the vascular wall.

Three stent devices have undergone a substantial amount of testing in the clinical setting: the Schneider WallStent, the Palmaz-Schatz stent (Johnson and Johnson), and the Gianturco-Roubin stent (Cook, Incorporated) (see Table 13–6). A balloon expandable device from Medtronic, Incorporated (the Wiktor stent) has just entered clinical testing, and another balloon expandable device from Cordis, Incorporated, has undergone preclinical evaluation. The following sections will focus on the first three devices that have undergone significant clinical testing at this time.

Intravascular Stents: Specific Devices

Schneider WallStent. Sigwart and colleagues reported the first clinical use of an intravascular stent in the coronary arteries (149). In collaboration with Medinvent SA, a company that had participated in earlier stent prototype development, Sigwart developed a multifilament stainless-steel self-expanding stent. The stent is made of several 600 micron-diameter stainless-steel interwoven strands. The stainless steel alloy that composes the

TABLE 13–6. Comparison of Coronary Stent Devices

	Schneider WallStent	Johnson & Johnson Palmaz-Schatz stent	Cook Gianturco-Roubinstent
Strut composition	Elastic, stainless steel	Stainless steel	Stainless steel
Strut thickness	600 microns	100 microns	150 microns
Strut configuration	Mesh	Slotted parallelogram	Coil
Expansion mode	Self-expanding	Balloon expandable	Balloon expandable
Expanded diameter	3–6 mm	2–6 mm	2–4 mm
Shortening during expansion	Moderate	Minimal	Moderate
Flexibility/trackability	++	++	+++
Potential for extraction before deployment	Excellent prior to sheath removal	Excellent prior to sheath removal	+/−
Anticoagulation regimen			
ASA/Persantine	Yes	Yes	Yes
Heparin	Yes	Yes	Yes
Dextran	Yes	Yes	+/−
Coumadin	Yes	Yes	Yes
Acute thrombosis	3.9%	~ 1.0%	~ 2.5%
Thrombosis 1 day–3 months	4.6%	~ 3%	N/A
Restenosis[a]	< 10%	15–50%	N/A

Flexibility/trackability is ranked on a + to ++++ scale.
[a]See text for discussion and references.

stent material has elastic properties that allow the overall diameter of the stent to be substantially reduced through elongation of the stent device. As the stent is deployed in an arterial vessel of suitable size, the residual elastic radial force of the collapsed stent leads to its expansion against the endoluminal vessel wall. The stent continues to dilate until an equilibrium is reached between the elastic resistance of the arterial wall and the elastic force of the stent itself.

Deployment of this stent device required the development of a novel catheter delivery technique. The stent is elongated along the distal portion of the delivery catheter, which is slightly smaller than 5 French in diameter. As the stent is elongated, it is held in place by a "constraining membrane." When the collapsed stent is in the proper position for deployment, the constraining membrane is pulled back and the radial elastic force of the stent causes its enlargement (Fig. 13–15). Stents with an extended diameter up to 6.5 mm can be mounted on the 5 French delivery device. A series of radiopaque markers on the distal portion of the catheter facilitate placement of the stent; the stent itself is radiolucent.

The initial animal, human peripheral, and human coronary experience with this device was described in 1987 (149). A total of 15 prostheses were implanted in experimental animal procedures. Seven of the devices were implanted in the coronary arteries, and eight, in the periphery. No chronic anticoagulation was given. Thrombosis was seen in two of the eight peripherally placed stents and in one of the seven intracoronary stents. Interestingly, there was no evidence of intimal hyperplasia in stented arterial segments. A thin neointimal layer approximately 450 microns thick was seen overlying the metallic stent material. Six patients with severe peripheral vascular atherosclerosis underwent placement of a total of ten stents in either femoral or iliac arteries. In this series of patients, stent diameters ranged from 6 to 12 mm. Patients were pretreated with aspirin and received 10,000 units of heparin during the implantation procedure. Following stent placement, patients were maintained on a coumarol agent (with prothrombin time 2.5 × control), aspirin, and dipyridamole for 3 months. At a mean follow-up of 6 months after placement, there was no evidence of restenosis based on symptoms, Doppler measurements of blood flow, or digital subtraction angiography. One patient required additional stent placement because of progression of atherosclerosis in nonstented femoral arterial segments at 3 months after initial treatment.

In this same report (149), patients underwent coronary stenting if they had restenosis following previous balloon angioplasty, if they had stenosis of a saphe-

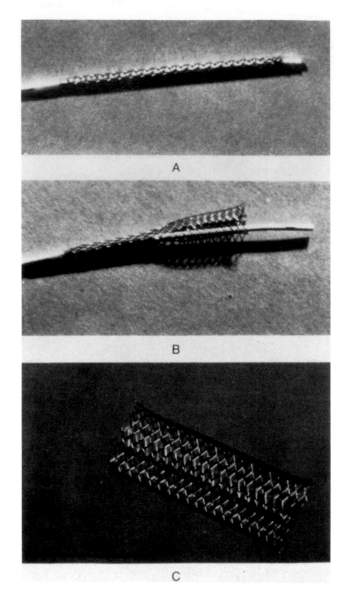

Fig. 13–15. Picture of the Schneider WallStent. In **panel A**, the stent is collapsed over the distal end of the deployment catheter. In **panel B**, the retaining membrane is partially withdrawn allowing the distal end of the WallStent to begin to expand. In **panel C**, the fully expanded WallStent is shown.

nous vein coronary bypass graft or if they had acute closure following initial balloon angioplasty. A total of 24 stents were placed in 19 patients. Actual deployment of this stent involved the use of the "exchange" guide wire technique. Stent diameters were chosen to be 15% larger than was the "reference" segment of the receiving coronary vessel. The entire length of the diseased coronary segment was treated. Following deployment of the stent, the treated arterial segment was "smoothed" by a brief balloon dilatation. Patients were pretreated with 1 g of aspirin the day before the procedure, and they received 15,000 units of heparin intravenously during the procedure. In addition, urokinase (50,000–100,000 units) was infused through the guiding catheter during the actual stent placement. Intravenous heparin was continued postoperatively until adequate anticoagulation was achieved with a coumarol agent. In addition, patients received calcium blocking agents, aspirin 330 mg, and dipyridamole 75 mg per day following stent placement. Thrombosis of the stent was documented in two of the 19 patients; in one patient, the thrombosis was successfully recanalized with intracoronary urokinase. A third patient died following emergency coronary bypass surgery for suspected stent failure. However, at the time of bypass surgery, the stent was found to be patent. The patient died the day following surgery, and at post-mortem, there was evidence of recent thrombus in the stent that was nonobstructing. Four patients were treated because of acute closure; they all experienced immediate relief of the closure following stent placement. Short-term follow-up was unremarkable in the remaining patients.

In a subsequent report (150), 27 patients were treated with the WallStent because of acute closure following conventional balloon angioplasty. Stenting was performed in 12 left anterior descending arteries, in 13 right coronary arteries, and in two circumflex arteries. Although there was a low incidence of temporary stent occlusion (7%) and distal embolization (3.5%), patency was restored in 26 of the treated patients and emergent surgery was necessary in only one. In a recent abstract, Serruys et al. described the angiographic follow-up that was available in 89 patients treated with the WallStent at a mean of 6.3 months following placement (151). Using a very strict quantitative angiographic definition, 29% of treated patients had evidence of hyperplasia (i.e., intimal thickening based on loss of absolute lumen diameter) within the stented segment. Sixteen percent of the patients met conventional restenosis criteria of $\geq$ 50% diameter stenosis in the stented segment. Further details of follow-up (such as necessity for repeat hospitalization, incidence of myocardial infarction, and need for coronary bypass surgery) have not been completely reported for this device.

At this time, several conclusions regarding the Medinvent WallStent are possible: 1) The device can be effectively deployed in elective and emergent settings during coronary angioplasty. 2) The device appears to be effective for relieving intimal dissection that leads to acute closure during balloon angioplasty procedures. 3) There is a suggestion that the WallStent may decrease the incidence of restenosis compared to conventional balloon angioplasty. Only a randomized trial will be able to answer this issue definitively. The

WallStent does have significant limitations including the need for a very aggressive anticoagulant regimen combining coumadin-type agents, aspirin, and dipyridamole. In addition, the device has limitations in trackability and can be deployed only in relatively accessible coronary artery or bypass graft segments. Finally, the technique involved in deployment of the stent must be quite careful and cautious; once the retaining membrane has begun to be removed, the distal end of the device is fixed within the arterial bed and significant shortening of the stent does occur. On balance, the WallStent has overcome some of the significant factors that have previously prevented clinical testing of intravascular stenting devices, and as such, this device has been the pacesetter in the new angioplasty field of clinical intravascular stent investigation.

Palmaz and Palmaz-Schatz stents. Palmaz developed a balloon expandible wire mesh stent in the mid-1980s (144). His colleague, Schatz, played an important role in the adaptation of the device for human coronary artery deployment. The Palmaz stent consists of a stainless-steel struts arranged in series of adjacent parallelograms. The filaments are 100 micron $\times$ 76 micron in size; fully expanded, the metal struts of the stent comprise about 10% of the total "stented" surface area (148). For coronary deployment, this stent is lengthened via the use of an articulated joint such that the total length of the device is 15 mm (Fig. 13–16). In preparation for delivery, the device is crimped onto a standard balloon angioplasty catheter prior to use. The balloon angioplasty catheter is then positioned across the stenosis using standard "over-the-wire" techniques. Once the device is properly placed across the lesion, the balloon catheter is inflated to 8–10 atm, deflated, and withdrawn, leaving the expanded stent adherent to the endoluminal surface of the treated vessel.

The Palmaz stent has been evaluated extensively in animal models. Twenty devices were placed in canine coronary arteries, and the animals were followed for periods up to 18 months. Initial anticoagulation consisted of aspirin and dipyridamole with heparin and low molecular weight dextran being given during the procedure. The animals were maintained on aspirin and dipyridamole for 3 months following the procedure. All stents remained patent for the duration of the study. Intimal thickening was assessed histologically and peaked at 8 weeks following implantation (148). The role of anticoagulation was assessed in another series of experimental observations (152). Using indium-labeled platelet imaging, intensity of platelet deposition 3 hr following stent implantation was assessed. The smallest amount of platelet deposition was

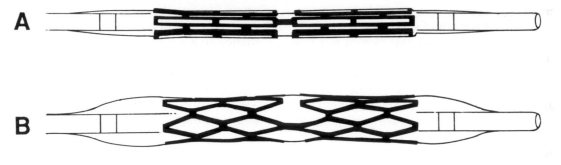

Fig. 13–16. Palmaz-Schatz stent. **A:** The stent is compressed onto the balloon.
B: The balloon is inflated, deploying the stent.

seen in animals treated with aspirin, dipyridamole, heparin, and dextran.

The Palmaz stent has been implanted in the iliac arteries of 31 patients (153). A total of 48 stents were placed. Claudication was improved in 90% of patients. One stent thrombosed and was reopened with urokinase and balloon dilatation. At 1 year, all 48 stents were patent.

Coronary implantation of the Palmaz stent began in the fall of 1987; soon thereafter routine use of the articulated Palmaz-Schatz stent for coronary implantation began. Patients were eligible for implantation if there was good collateral flow to the artery to be stented. In the majority of cases, patients had either total occlusion or very high grade stenosis such that high-grade collaterals could develop (154). Patients were pretreated with aspirin 325 mg and dipyridamole 75 mg t.i.d.. At the time of stent placement, patients received 10,000 units of intravenous heparin and a dextran infusion beginning at the time of placement and lasting for 24 hr. In the first 45 patients in whom stent placement occurred, there was no acute closure of the stented arterial segment during the procedure. Subacute closure occurred in 16% of treated patients, however, and documented myocardial infarction occurred in 13%; urgent coronary bypass surgery was necessary in 4.4% of patients (155). Because of these complications, warfarin therapy for 3 months following stent placement was added to chronic aspirin and dipyridamole therapy. An additional 245 patients have been treated according to the new anticoagulation protocol. In this second series of patients, there was no acute closure of the stented arterial segments. The incidence of subacute closure (2.8%) and myocardial infarction (2.8%) were significantly reduced. Six month follow-up data has been accumulated in 90 patients, and angiographic evaluation of lesion patency is available in 87 (96%) (156). All angiograms have been reviewed in a central laboratory. Restenosis (defined as $\geq$ 50% stenosis by caliper measurement) was present in 35% of treated lesions. The restenosis rate was significantly related to diameter of the treated vessel and to the number of stents placed. In vessels $\geq$ 3.2 mm diameter (reference segment) treated with a single stent, the restenosis rate was 16%. In vessels with a reference segment < 3.2 mm diameter treated with multiple stents, the restenosis rate was 100%. In several subgroups of patients previously considered to be at high risk for restenosis (e.g., patients with chronic total occlusion of the LAD) treated with a single stent, the catheter rate appeared surprisingly low ($\sim$ 20%). The investigators concluded that intracoronary stenting appeared promising for reducing restenosis risk in patients treated with one stent per lesion as long as the lesion was present in a reasonably large diameter vessel.

The majority of clinical experience with the Palmaz-Schatz stent has been obtained in the setting of elective treatment of coronary lesions; thus, this stent differs from the Schneider WallStent and the Gianturco-Roubin stent that have been tested in a significant number of patients suffering acute closure following conventional balloon angioplasty. As is the case with other stents, the early reports of the Palmaz-Schatz stent experience emphasize the necessity for a very aggressive anticoagulation regimen following stent placement to prevent thrombosis. Early follow-up reports suggest that a strategy of treating lesions in reasonably large diameter vessels with single stents may result in a lower risk of restenosis compared to treatment with conventional balloon angioplasty. Finally, though clinical experience is accumulating rapidly with this and other stent designs, conclusions about the safety and efficacy of the Palmaz-Schatz stent relative to other clinically evaluated stents remains to be determined.

Gianturco-Roubin stent. Gianturco and colleagues began evaluating designs for endovascular stents in the mid-1980s (143). Although the initial designs were found to be suboptimal, a stainless-steel coiled stent design was found to be much more promising (157). The stent is made of surgical stainless-steel suture 150 microns in diameter that is wrapped in a series of overlapping "U" shapes (Fig. 13–17). This stent is compressed over a conventional balloon angioplasty catheter. Stents can be made to have an expanded diameter of 2–4 mm and come in lengths of 1.5–3.0 cm. The balloon catheter on which the coil stent is placed must tolerate high inflation pressures. A particularly attractive aspect of this design is its inherent flexibility. Flexion testing of the coiled stent's ability to tolerate repetitive flexion-extension test was carried out (158). Uninterrupted cycling of flexion-extension that approximated 1 month's placement in a coronary vessel demonstrated no evidence of weakening or corrosion of the stainless-steel wire.

The stent is placed in a relatively conventional manner for angioplasty. The lesion is crossed with a conventional guide wire, and the lesion is predilated using a conventional balloon catheter; using the exchange technique, the delivery balloon catheter is then advanced over the wire to the lesion being treated. At the site of the lesion, initial inflation to 5–6 atm is carried out. To further imbed the coiled stent into the subintimal layers of the arterial wall, higher inflation pressures that expand the compliant delivery balloon to larger diameters are then used.

The coiled stent has been tested in experimental animal models. In initial testing in canine coronary

arteries, several animals died within 5 weeks of initial stent placement because of thrombosis within the stented segment. The animals were treated with warfarin; however, it was very difficult to maintain reasonable control over prothrombin levels in this animal species (159). A second series of animals were treated with aspirin and dipyridamole instead. There was no incidence of premature death due to thrombolytic occlusion in this series of animals. Serial histologic studies demonstrated endothelialization at 2 weeks following stent placement. At 6 months following placement, a completely normal appearing endothelial layer was present (158). Another series of experiments were carried out in the rabbit model of iliac atherosclerosis (160). One atherosclerotic iliac artery was treated with a conventional 2 mm balloon catheter, whereas the other was treated with the coiled stent. Both acutely and at 4 weeks following initial angioplasty, angiography demonstrated a larger diameter in stented segments compared to the balloon-treated segments. Morphometric analysis confirmed this finding; however, there was a slight attenuation of the medial wall thickness in the stented segments compared to control segments. Interestingly though, there was still evidence of some (albeit less) intimal proliferation in the stented arterial segments; however, the vessel lumen was preserved because of its larger initial opening in stented vessels. In this same report, serial scanning electron microscopy was used to evaluate the time course of reendothelialization. Immediately following stent deployment, there was partial deendothelialization in the stented segment with platelets and white cells attaching to the exposed intima and elastic lamina. At 1 week after stent placement, the endothelial layer was "nearly" restored and the process appeared completed at 2 weeks. Thus, the time course of reendothelialization appears similar in both the dog and rabbit species.

The initial clinical experience with the Gianturco-Roubin stent was acquired in patients suffering acute closure following conventional balloon angioplasty (161). Eleven patients had the stent successfully deployed. According to the protocol design, all patients then underwent coronary bypass surgery. Stent deployment resulted in reestablishment of blood flow through the acutely closed arterial segment in all cases. The patients were described as being "stable" in their transfer to surgery. There was no Q wave myocardial infarction documented; however, one patient died postoperatively. As reported by Roubin in March 1990 (personal communication), this stent has been deployed in more than 170 patients. Current protocols for use of this stent include a Phase 2 study for acute closure or threatened acute closure due to arterial

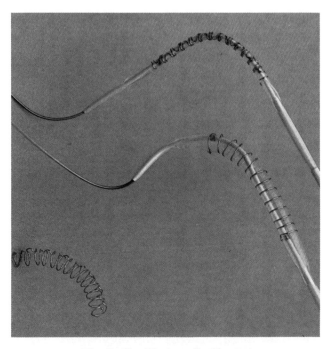

Fig. 13–17. Gianturco-Roubin stent.

dissection in small to medium-size vessels. According to this protocol, emergency coronary bypass surgery is not mandatory if adequate treatment of the acute closure is achieved by stent placement. A Phase 3 study allows the use of this stent as a primary angioplasty procedures such that both the acute outcome of the stent placement procedure and the long-term follow-up following stent placement to evaluate restenosis rates can be observed. As is the case with the WallStent and the Palmaz-Schatz stent, anticoagulation with aspirin, dipyridamole, heparin, and dextran is necessary at the time of implantation. Coumadin and antiplatelet therapy is continued for 3 months postimplantation.

The Gianturco-Roubin stent is at an earlier stage of clinical evaluation compared to the Medinvent WallStent and the Palmaz-Schatz stent. Nonetheless, it appears that this device is effective for the treatment of acute closure that occasionally complicates conventional balloon angioplasty procedures. The design of this device gives it a theoretical advantage over the other two clinically tested stents in regard to flexibility; whether this theoretic advantage will be practically important remains to be seen. As with the other stent devices, the short- and long-term follow-up evaluating risk of sudden reocclusion, subacute thrombosis, risk of restenosis, and other adverse events is the subject of ongoing investigation.

Summary of Intracoronary Stent Devices

Intracoronary stents have been placed in almost 1,000 patients as of March 1990 and this experience is increasing rapidly. Table 13–5 provides a summary of structural characteristics and clinical experience with the three stents reviewed here. From the initial experience with these stents, several beneficial attributes are identifiable: 1) It appears that appropriately placed stents can restore patency in the setting of acute closure complicating conventional balloon angioplasty, and 2) initial follow-up reports suggest that stenting may have some beneficial impact on the risk of restenosis following angioplasty procedures. Beyond these beneficial attributes, however, significant limitations of stenting must be acknowledged. There is a finite risk of thrombosis immediately and for several months following stent placement; very aggressive anticoagulation treatment regimens are necessary to minimize this risk. Placement of the current generation of stents is often difficult because of the poor visibility of the devices, their relative lack of flexibility and trackability, and, in some cases, the

stent shortening that occurs during deployment involves the permanent implantation of a prosthetic device. The long-term response to this prosthetic material remains to be determined. Further modifications of the current generations of stent devices may address some of these limitations; for instance, bonding of heparin molecules to stent materials may decrease risk of thrombosis. The radiopacity of stents can be improved by altering the alloys used for the stent strut material. Therefore, it is anticipated that further improvements in stent design will occur and that these improvements may favorably impact current limitations that have been observed.

It must also be recognized that we are in the first generation of intracoronary stenting. Several investigators have already suggested the potential usefulness of polymers for stenting (162,163). Beyond the simple mechanical scaffolding and support that current stents offer, it is quite possible that future generations of stents may serve as very useful drug delivery systems. Finally, it is possible that stents may serve as "platforms" for the implantation of genetically engineered endothelial cells that will serve as the source of specific biologically active substances. Preliminary feasibility studies involving implantation of endothelial cells on vascular graft material (164) and intravascular stents (165) have been conducted. Thus, the future of intracoronary stenting appears extremely promising. The potential to combine mechanical structural support with local drug delivery aimed at biologic processes holds the promise of providing intravascular stenting with a truly unique and important position in the field of angioplasty.

SUMMARY

As one can appreciate from this chapter, there has been a veritable explosion of new technologies during the last several years, all intended to improve the short- and/or long-term efficacy of catheter-based revascularization. This field is moving very rapidly, so that any review provides only a snapshot of the state of the technology at one point in time. Bearing that limitation in mind, it is worthwhile to speculate about the future of these new technologic approaches to the treatment of coronary artery disease. It is likely that the further evolution of the technology described in this chapter will ultimately improve the safety and expand the applicability of catheter-based revascularization procedures. Many patients who now must undergo coronary artery bypass grafting may soon be reasonably treated by less invasive techniques utilizing these new devices. It is unlikely that any single device will fulfill the needs of every clinical situation. It is more likely that various devices will eventually be shown to have utility in certain niches, such as total occlusions (e.g., lasers or ultrasonic ablation catheter), treatment of ostial lesions (e.g., retrograde atherectomy), and treatment of intimal dissection and abrupt coronary closure after PTCA (e.g., stents, atherectomy, or laser ther-

mal balloon). The ability of any of these devices to decrease restenosis remains uncertain. It should be acknowledged that the comparison(s) of various devices in this chapter is based, in part, on a subjective evaluation of each device based on relatively limited data. Ultimately, large randomized comparative clinical trials will be required to define the role(s) of each of these new technologies compared to "plain old" balloon and coronary artery bypass graft surgery, as well as to each other.

APPENDIX I
CASE PRESENTATIONS

CASE NUMBER 1

Clinical

73-year-old woman with abrupt onset of unstable angina, admitted to the hospital with evidence of an inferior myocardial infarction; resolution with IV nitroglycerin, but continued pain

Angiography

RCA: long area of severe disease culminating in 95% narrowing in proximal third and tandem lesions of 80% in midzone
LMain: normal
LAD: minimal irregularity
LCX: moderate disease
LV: normal

Equipment

Guide	Dilatation Catheter	Wire
FR4 SH	2.5 mm ACX; 3 mm ACX	0.014 HTF

Strategy and Procedure

This was done as an ad hoc procedure because of the patient's clinical instability. An FR4 guide damped, and an FR4 guide with side holes was used with no problems and coaxial seating. The wire was passed carefully across the eccentricity of the lesions in the left lateral projection (C). Balloon inflations were carried out first at the proximal lesion because the balloon shaft would not cross the lesion prior to inflation. This facilitated passage across the distal lesion, and this was then dilated (E,F). The balloons were inflated to 10 atm at both sites of disease, and less than adequate lumens were achieved. The wire was extended, a 3.0 mm ACX balloon positioned at the lesions, and inflations at 7 atm for 1 min $\times 2$ at each area carried out. This gave an excellent angiographic result, and the patient has done well clinically 1 year postprocedure.

136

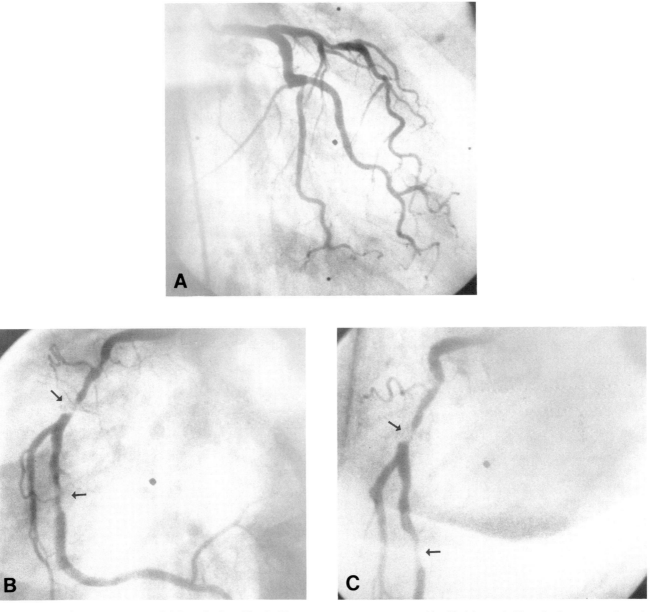

Case 1. A: Left coronary artery, RAO projection. No significant disease is seen in the left coronary system. **B:** Right coronary artery, LAO projection. Severe tandem lesions in the midzone of the right coronary artery are identified (arrows). There is also an area of proximal narrowing that measured no more than 50% on three views. **C:** Right coronary artery, left lateral projection. See above.

Scc following pages for continuation of figures.

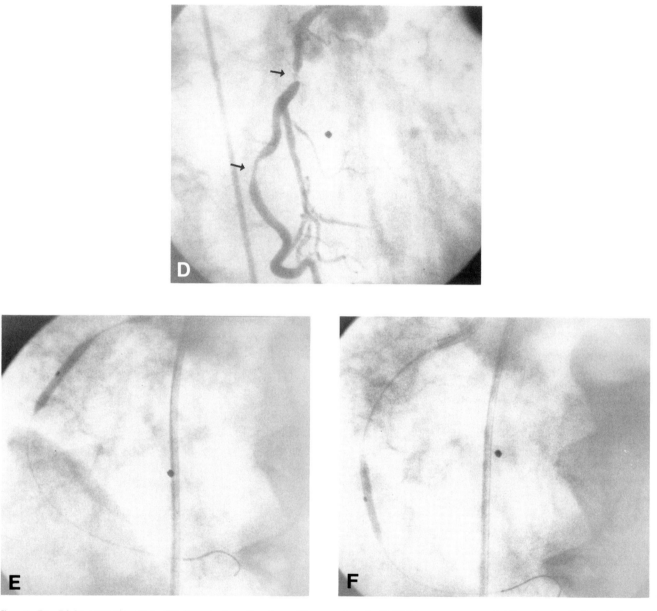

Case 1. D: Right coronary artery, RAO projection. See above. **E:** Right coronary artery, LAO projection. Balloon inflated at proximal stenosis. **F:** Right coronary artery, LAO projection. Balloon inflated at distal stenosis.

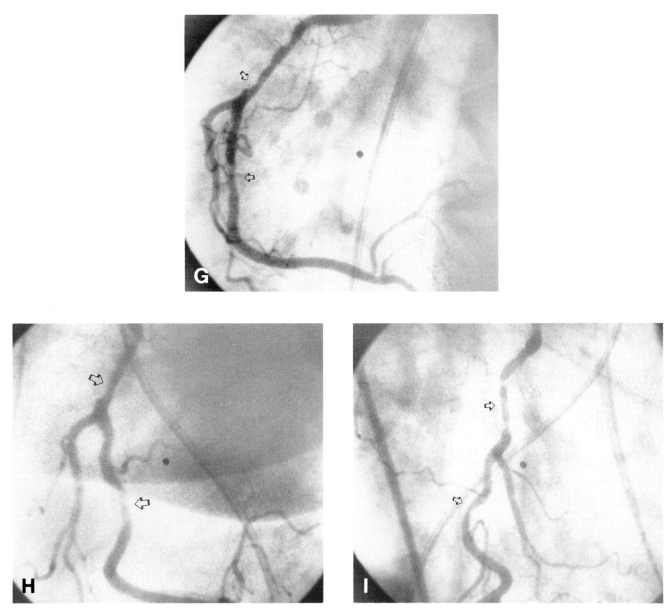

Case 1. G: Right coronary artery, LAO projection. Postangioplasty angiography shows adequate lumen improvement and excellent distal flow (arrows). **H:** Right coronary artery, left lateral projection. See above. **I:** Left coronary artery, RAO projection. See above.

CASE NUMBER 2

Clinical

45-year-old mailman who first presented at age 40 with exertional accelerating angina and positive treadmill; angiography showed an apparent 80% proximal LAD lesion (A), but following intracoronary nitroglycerin, no pressure gradient was demonstrated across the lesion and no balloon inflations were carried out when the lesion appeared to be less than 50% stenotic (B); he was treated with medication and was pain-free for 6 years and now presents again with exertional angina, and thallium treadmill is positive anteriorly

Angiography

RCA:	normal
LMain:	normal
LAD:	80% irregular proximal third lesion, not resolving with IC nitro
LCX:	normal
LV:	normal

Equipment

Guide	Dilatation Catheter	Wire
JL4	3 mm Profile Plus 3.5 mm Profile Plus	0.014 FS

Strategy and Procedure

Because of the previous experience with this patient, intracoronary nitroglycerin was given and the lesion did not resolve (C,D). The flexible steerable wire was passed easily across the lesion, and 3 mm balloon inflations carried out to 8 atm for as long as 40 sec ×3. There was continued narrowing of that area, and the wire was extended and the balloon replaced with a 3.5 mm Profile Plus, which was inflated to 7 atm pressure. Postangioplasty angiography shows an excellent luminal result (F). The patient has done well clinically for 2 years postprocedure.

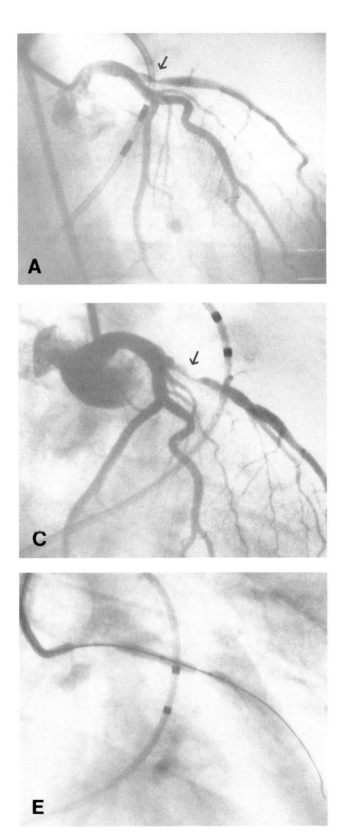

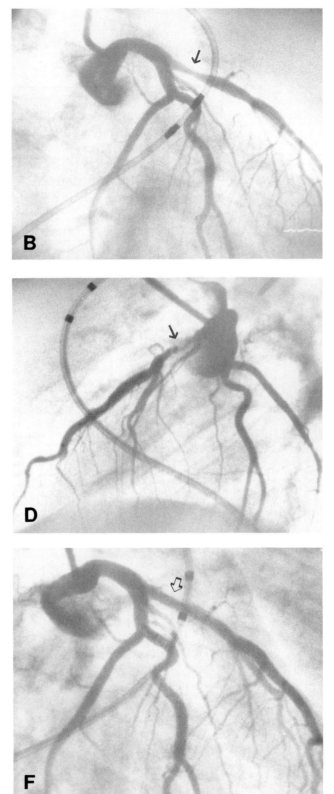

Case 2. A: Left coronary artery, RAO projection, 1984. This initial injection suggests the presence of a severe localized stenosis in the proximal LAD (arrow). **B:** Left coronary artery, RAO projection, 1984. Following intracoronary nitroglycerin, the lumen markedly improved, and no gradient was demonstrated across the proximal area of the LAD (arrow). No balloon inflations were carried out. **C:** Left

coronary artery, RAO projection, 1988. The proximal LAD (arrow) again appears severely stenotic and is now diffusely irregular. Intracoronary nitroglycerin did not change this lesion. **D:** Left coronary artery, left lateral projection. See C. **E:** Left coronary artery, RAO projection. Balloon inflated at lesion. **F:** Left coronary artery, RAO projection. Postangioplasty (arrow).

CASE NUMBER 3

Clinical

75-year-old man admitted in 1987 with inferior wall myocardial infarction and continuing postinfarction angina, which led to his first angiography and angioplasty procedures; 2 years later, the return of symptoms led to restudy and the finding of a new lesion in the proximal LAD, treated as documented below

Angiography

	1987	1990 (Video Tape)
RCA:	90% midzone	localized 80% midzone
	70% midzone	
	90% origin PDA	
LMain:	normal	normal
LAD:	90% midzone	new 90% proximal lesion, good results in midzone
LADD:	90% origin	widely patent
LCX:	90% proximal third	good lumen with local aneurysm
LV:	mild inferobasal hypokinesia	mild inferobasal hypokinesia

Equipment

Guide	Dilatation Catheter		Wire	
	1987	1990	1987	1990
JR4/JL4	2.0 mm	3.0 mm	0.014 FS	0.014
	3.0 mm ACX	3.5 mm ACX		high-torque floppy

Strategy and Procedure

At the time of the initial diagnostic study (A–C), it was decided to go ahead with an ad hoc angioplasty of the right coronary artery. The wire was passed across all lesions, and it was necessary to dilate the midzone lesion with a 2 mm balloon in order to get the balloon shaft profile across the area of the midzone disease (D). The distal lesion was then dilated with a 2 mm balloon (E). The wire was extended, and a 3 mm balloon used to inflate the midzone diseased area (F). Guiding catheter injections showed good result in midzone and dissection or spasm in the posterior descending branch (G). The 2 mm balloon was again used to dilate the segment (H); and a good result obtained (I–L). The patient was returned to the laboratory 2 days later, and the results of the right coronary artery dilatations appeared adequate (M). The circumflex was then approached (N), and using an FL4 guide and a 2.5 mm balloon with a 0.014 wire across the lesion, inflations were carried out at up to 9 atm pressure for as long as 45 sec. An initial large pressure gradient across this area was obliterated, and guiding injections showed excellent patency procedure (P). The tandem lesions in the LAD and the origin lesion in the LADD were then approached (Q). A wire was passed across all lesions, and the distal lesion in the LAD dilated first (R). The proximal lesion was then

142

dilated (S), and the origin of the LADD also dilated with the same 2 mm balloon. The final result of angioplasty appeared excellent (T). The patient returned 2 years later with unstable angina. Left coronary injections showed a new lesion in the proximal third of the right coronary artery that had had no significant stenosis in previous studies (U). The circumflex had healed with an adequate lumen and a small aneurysmal dilatation in the area of previous angioplasty (U). The results in the mid and distal LAD and at the origin of the major diagonal branch appeared excellent (V). The right coronary artery appeared adequately patent (W), and there were early collaterals to the LAD. The LAD lesion was crossed with a 0.014 FS wire and dilated with a 3 mm balloon (X). Note the aneurysmal dilatation of the artery just distal to the area of balloon dilatation. The wire is in the major diagonal branch. The wire was extended and replaced with a 3.5 mm balloon that was inflated in the proximal lesion (Y). An excellent tubular lumen was then achieved at the area of previous severe stenosis proximal to the area of ectasia (AA). Six weeks later, the patient returned with recurrent angina. The LAD appeared to be adequately patent (BB,CC). The right coronary artery continued to show an area of 80% proximal third stenosis, and a thallium treadmill showed inferior reversible ischemia (DD). Angioplasty was then undertaken with a 3.0 mm balloon (FF), and an adequate lumen was achieved, with relief of the patient's symptoms (GG).

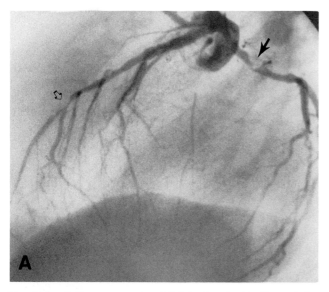

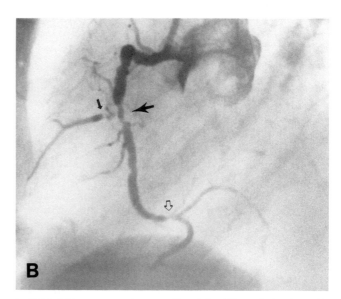

Case 3. A: Left coronary artery, left lateral projection. Severe lesion in midzone of LAD (open arrow), and in proximal circumflex (solid arrow). **B:** Right coronary artery, left lateral projection. Severe proximal disease in midzone of right coronary artery (large solid arrow) and in distal right coronary artery near the origin of the posterior descending branch (open arrow). The small solid arrow denotes slow flow into a right ventricular branch originating from the proximal area of severe disease. Note ectasia of vessel.

See following pages for continuation of figures.

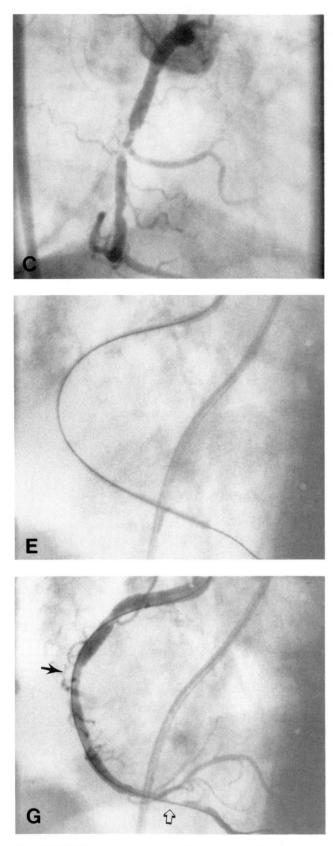

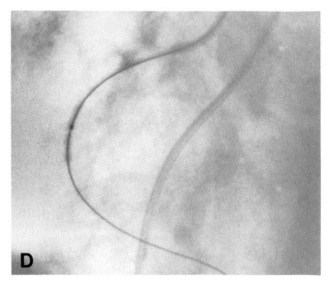

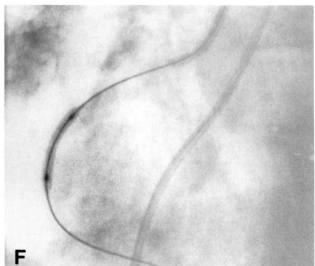

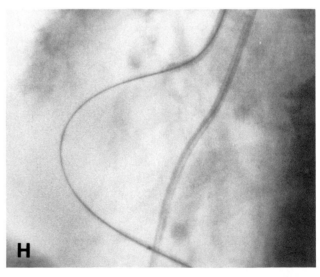

Case 3. C: Right coronary artery, RAO projection. **D:** Right coronary artery, LAO projection. Two millimeter balloon inflated at area of stenosis. **E:** Right coronary artery, LAO projection. Two millimeter balloon inflated at distal lesion. **F:** Right coronary artery, LAO projection. Three millimeter balloon inflated at proximal lesion. **G:** Right

coronary artery, LAO projection. Improvement in lumen at proximal lesion (solid arrow) and severe stenosis/dissection/spasm in posterior descending branch (open arrow). **H:** Right coronary artery, LAO projection. Two millimeter balloon inflated at area of distal concern.

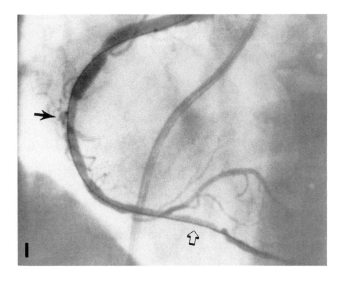

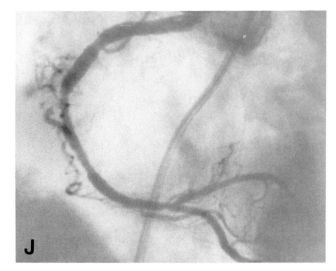

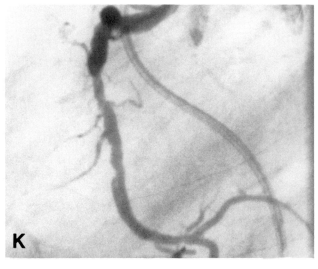

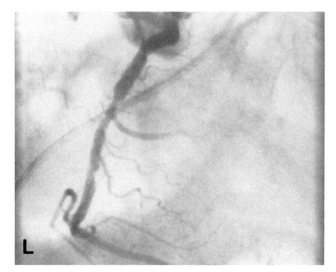

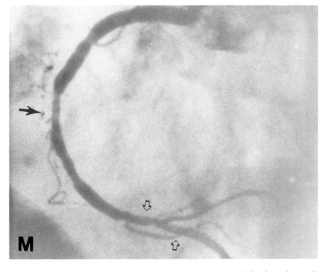

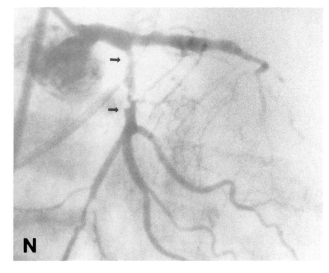

Case 3. I: Right coronary artery, LAO projection. Injection through guide with wire still across all lesions. Open arrow shows good result in proximal posterior descending branch, and solid arrow shows good result in the midzone of right coronary artery. Note that flow in right ventricular marginal branch is not present. **J:** Right coronary artery, LAO projection. Postangioplasty angiogram demonstrating good result in midzone of right coronary artery and in distal vessel. There is again slow flow in the right ventricular branch. **K:** Right coronary artery, left lateral projection. Postangioplasty. **L:** Right coronary artery, RAO projection. Postangioplasty. **M:** Right coronary artery, LAO projection. This injection done 2 days later at second stage of procedure shows persistent good result in midzone of right coronary artery (solid arrow) and in distal vessel (open arrows). **N:** Left coronary artery, RAO projection. Long area of severe disease in proximal circumflex artery (arrows).

See following pages for continuation of figures.

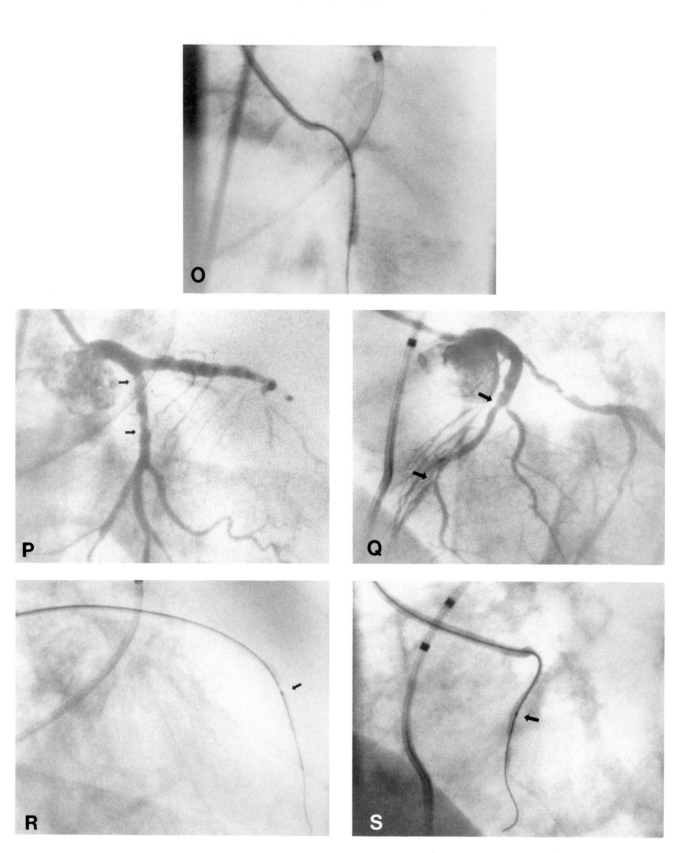

Case 3. O: Left coronary artery, RAO projection. Balloon inflation across area of long disease in circumflex. **P:** Left coronary artery, RAO projection. Lumen achieved with 3 mm balloon in proximal circumflex coronary artery. **Q:** Left coronary artery, LAO projection. Proximal third- and midzone lesions in LAD demonstrated by arrows. LADD origin lesion seen. **R:** Left coronary artery, RAO projection. Balloon inflated at distal lesion (arrow). **S:** Left coronary artery, LAO projection. Balloon inflated at proximal lesion (arrow).

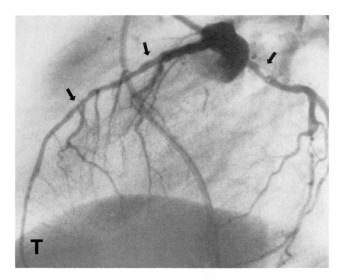

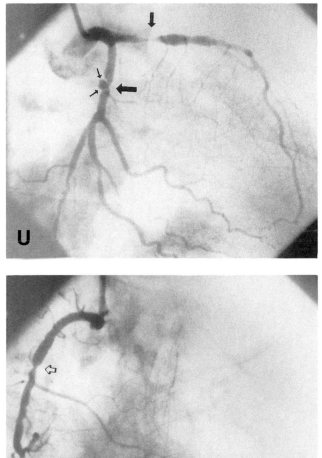

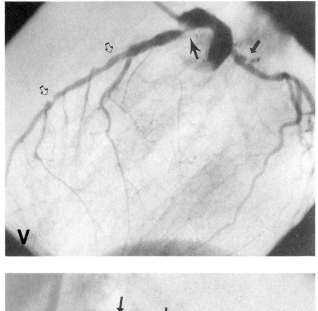

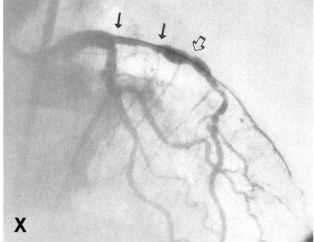

Case 3. T: Left coronary artery, left lateral projection. Results of angioplasty in tandem lesions in LAD and in the proximal circumflex artery (arrows). **U:** Left coronary artery, RAO projection. This demonstrates new lesion in proximal LAD (top arrow) 2 years later. The circumflex has healed with an apparent small aneurysmal dilatation (small arrows), but an excellent lumen with good flow into the distal vessel (large bottom arrow). **V:** Left coronary artery, left lateral projec-tion. New lesion in proximal LAD and results of previous angioplasty seen in proximal third and midzone LAD. **W:** Right coronary artery, RAO projection. Results of angioplasty 2 years prior demonstrated by arrows. Note collaterals through septum to LAD. **X:** Left coronary artery, RAO projection. Long area of tubular narrowing following dilatation with 3 mm balloon (solid arrows). Note ectasia of proximal third of LAD (open arrow).

See following pages for continuation of figures.

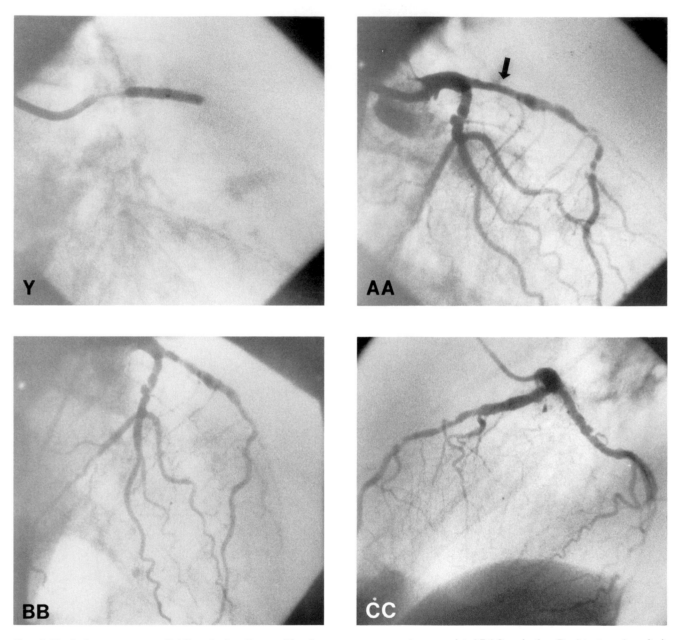

Case 3. Y: Left coronary artery RAO projection: Repeat dilatation with 3.5 mm balloon. **AA:** Excellent tubular opening of severe proximal LAD lesion (arrow). Note ectasia distal to the area of repair. **BB:** Left coronary artery, angulated RAO projection. Persistent good results in left anterior descending coronary artery 6 weeks later. **CC:** Left coronary artery, left lateral projection.

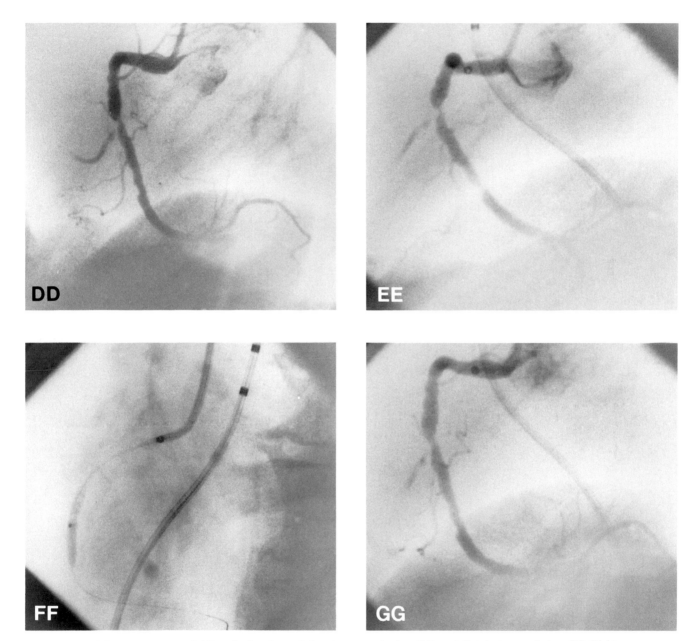

Case 3. DD: Right coronary artery, LAO projection. Severe lesion at junctions of proximal and middle thirds, with slow flow into right ventricular branch and ectasia throughout the vessel. **EE:** Right coronary artery, left lateral projection. **FF:** Right coronary artery, LAO projection. Balloon inflated at severe lesion. **GG:** Right coronary artery, left lateral projection. Results of angioplasty in right coronary artery.

CASE NUMBER 4

Clinical   75-year-old man with chronic stable angina for years, recently unstable, and thallium treadmill test with diffuse reversible defects

Angiography

RCA: "dominant" with 90% proximal third lesion
LMain: normal
LAD: 90% proximal third
LCX: 80% main; 90% OM
LV: normal

Equipment

Guide	Dilatation Catheter	Wire
RCA: JR4	2.5 mm ACX; 3.0 mm ACX	0.014 HTF
LCX: JL4	2.5 mm SULP	0.014 HTF
LAD: Amplatz left II	2.5 mm SULP	0.014 HTF

Strategy and Procedure

Angiography showed multiple-vessel disease (A,B) in a patient who refused elective surgery. The RCA was approached first because of the severity of the lesion and the large amount of myocardium affected (B,C). The JR4 guide seated nicely, and the 0.014 HTF wire passed easily across the lesion and into the distal vessel. Balloon inflations at the lesion with the 2.5 mm balloon to 10 atm for 45 sec several times. Injection showed some distal narrowing that cleared with IC nitroglycerin. Further balloon inflations resulted in haziness. The wire was extended and the balloon replaced with a 3.0 mm ACX balloon, which was inflated at low pressures 4–5 atm for up to 2 minutes (F). An adequate lumen was achieved (G,H). Because of the amount of contrast used, it was decided to stage the procedure, and the next day he was returned to the laboratory and a good persistent result in the RCA was demonstrated. The LCX was then approached, and the OM branch first dilated with a 2.5 mm SULP at 7 atm for 45 sec several times. This looked good on guiding catheter injections, and the balloon and wire were withdrawn into the proximal LCX and then the ongoing LCX wired and the balloon inflated to 4 atm with a good result. Injections then showed some further narrowing of the OM branch, and this was rewired and remolded with 4 atm, 2 min inflations ×2. Postangioplasty angiograms demonstrated a good result in the LCX (K). The patient was then returned to the laboratory 3 weeks later, and good persistent results in the RCA and LCX were demonstrated and the long area of disease in the LAD approached (L). Attempts to get the wire into the LAD were not successful with the JL4 guide. An Amplatz left II guide directed itself into the ostium of the LAD, and the vessel was easily wired and the balloon inflated to 7 atm pressure × one min several times. A good angiographic result was achieved (M). The patient had a return of symptoms 2 months later, and repeat angiography showed a good persistent result in the LAD, RCA, and main circumflex, but a recurrent lesion in the OM circumflex (N). Using a JL4 guide and a 2 mm ACX

150

balloon over a 0.014 HTF wire, the lesion was carefully wired in its eccentric lumen (15° RAO, 15° caudal view) and inflations carried out (O) to 8 atm for 1 min ×3. The result was an excellent lumen in that vessel (P). He has continued to do well clinically for 6 months postprocedure.

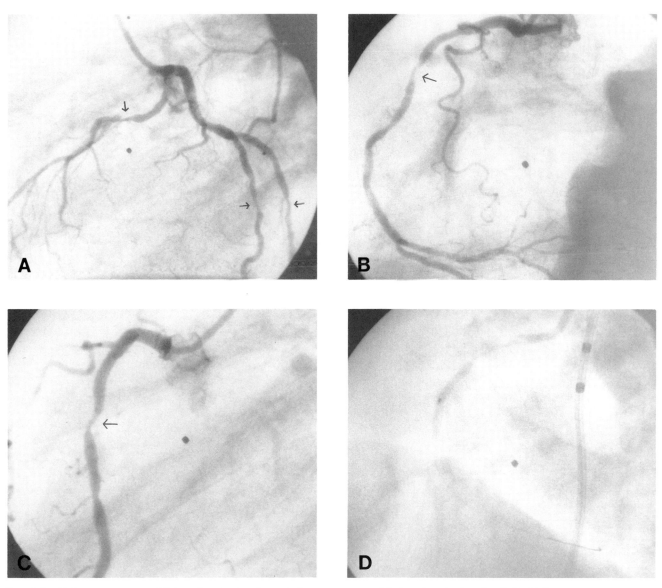

Case 4. A: Left coronary artery, left lateral projection. Severe lesions in LAD, main LCX, and OM LCX (arrows). B: Right coronary artery, LAO projection. Severe proximal lesion (arrow). C: Left coronary artery, left lateral projection. See B. D: Right coronary artery, LAO projection. Balloon inflation.

See following pages for continuation of figures.

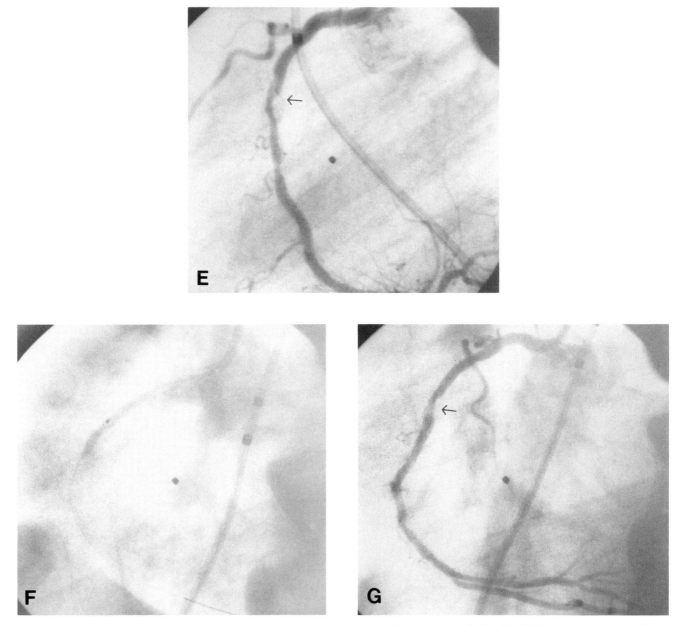

Case 4. E: Right coronary artery, left lateral projection. Postangioplasty with dissection (arrow). **F:** Right coronary artery, LAO projection. Molding balloon inflation. **G:** Right coronary artery, LAO projection. Postangioplasty (arrow).

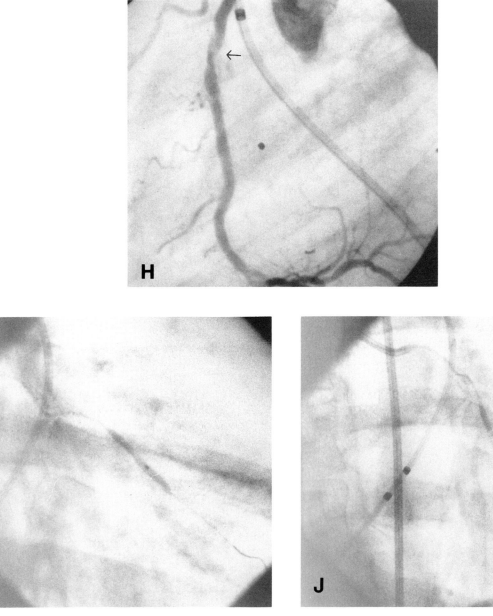

Case 4. H: Right coronary artery, LAO projection. Postangioplasty (arrow). **I:** Left coronary artery, RAO projection. Balloon inflation in OM LCX. **J:** Left coronary artery, RAO projection. Balloon inflation in LCX.

See following pages for continuation of figures.

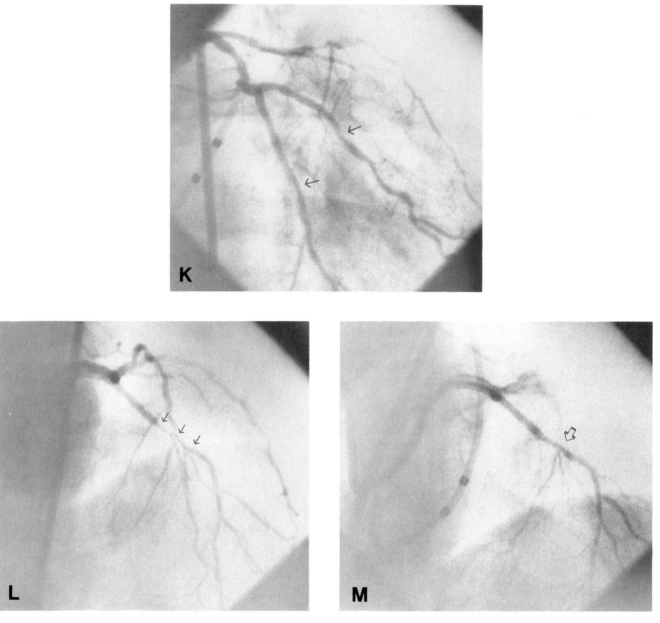

Case 4. K: Left coronary artery, RAO projection. Postcircumflex angioplasties (arrows). **L:** Left coronary artery, angulated RAO projection. Long area of disease in LAD (arrows). **M:** Left coronary artery, angulated RAO projection. Post LAD angioplasty (arrow).

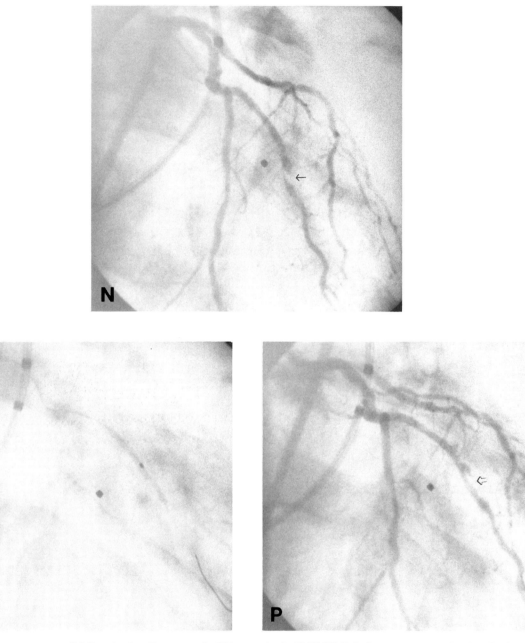

Case 4. N: Left coronary artery, RAO projection. Recurrence in OM LCX (arrow). **O:** Left coronary artery, RAO projection. Balloon infla- tion in OM LCX. **P:** Left coronary artery, RAO projection. Postangio- plasty of OM LCX (arrow).

CASE NUMBER 5

Clinical	74-year-old man with accelerating angina and positive treadmill test

Angiography

RCA: tandem 80–90% proximal third; 95% midzone
LMain: normal
LAD: normal
LCX: tandem 80% in OM

Equipment

Guide	Dilatation Catheter	Wire
LCX: JL4	2.0 mm mini	0.014 FS
RCA: JR4 SH	2.5 mm mini; 3.0 mm mini	0.014 FS

Strategy and Procedure

The OM branch was approached first. Tandem lesions were easily wired and balloon inflations carried out with 2.0 mm balloon to 7 atm pressure for 45 and 60 sec, each lesion. Excellent angiographic result achieved (B). RCA then approached wide side-hole catheter because of proximity of first lesion (C). The wire was passed easily across the proximal tandem lesions, and the midzone lesion was wired in the lateral projection because of its eccentricity (D). A 2.5 mm balloon was passed across all lesions, and the distal lesion dilated first, then the proximal tandem lesions, all at 8 atm pressure for 60 sec each. The wire was then extended, and a 3.0 mm balloon positioned across all lesions and back dilatations done in all three areas. The postangioplasty angiograms (E,F) were performed with the wire still in place as a brace to prevent the guide from disrupting the area of proximal balloon inflation. The patient has done well clinically with no recurrence at 18 months.

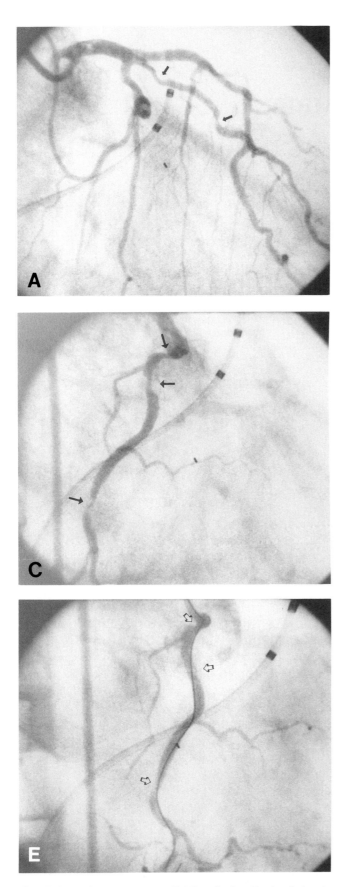

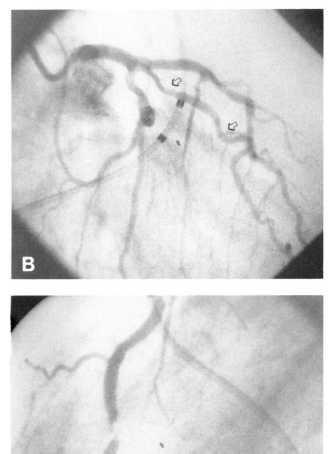

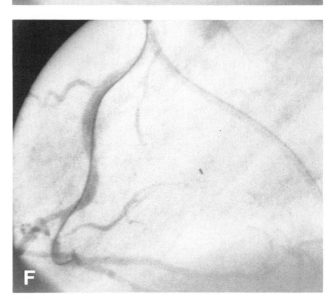

Case 5. A: Left coronary artery, RAO projection. Tandem lesions in obtuse marginal circumflex (arrows). **B:** Left coronary artery, RAO projection. Postangioplasty (arrows). **C:** Right coronary artery, RAO projection. Three lesions in right coronary artery (arrows). **D:** Right coronary artery, left lateral projection. Preangioplasty. **E:** Right coronary artery, RAO projection. Postangioplasty (arrows). **F:** Right coronary artery, left lateral projection. Postangioplasty.

CASE NUMBER 6

Clinical   45-year-old man first seen with unstable angina in 1984, with subsequent episodes of reonset angina in 1986 and 1989

Angiography

	1984	1986	1989
RCA:	40% proximal	90% proximal	10% proximal
LMain:	normal	normal	normal
LAD:	95% midzone	normal	90% proximal (new lesion)
			midnormal
LCX:	50% main	80% mid	10% main
LV:	normal	normal	normal

Equipment

	Guide	Dilatation Catheter	Wire
1984:	JL4/JR4	2.5 mm LPS	0.014 FS
1986:	JL4/JR4	3.0 mm LPS	0.014 FS
1989:	JL4	3.0 mm Profile Plus	0.014 FS

Strategy and Procedure

In 1984, the LAD lesion was obviously severe and was approached first. A 2.5 mm LPS balloon catheter was positioned at the lesion, and inflations carried out to 6 atm for as long as 40 sec several times (B). This achieved an excellent lumen in the LAD (C). The severity of the lesions in the circumflex and right coronary arteries was not angiographically clear, so pressure gradients were measured across both lesions with the 2.5 mm LPS balloon. A 6 mm drop in pressure was measured across the circumflex lesion (D), and a 10 mm pressure drop across the right coronary artery lesion (F) was seen. No balloon inflations were carried out in the RCA or LCX at that time. The patient, a very athletic man, returned with exertional angina in 1986. The study then showed that the lumen achieved in 1984 in the midzone of the LAD continued to be widely patent (G), but the lesions in both the LCX and RCA had progressed (G,H). The RCA lesion was approached first as an ad hoc procedure with a JR4 guide with side holes, and a 3 mm LPS balloon was passed over a 0.014 FS wire and a 60 mm gradient now measured. Balloon inflations were carried out at up to 10 atm for as long as 30 sec. The balloon was still indented at 9 atm and opened at 10 (I). Luminal improvement was achieved (J). The LCX was then approached with a JL4 guide and the same 3 mm LPS balloon. A 65 mm pressure gradient was measured across the circumflex lesion, and inflations were carried out at 7 atm for 60 sec several times. The pressure gradient was reduced to 0 (K). A good angiographic result was achieved. The patient again returned with exertional angina in 1989, and initial injections in the RCA showed a good persistent result (M). The circumflex was also widely patent, but a new lesion had developed in the proximal third of the LAD (N), while the midzone of the LAD initially treated in 1984 remained widely patent. Repeat angioplasty was performed utilizing a JL4 guide and a 3.0 mm mini profile balloon with a 0.014 FS wire. The balloon was inflated at 8 atm or as long as 45 sec ×3 and an excellent lumen achieved. A small crack was evident in the superior aspect of the area of dilatation (P,Q). The patient has continued to do well with no further symptoms and a normal thallium treadmill 18 months following his last procedure.

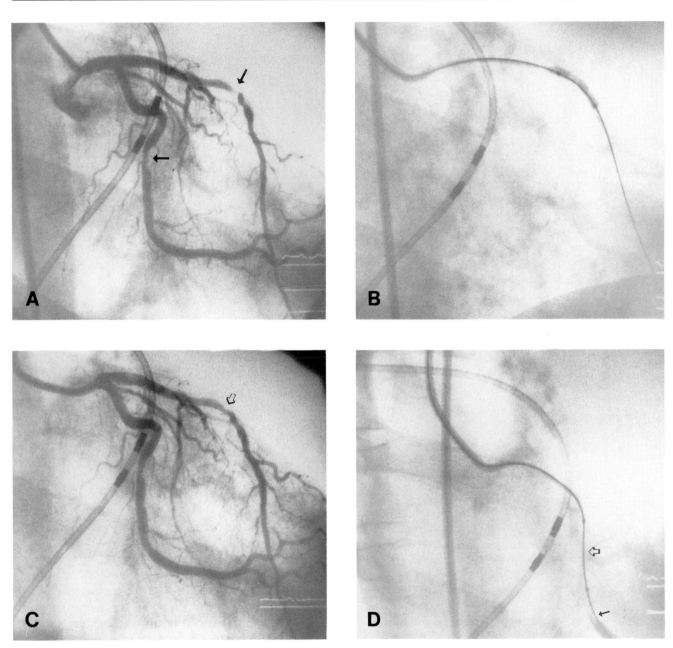

Case 6. A: Left coronary artery, RAO projection, 1984. Severe lesion in LAD and narrowing in circumflex (arrows). **B:** Left coronary artery, RAO projection, 1984. Balloon inflation. **C:** Left coronary artery, 1984. Postangioplasty of LAD (arrow). **D:** Left coronary artery, RAO projection, 1984. Pressure gradient measurement across circumflex lesion (open arrow). Distal injection through balloon catheter (solid arrow).

See following pages for continuation of figures.

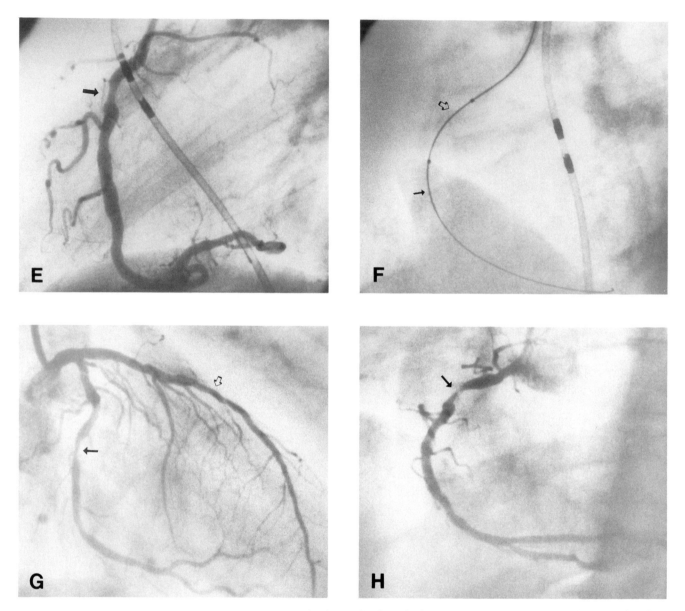

Case 6. E: Right coronary artery, LAO projection, 1984. Proximal area of stenosis (arrow). **F:** Right coronary artery, LAO projection. Pressure gradient measurement across right coronary lesion (open arrow). Tip of balloon catheter at solid arrow. **G:** Left coronary artery, RAO projection, 1986. Long-term patency of LAD lesion (open arrow). Worsening of circumflex lesion (solid arrow). **H:** Right coronary artery, LAO projection, 1986. Worsening of proximal stenosis in right coronary artery (arrow).

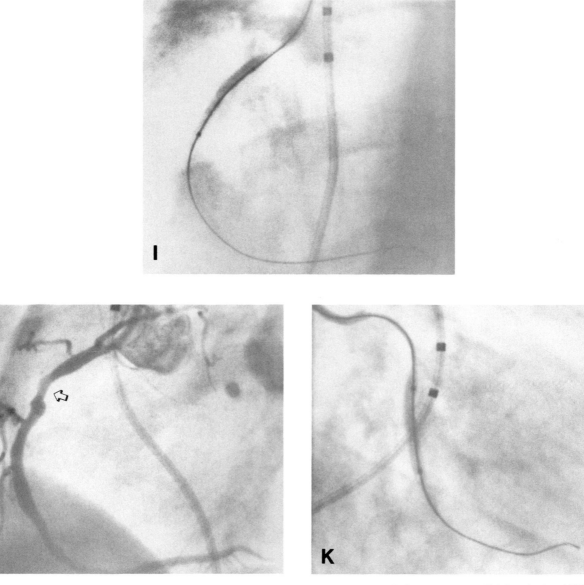

Case 6. I: Right coronary artery, LAO projection, 1986. Balloon inflation. **J:** Right coronary artery, LAO projection, 1986. Postangio-plasty (arrow). **K:** Left coronary artery, RAO projection, 1986. Balloon inflation in circumflex.

See following pages for continuation of figures.

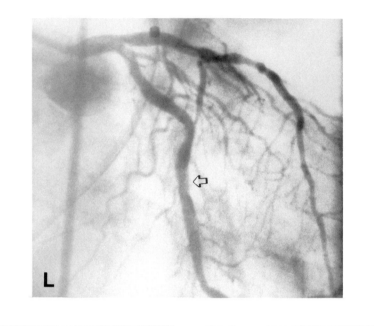

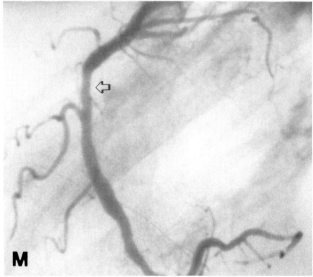

Case 6. L: Left coronary artery, RAO projection, 1986. Post circumflex angioplasty (arrow). **M:** Right coronary artery, left lateral projection, 1989. Long-term patency of proximal right lesion (arrow). **N:** Left coronary artery, RAO projection. Long-term patency of LAD lesion and circumflex lesion, previously dilated (open arrows). New proximal lesion in LAD (solid arrow).

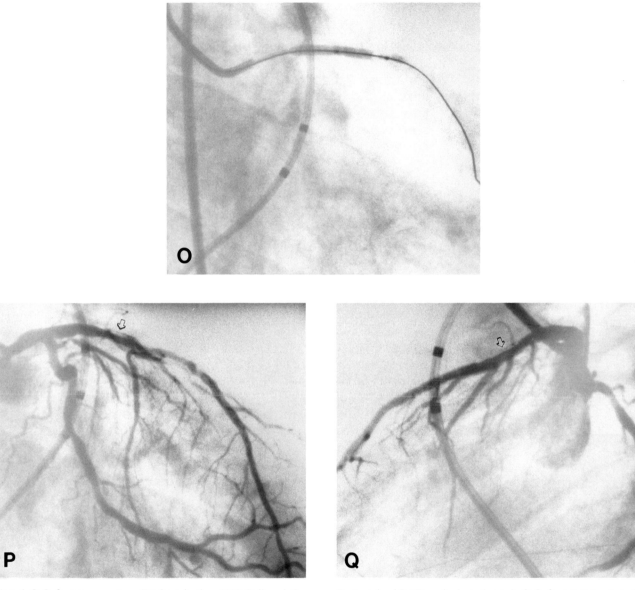

Case 6. O: Left coronary artery, RAO projection, 1989. Balloon inflation in proximal LAD. P: Left coronary artery, RAO projection, 1989.

Postproximal LAD angioplasty (arrow). Q: Left coronary artery, left lateral projection, 1989. Postangioplasty (arrow).

CASE NUMBER 7

Clinical   70-year-old man with chronic stable angina, recently becoming unstable, with positive EKG treadmill in anterior leads

Angiography
RCA: "dominant," normal
LMain: normal
LAD: tandem lesions 90% proximal third, 90% midzone
LCX: no disease
LV: normal

Equipment

Guide	Dilatation Catheter	Wire
JL4	2.0 mm ACX; 3.0 mm ACX	0.014 FS

Strategy and Procedure

The wire was passed easily across both lesions utilizing particularly the lateral and LAO views to identify the route of the wire (B,C). The 2 mm balloon would not easily cross the proximal lesion, and inflations were carried out there first to facilitate distal passage (D). The inflations at the distal lesion conformed nicely to the curve of the artery (E). The first lesion was inflated at 8 atm for 45 sec, and the second at 7 atm for 45 sec ×3. The wire was extended and this balloon removed and a 3.0 mm balloon inflated proximally because of an apparent inadequate lumen with a 2 mm balloon (F–H). A 3 mm balloon was inflated to 6 atm to achieve full balloon inflation, and molding inflations at 7 atm, to achieve full balloon inflation. Molding inflations at 7 atm were carried out several times. Angiography then showed some haziness in the proximal lesion, and an excellent result distally (I,J). Because of some concern about the proximal lesion, he was returned to the laboratory 2 days later, and, angiographically, the area appeared fully patent (K). The patient's treadmill normalized, and he continues to do well 8 months postprocedure.

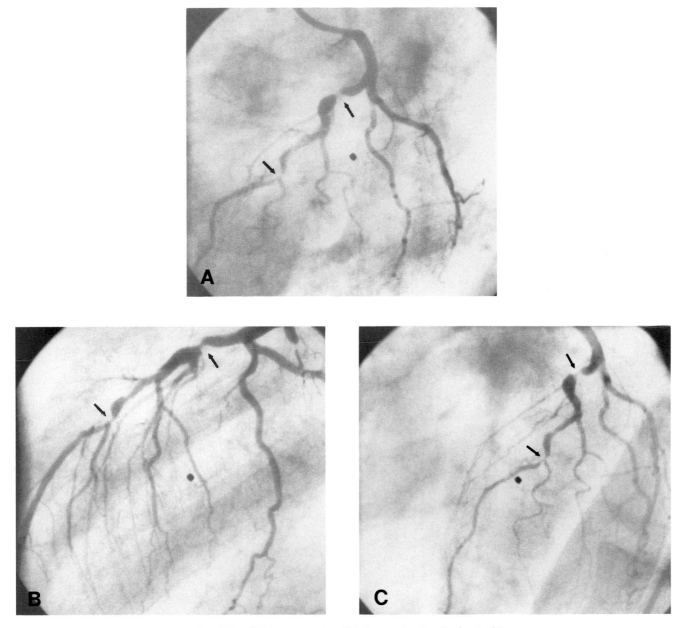

Case 7. A: Left coronary artery, LAO projection. Proximal and mid-zone LAD lesions (arrows). **B:** Left coronary artery, left lateral projection. See A. **C:** Left coronary artery, shallow LAO projection. See A.

See following pages for continuation of figures.

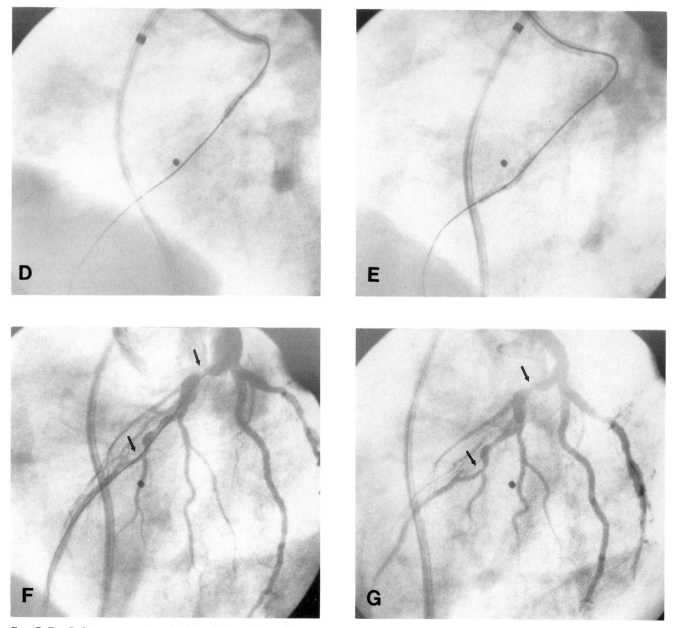

Case 7. D: Left coronary artery, LAO projection. Two millimeter balloon inflated at proximal lesion. **E:** Left coronary artery, LAO projection. Two millimeter balloon inflated at midzone lesion. **F:** Left coronary artery, LAO projection. Post 2 mm balloon angioplasty (arrows). **G:** Left coronary artery, LAO projection. Post 2 mm balloon angioplasty (arrows).

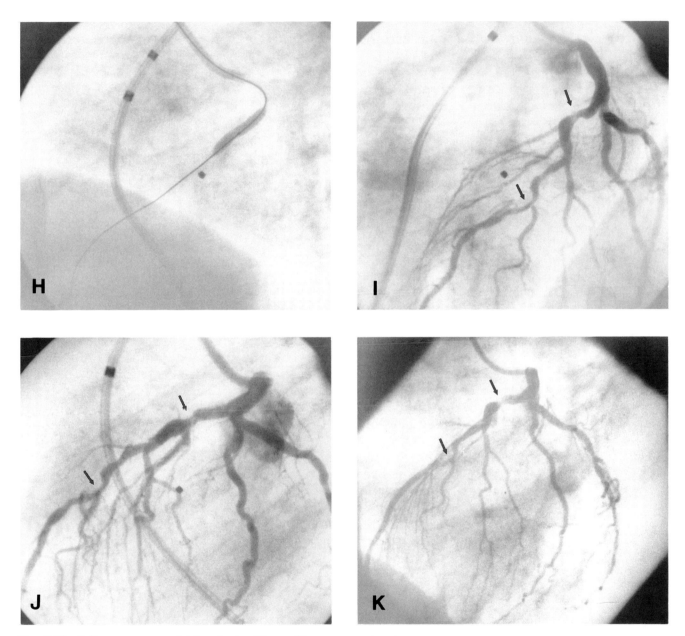

Case 7. H: Left coronary artery, LAO projection. Three millimeter balloon inflation at proximal lesion. **I:** Left coronary artery, LAO projection. Postangioplasty (arrows). **J:** Left coronary artery, left lateral projection. Postangioplasty (arrows). **K:** Left coronary artery, LAO projection. Two days postangioplasty (arrows).

CASE NUMBER 8

Clinical   66-year-old man with recent onset angina and positive treadmill test

Angiography

RCA:	"dominant" 90% proximal third lesion
LMain:	normal
LAD:	subtotal obstruction proximal third with slow distal flow
LCX:	90% proximal lesion with 90% lesion at origin of OM
LV:	normal

Equipment

Guide	Dilatation Catheter	Wire
LAD: JL4	2.0 mm ACX	0.014 FS; 0.014 intermediate
RCA: JR4	3.0 mm ACX	0.014 HTF
LCX: JL4	2.0 mm ACX	0.014 HTF

Strategy and Procedure

Following review of the diagnostic angiograms, it was decided that if the LAD could be successfully opened then angioplasty could probably be done of the other vessels with relative certainty. The LAD was therefore approached first. A JL4 guide seated well, and a 2 mm balloon with a 0.014 FS wire was used initially. The wire continually buckled and was replaced with a 0.014 intermediate wire. In the LAO view, this wire was seen to begin to traverse the obvious tract in the LAD (C) and would not cross without bringing the balloon down to stiffen the wire (D). The wire was then passed across this lesion (E,F), and forward inflations of the balloon catheter were made (G). This opened a fairly good lumen in the vessel (H,I), and there was an apparent lesion downstream in the LAD once antegrade flow had been reestablished (I). Further balloon inflations in that area were carried out at 10 atm, and good molding inflations made. An excellent angiographic result was achieved (K). The right coronary was then approached at the same sitting, and an FR4 guide with side holes was used, along with a 3 mm balloon and a 0.014 HTF wire. There was dimpling of the balloon up to 5 atm, and molding inflations were carried out at 7 atm several times. A good angiographic result was achieved (O,P). Three weeks later, the patient was returned to the laboratory to check the results of these angioplasties. The LAD remained widely patent (Q,R), and the RCA was also widely opened. Attempts to get the wire across the obtuse marginal branch resulted in the inability to advance the wire into the distal vessel, and the manipulation in that area resulted in slow flow in the OM branch. The patient was stable, and the wire was then passed across the main circumflex lesion into the distal vessel and balloon inflations carried out (S). The final result in the circumflex showed a good lumen in the main vessel and slow flow in the OM branch. The patient remained stable, had no EKG or enzyme changes, and has done well clinically for 8 months following the procedures.

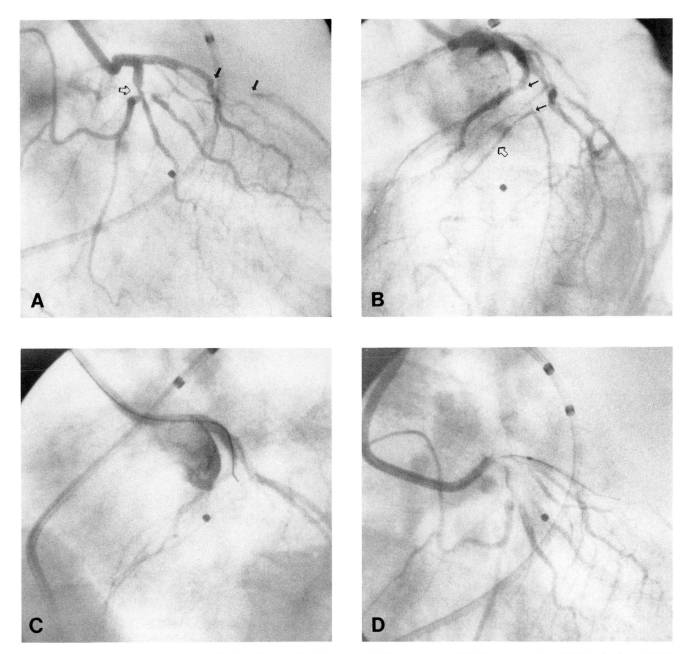

Case 8. A: Left coronary artery, RAO projection. Near-total occlusion of the proximal LAD with slow flow into the distal vessel (solid arrows). Severe disease in the proximal circumflex (open arrow). **B:** Left coronary artery, LAO projection. Solid arrows denote severe proximal disease in LAD with slow flow into the distal vessel indi-

cated by open arrow. **C:** Left coronary artery, LAO projection. A 0.014 intermediate wire is heading into severe stenosis in LAD. **D:** Left coronary artery, RAO projection. Guiding catheter injection confirms wire traversing desired path toward distal vessel.

See following pages for continuation of figures.

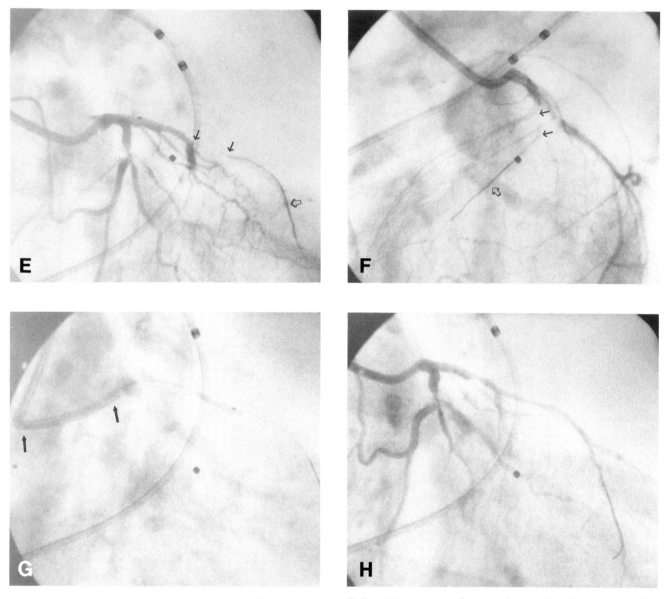

Case 8. E: Left coronary artery, RAO projection. A 0.014 intermediate wire is across lesion (solid arrows) and in distal vessel (open arrow). **F:** Left coronary artery, LAO projection. Tip of wire in distal LAD (open arrow) and across severe proximal stenosis (solid arrows). **G:** Balloon inflated at area of near-total obstruction. Note power position of femoral guide needed to force balloon across lesion (arrows). **H:** Left coronary artery, RAO projection. Improved patency of proximal vessel with wire in distal LAD.

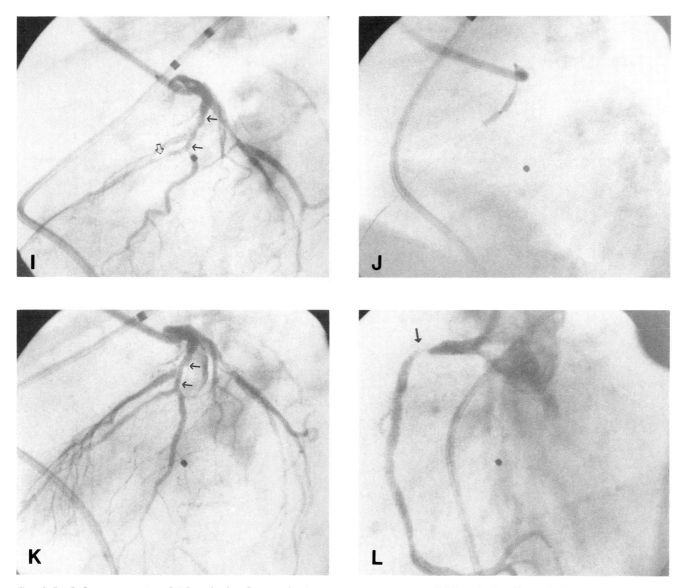

Case 8. I: Left coronary artery, LAO projection. Improved patency of proximal LAD (solid arrows) with apparent lesion in LAD distal to major diagonal branch (open arrow). **J:** Left coronary artery, LAO projection. Balloon inflation across lesion in middistal LAD. **K:** Left coronary artery, LAO projection. Postangioplasty. Patency of proximal LAD with good flow into distal vessel (arrows). **L:** Right coronary artery, LAO projection. Severe proximal stenosis (arrow).

See following pages for continuation of figures.

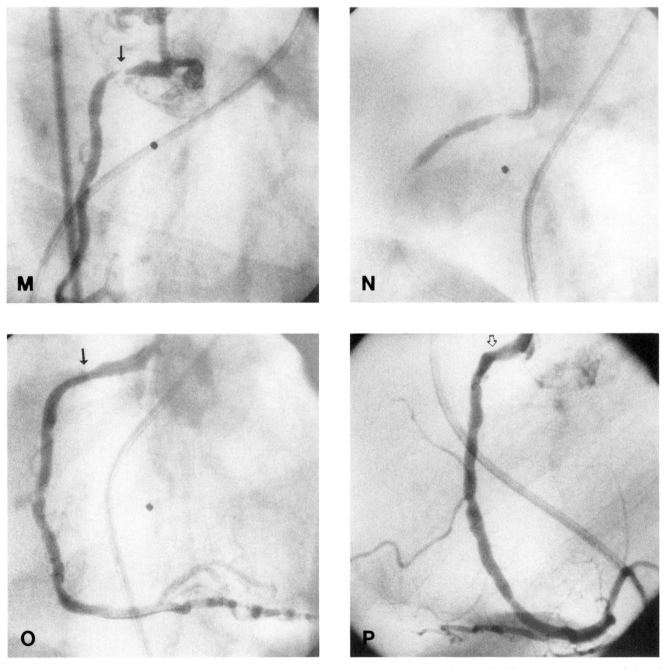

Case 8. M: Right coronary artery, RAO projection. Severe proximal stenosis (arrow). **N:** Right coronary artery, LAO projection. Balloon inflated across proximal lesion. **O:** Right coronary artery, LAO projec-

tion. Postangioplasty (arrow). **P:** Right coronary artery, left lateral projection. Four weeks postangioplasty (arrow).

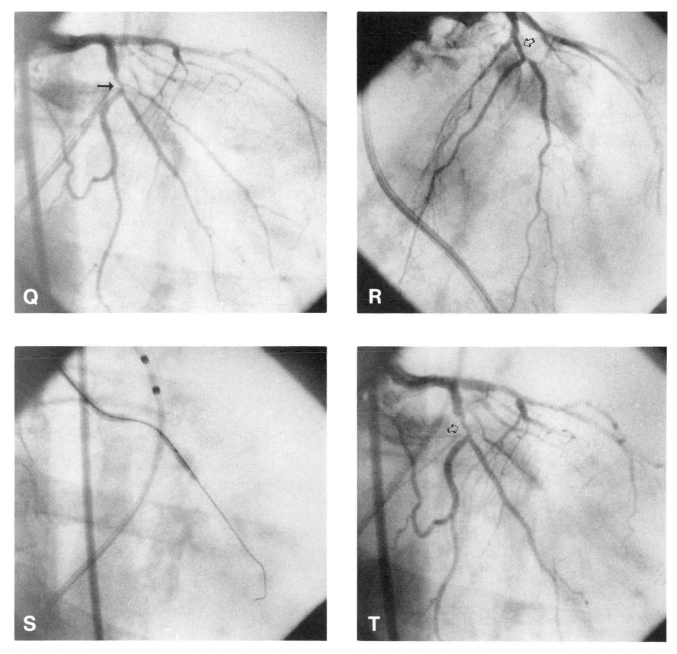

Case 8. Q: Left coronary artery, RAO projection. Continued patency of LAD with severe stenosis in circumflex (arrow). **R:** Left coronary artery, LAO projection. Continued patency of proximal LAD (arrow). **S:** Left coronary artery, RAO projection. Two millimeter balloon in-flated in circumflex. **T:** Left coronary artery, RAO projection. Improved patency of main circumflex lesion with slow flow in first obtuse marginal branch (arrow), originating from the lesion postangioplasty.

CASE NUMBER 9

Clinical

73-year-old, blind, diabetic woman with onset of chest pain in 1988; underwent successful angioplasty of LAD and RCA at that time and then had recurrent pain in 1989

Angiography

	1988	1989
RCA:	90% proximal third	minimal narrowing
LMain:	normal	normal
LAD:	total occlusion in proximal third	minimal narrowing
LCX:	moderate disease in midzone	severe stenosis at bifurcation with OM
LV:	normal	normal

Equipment

Guide	Dilatation Catheter	Wire
RCA: FR4 SH	3 mm Profile Plus	0.014 FS
LAD: JL4	3 mm Profile Plus	0.014 FS
LCX: JL4	2 mm SULP	0.014 HTF

Strategy and Procedure

The patient's first presentation was with a totally occluded LAD and severe lesion in the proximal RCA. It was decided to do the LAD first because this was believed to be the least likely vessel to succeed. The 0.014 FS wire was passed quite easily across the area of total obstruction and into the distal vessel. Balloon inflations were carried out through the area of total occlusion (D), and a patent vessel but with some apparent dissection was demonstrated (E,F). Because of the dissection, the patient was kept on heparin for 3 days and then returned to the laboratory, and a good persistent result of the LAD angioplasty was ascertained.
Attention was then turned to the right coronary artery, and an FR4 guide with side holes was used, with a 3 mm balloon over a 0.014 FS wire (H). A good angiographic result was achieved (I). The patient did well for 9 months and then had some pain and was restudied, and good results in all areas were ascertained. She had further pain 1½ years after the first angioplasty, and was restudied and found to have progression of disease in the LCX, with good persistent results in the RCA and LAD (J,K). Because of the bifurcation of the LCX, a kissing balloon angioplasty of that vessel was the procedure of choice. An FL4 guide was used, and two 2.0 mm SULP balloon catheters were advanced over two HTF 0.014 wires. The OM branch artery was wired first, and the main circumflex, second. The balloon was passed into the OM branch first and inflations carried out at 7 atm for 45 sec, and then the balloon was withdrawn and injection showed a good result in that vessel. The balloon was then advanced into the ongoing circumflex and inflations carried out (N). Postangioplasty angiography showed good results in all views (O,P). She has done very well clinically for 1 year postprocedure.

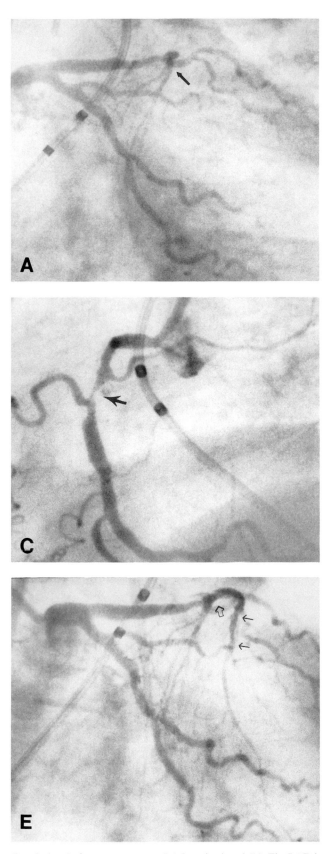

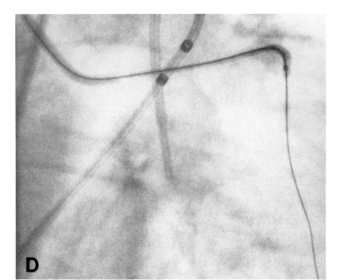

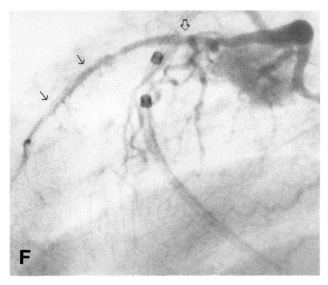

Case 9. A: Left coronary artery, RAO projection, 3/88. The LAD is totally occluded in its proximal third (arrow). B: Left coronary artery, LAO projection, 1988. The total occlusion of the LAD is seen (solid arrow), and there is some distal filling of the midzone of the LAD (open arrow). C: Right coronary artery, left lateral projection, 1988. Severe proximal stenosis (arrow). D: Left coronary artery, RAO projection.

Balloon inflated in total occlusion. E: Left coronary artery, RAO projection. Antegrade flow in LAD postangioplasty. The area of total occlusion (open arrow) is followed by a long area postdilatation (small arrows) that appears to be dissected. F: Left coronary artery, left lateral projection. Postangioplasty (see E).

See following pages for continuation of figures.

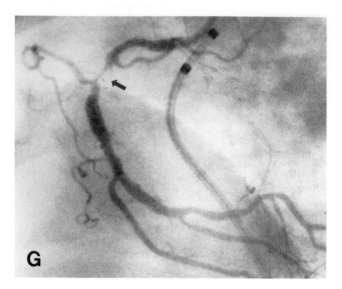

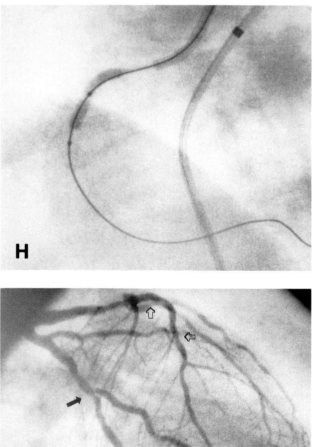

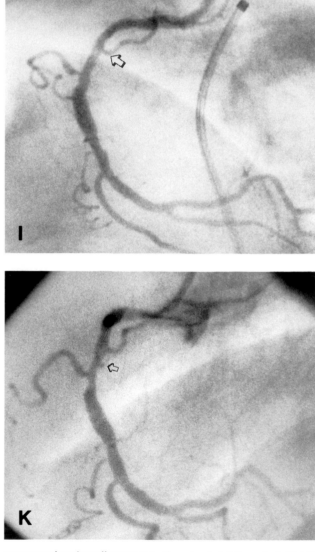

Case 9. G: Right coronary artery, LAO projection. Severe proximal lesion (arrow). **H:** Right coronary artery, LAO projection. Balloon inflated at lesion. **I:** Right coronary artery, LAO projection. Postangioplasty (arrow). **J:** Left coronary artery, RAO projection, 9/89. Demon-strates continued excellent patency of previously totally occluded LAD (open arrows) and new severe disease in the circumflex (solid arrow). **K:** Right coronary artery, LAO projection, 9/89. Continued excellent patency of the proximal right coronary artery (arrow).

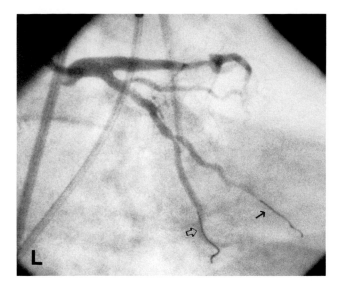

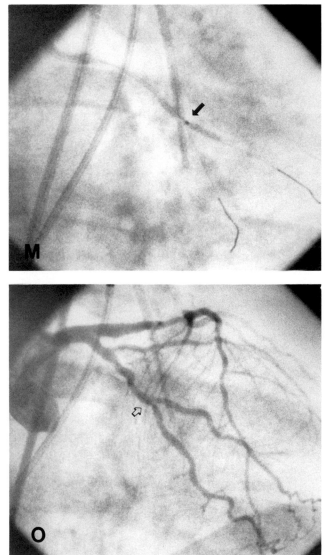

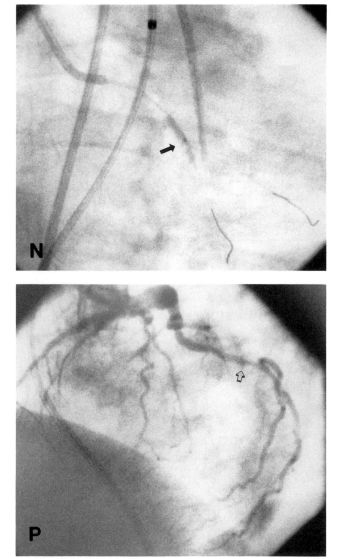

Case 9. L: Left coronary artery, RAO projection. Two-wire systems in circumflex with wires in both the obtuse marginal branch (solid arrow) and the main circumflex (open arrow). M: Left coronary artery, RAO projection. Balloon inflated in obtuse marginal branch (arrow).

N: Left coronary artery, RAO projection. Balloon inflated in main circumflex (arrow). O: Left coronary artery, RAO projection. Postangioplasty (arrow). P: Left coronary artery, LAO projection. Postangioplasty (arrow).

CASE NUMBER 10

Clinical
61-year-old man with unstable angina and a positive thallium treadmill with anterior reversible defect

Angiography

RCA:	normal
LMain:	normal
LAD:	90% narrowing in proximal third involving the origin of the first diagonal branch
LCX:	normal
LV:	normal

Equipment

Guide	Dilatation Catheter	Wire
8.3 F medium brachial JL3.5	2.5 SULP; 2.0 SULP	0.014 FS

Strategy and Procedure

The severe proximal lesion in the LAD involved the origin of the major diagonal branch (A). It was believed that the diagonal branch was borderline, but probably big enough to bypass and therefore should be protected. The brachial-femoral approach was used. For both vessels, 0.014 FS wires were used, and the LADD was wired with a 2.0 balloon, the LAD with a 2.5 balloon through the brachial guide (B). Balloon inflations in the LAD were carried out first to 7 atm and then the balloon withdrawn into the brachial guide (C,D). The balloon was then advanced into the LADD and inflations at 7 atm carried out (D). Guiding catheter injections then showed adequate flow in the LAD, but poor flow in the LADD (E). Repeat dilatations were carried out in the same sequence at 7 atm for 1 min each (F,G). Subsequently, guiding catheter injections showed adequate flow in the LAD and no flow in the LADD (H). A 5 atm inflation was then carried out in the LAD with the uninflated balloon in the LADD to act as a stent during the inflation in the LAD (I). This restored some flow in the LADD (J,K). The wire was then withdrawn from the minor vessel (LADD) and a 4 mm, 1 min inflation carried out in the LAD (L). Subsequent injections showed good flow in the LAD and very slow and poor flow in the LADD (M,N). The patient was clinically stable with no chest pain and no EKG changes, and it was believed that the diagonal branch was not important enough to consider sending the patient to surgery in the face of a patent LAD. Three months later, the patient returned with recurrent angina. He was studied and found to have a recurrence in the LAD. Of interest is the fact that the LADD again had flow in it (O,P). Because of the previous experience with the LADD, it was decided just to dilate the LAD with a 3 mm balloon, which was carried out (Q) with excellent angiographic results (R,S,T). It is of further interest that flow did continue in the LADD in spite of no protection of the vessel at this second procedure.

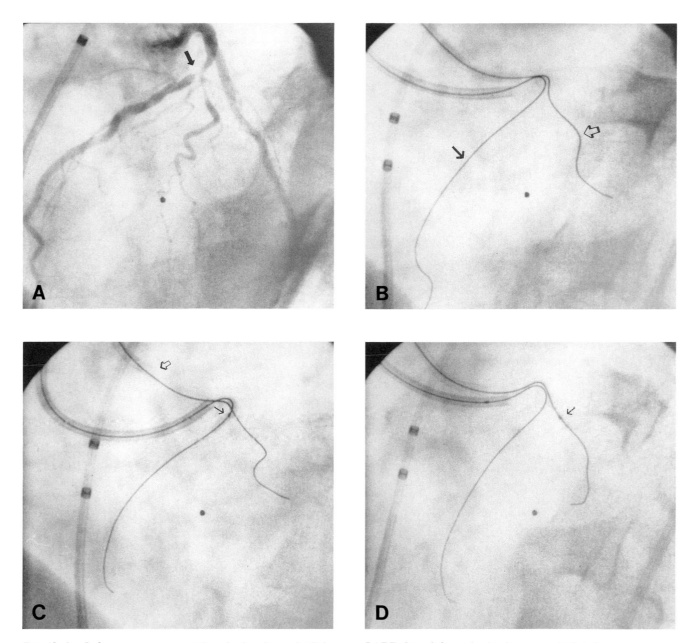

Case 10. A: Left coronary artery, LAO projection. Severe LAD lesion at bifurcation of major diagonal branch involving the origin of LADD (arrow). **B:** Left coronary artery, LAO projection. A 0.014 wire is in LAD through brachial guide (solid arrow). A 0.014 wire is in LADD through femoral guide (open arrow). **C:** Left coronary artery, LAO projection. Balloon inflated in LAD (solid arrow). Note withdrawn femoral guide tip (open arrow). **D:** Left coronary artery, LAO projection. Balloon inflated in LADD (arrow).

See following pages for continuation of figures.

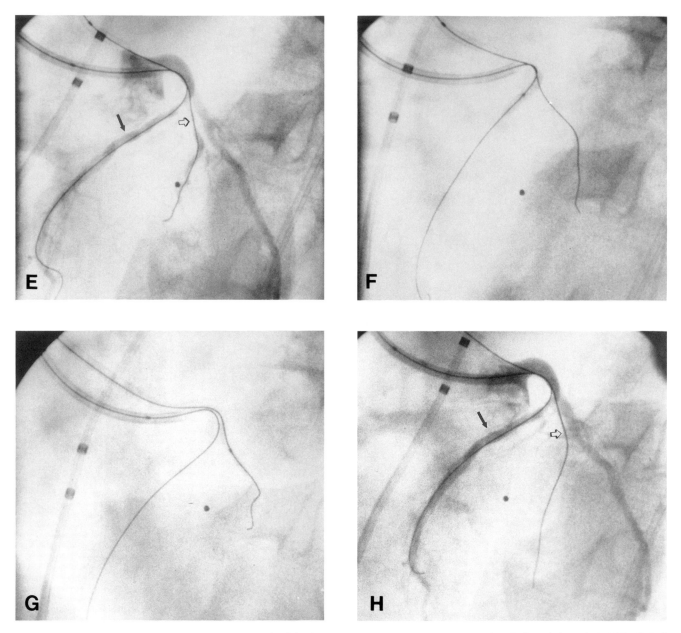

Case 10. E: Left coronary artery, LAO projection. Guide injection through brachial guide shows adequate flow in LAD (solid arrow) and area of spasm/dissection in proximal LADD (open arrow). **F:** Left coronary artery, LAO projection. Balloon inflated in LAD. **G:** Left coronary artery, LAO projection. Balloon inflated in LADD. **H:** Left coronary artery, LAO projection. Guiding catheter injection through brachial guide shows adequate flow in LAD (solid arrow) and no flow in LADD (open arrow).

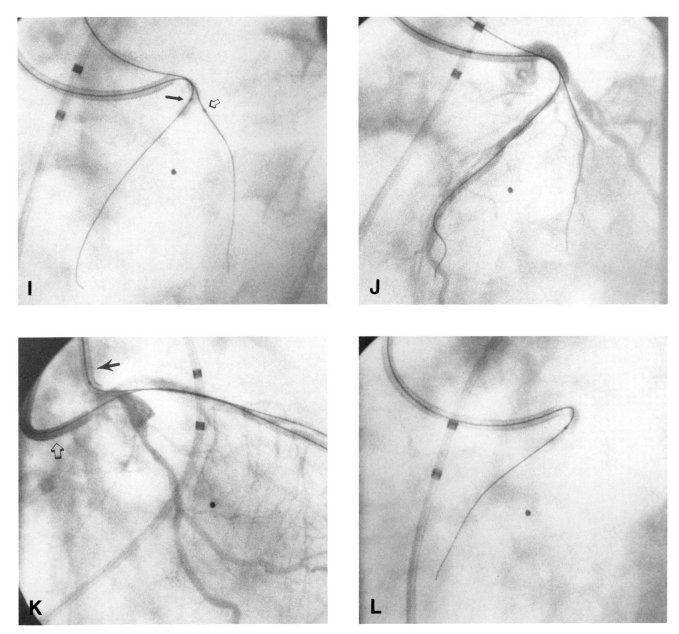

Case 10. I: Left coronary artery, LAO projection. Balloon inflated in LAD (solid arrow), with uninflated balloon in LADD as stent (open arrow). **J:** Left coronary artery, LAO projection. Adequate flow in LAD and better flow in LADD. **K:** Left coronary artery, RAO projec- tion. Injection through femoral guide (solid arrow). Note withdrawn position of brachial guide (open arrow). **L:** Left coronary artery, LAO projection. Wire withdrawn from LADD and balloon inflated in LAD.

See following pages for continuation of figures.

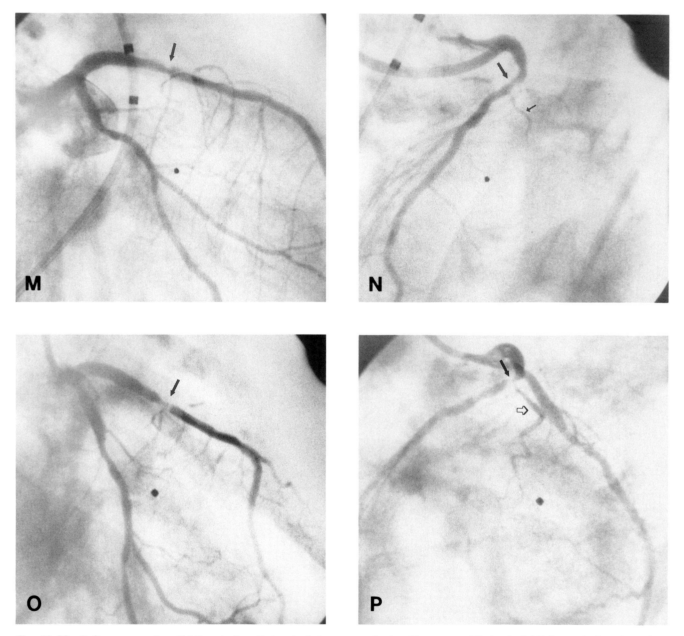

Case 10. M: Left coronary artery, RAO projection. Postangioplasty lumen in LAD (arrow). **N:** Left coronary artery, LAO projection. Postangioplasty view with adequate flow in LAD (large arrow) and minimal flow in LADD (small arrow). **O:** Left coronary artery, RAO projection. Recurrence of lesion in LAD 3 months later (arrow). **P:** Left coronary artery, LAO projection. Recurrence in LAD (solid arrow) and returned flow in LADD (open arrow).

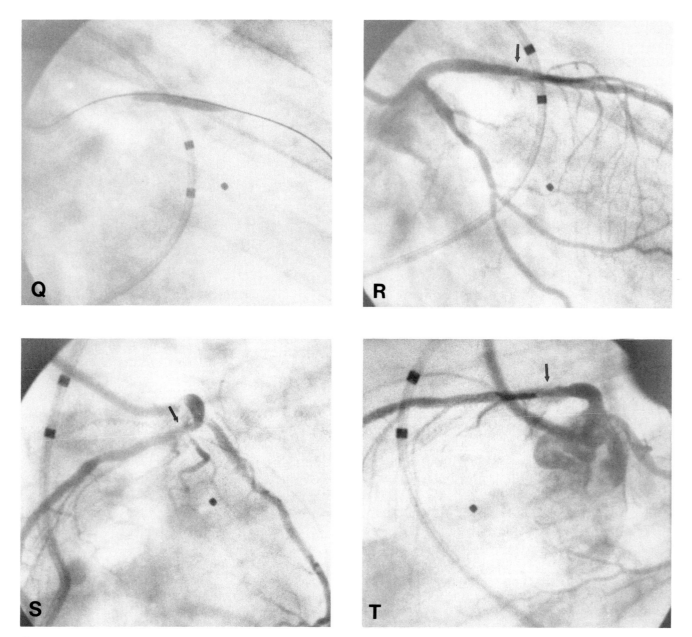

Case 10. Q: Left coronary artery, RAO projection. Three millimeter balloon inflated at LAD lesion. **R:** Left coronary artery, RAO projection. Postangioplasty (arrow). **S:** Left coronary artery, LAO projection. Postangioplasty (arrow). **T:** Left coronary artery, left lateral projection. Postangioplasty (arrow).

CASE NUMBER 11

Clinical   45-year-old man with chronic stable angina and positive treadmill at low workload

Angiography   RCA: total occlusion midzone; collateral filling of distal vessel from left coronary system
                      LMain: normal
                      LAD: total occlusion proximal third with collateral filling at distal vessel
                      LCX: normal
                      LV: normal

Equipment

Guide	Dilatation Catheter	Wire
RCA: JR4, Amplatz left II	2.0 mm SULP: 2.5 mm SULP	0.014 FS
LAD: JL4	2.0 mm SULP; 2.5 mm SULP; 3.0 mm SULP	0.014 FS

Strategy and Procedure

Diagnostic angiography showed total obstructions of both the RCA and the LAD, with good collateral filling of the distal vessels (A G). The RCA was approached first. A standard JR4 guide did not give appropriate backup, and an Amplatz left II guide was used to provide appropriate backup. The 0.014 USCI Flex-J wire was passed across the lesion with considerable backup and with stiffening of the tip of the wire with the balloon catheter. The 2.0 mm balloon catheter was inflated throughout the area of disease in an antegrade manner, and considerable difficulty was encountered in advancing the balloon catheter throughout the area of disease. There was indentation in the proximal area of total disease (H) until 12 atm was used. The balloon then crossed the entire lesion, and inflations were carried out throughout the area of disease, the wire extended and replaced with a 2.5 mm balloon, and further inflations carried out. Twenty-eight separate balloon inflations were carried out to achieve antegrade flow in this vessel (I–K). Ten days later, the patient was returned to the laboratory, and injections in the right coronary artery confirmed the presence of a good long-term result (L). The LAD was then approached. A JL4 guide was used, and the total occlusion in the LAD was crossed with a 0.014 FS wire, with considerable difficulty. The total occlusion was finally crossed by stiffening the tip of the wire with the balloon catheter. The 2.0 mm SULP balloon was passed into the region of total stenosis, and antegrade inflations of 4–7 atm for 45 sec each were used to completely open the vessel. The wire was then extended, and a 2.5 mm balloon utilized with inflations at 6 atm throughout the area. The extension wire was again used and the 2.5 mm balloon replaced with a 3.0 mm SULP and nine dilatations performed at 6 atm for 45–120 sec. Following this, an excellent antegrade lumen was achieved and good antegrade flow seen in the LAD (Q,R). The patient has continued to do well clinically with a normal thallium treadmill test 18 months following the procedures.

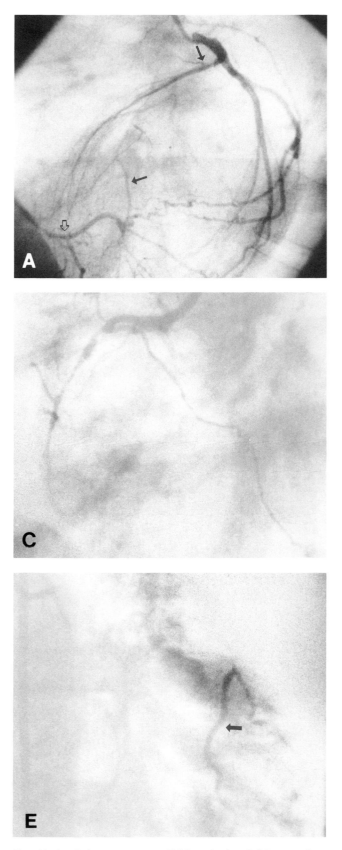

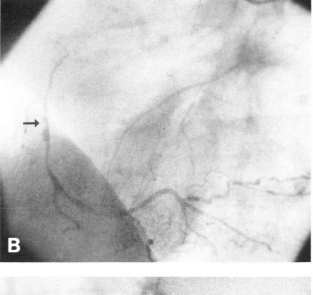

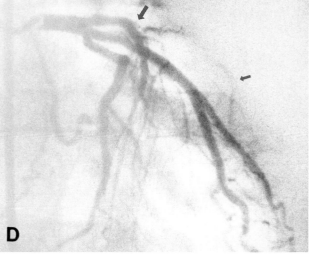

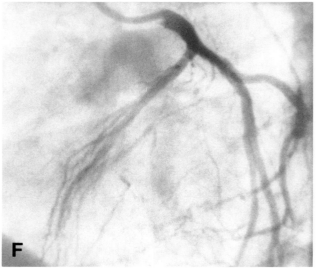

Case 11. A: Left coronary artery, LAO projection. Solid arrows show total occlusion of LAD and proximal third, with collateral filling of distal LAD. Collateral filling of distal right coronary is seen (open arrow). **B:** Left coronary artery, LAO projection. Late phase of injection shows collateral filling of RCA (arrow). **C:** Right coronary artery, LAO projection. Long segmental disease culminating in total occlu- sion. **D:** Left coronary artery, RAO projection. Total occlusion of LAD at proximal (large arrow), with faint collateral filling of distal vessel (small arrow). **E:** Left coronary artery, RAO projection. Late phase of D. Collateral filling of distal LAD (arrow). **F:** Left coronary artery, LAO projection.

See following pages for continuation of figures.

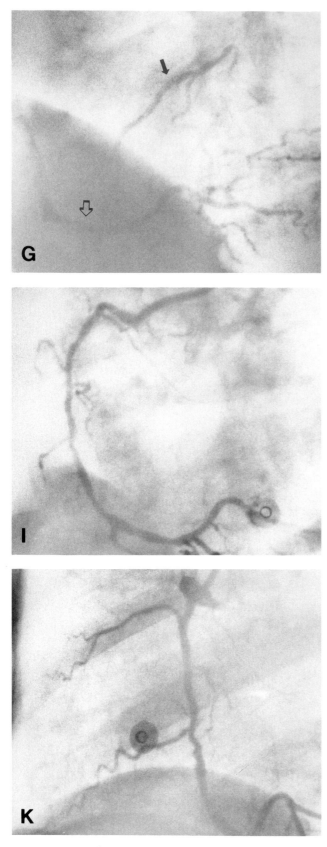

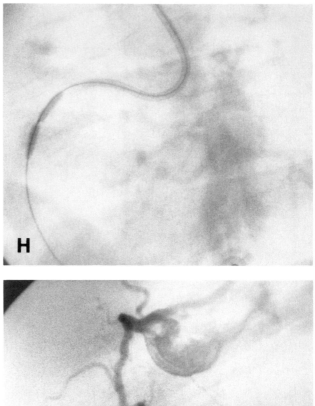

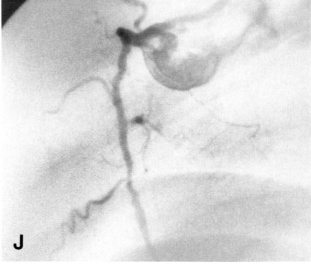

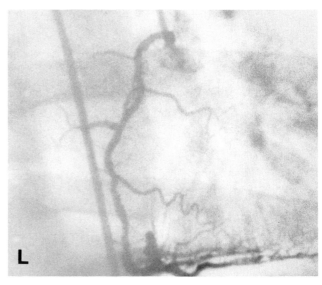

Case 11. G: Left coronary artery, LAO projection. Late phase of F, showing collateral filling of distal LAD (solid arrow) and right coronary artery (open arrow). **H:** Right coronary artery, LAO projection. Amplatz guide and initial balloon inflation in right coronary artery showing indentation. **I:** Right coronary artery, LAO projection. Post- angioplasty, with reestablished antegrade flow. **J:** Right coronary artery, left lateral projection. Postangioplasty. **K:** Right coronary artery, left lateral projection. Four weeks postangioplasty. **L:** Right coronary artery, RAO projection. Four weeks postangioplasty.

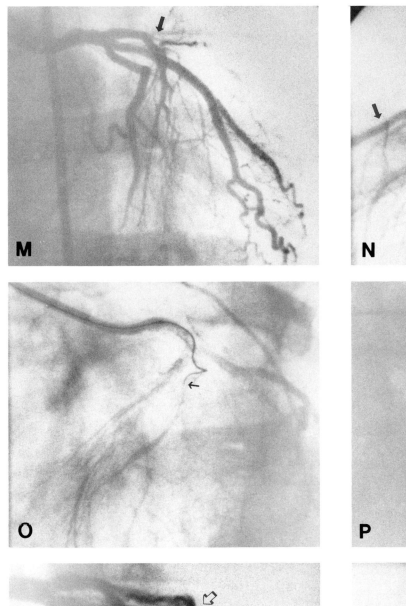

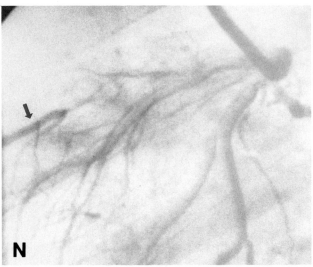

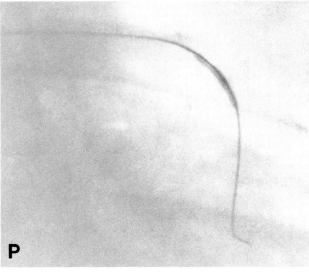

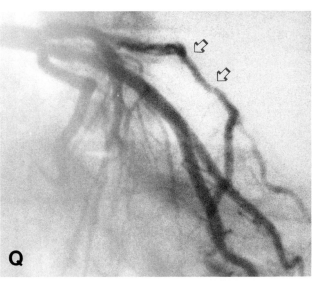

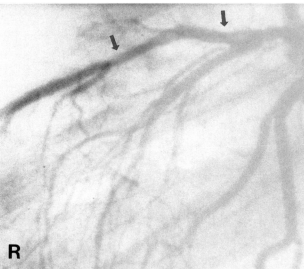

Case 11. M: Left coronary artery, RAO projection. Total occlusion of LAD (arrow). **N:** Left coronary artery, left lateral projection, late phase. Collateral distal filling of LAD seen (arrow). **O:** Left coronary artery, LAO projection. A 0.014 wire tip has nearly traversed total occlusion (arrow). **P:** Left coronary artery, RAO projection. Wire across total occlusion in distal vessel with balloon inflated. **Q:** Left coronary artery, RAO projection. Recanalization of previous long area of total occlusion (arrows). **R:** Left coronary artery, left lateral projection. See Q.

CASE NUMBER 12

Clinical

51-year-old man with first angiogram in 1984 following an anterior myocardial infarction that showed diffuse disease in the LAD and no significant disease elsewhere, treated medically; return admission in 1989 for severe exertional angina and positive treadmill

Angiography

	1984	1989
RCA:	minor distal disease	95% mid right
LMain:	normal	normal
LAD:	50% mid lesion	total occlusion proximal third; collateralization distal vessel
LADD:	diffuse disease, slow flow	
LCX:	moderate lesions	95% LCX; 80% OM
LV:	anterior hypokinesia	anterior hypokinesia

Equipment

Guide	Dilatation Catheter	Wire
RCA: JR4	3.0 mm ACX; 3.5 mm ACX	0.014 HTF
LCX: JL4	2.0 mm SULP; 2.5 mm SULP	0.014 HTF

Strategy and Procedure

The current study shows progression of disease from the 1984 angiograms (A–F). It was decided that each lesion was independently treatable with angioplasty, other than the totally occluded LAD that supplied an area of infarcted myocardium. RCA was approached first with an FR4 guide. This seated coaxially, and at this stage, and the subsequent stage, an intraaortic balloon pump was in the room and available and a 6 French arterial sheath was positioned in the left femoral artery for immediate access. The RCA was first dilated with a 3 mm ACX balloon over a 0.014 HTF wire, two inflations at 7 atm for 60 sec were carried out, and the balloon exchanged for a 3.5 mm ACX balloon with which two more inflations of 7 atm for 60 sec were carried out. Postdilatation angiography showed an excellent result (H,I). The patient was returned to the laboratory the next day, and following sterile exchange of the sheath, an injection confirmed an excellent result in the RCA. An FL4 guide was used and a 2 mm SULP balloon catheter advanced into the main circumflex and inflations at 7 atm for 45 sec carried out several times (K). A good result in the ongoing circumflex was obtained (L), and the same wire was then passed across the OM branch and a 2.5 mm SULP balloon positioned at the lesion. Inflations were carried out at 7 atm for as long as 1 min several times and injection showed good flow and patency. The postangioplasty angiography demonstrated good results in both circumflex vessels (N). The patient has done well clinically for 1 year postprocedure.

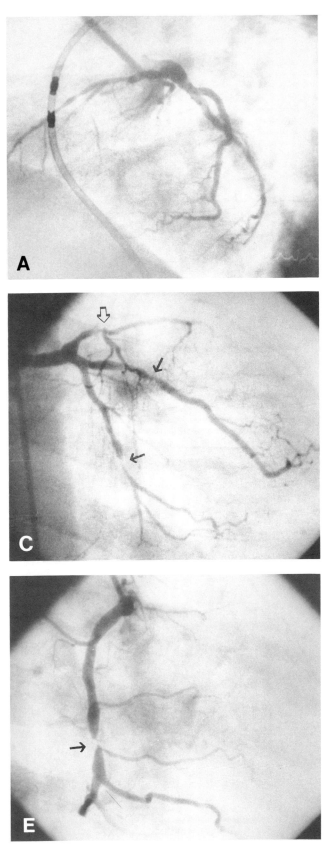

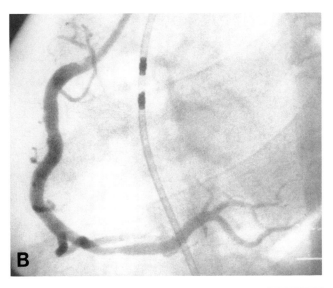

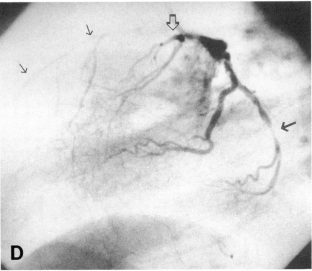

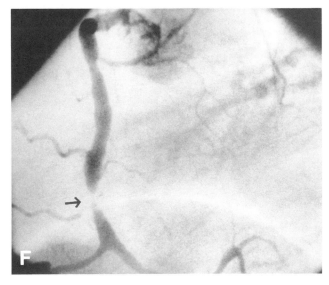

Case 12. A: Left coronary artery, left lateral projection, 1984. **B:** Right coronary artery, LAO projection, 1984. **C:** Left coronary artery, RAO projection, 1989. Severe stenosis in circumflex coronary artery (bottom solid arrow) and first obtuse marginal branch of circumflex coronary artery (top solid arrow), and total occlusion of the LAD (open arrow). **D:** Left coronary artery, left lateral projection. Severe lesion in circumflex (large solid arrow), total occlusion of LAD (open arrow), and collateral filling of distal LAD (small arrows). **E:** Right coronary artery, 1989. New severe lesion in right main trunk (arrow). **F:** Right coronary artery, 1989, left lateral projection. See E.

See following pages for continuation of figures.

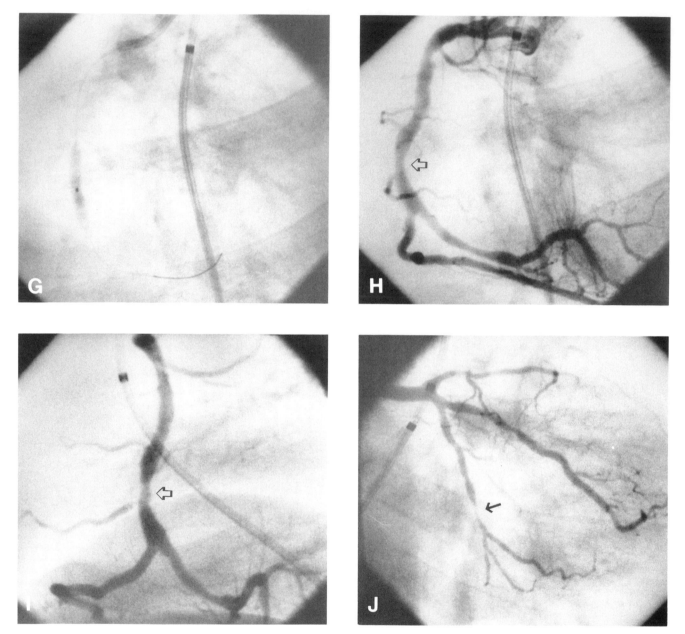

Case 12. G: Right coronary artery, LAO projection. Balloon inflated in lesion. **H:** Right coronary artery, LAO projection. Postangioplasty (arrow). **I:** Right coronary artery, left lateral projection. Postangio- plasty (arrow). **J:** Left coronary artery, RAO projection. Circumflex lesion preangioplasty (arrow).

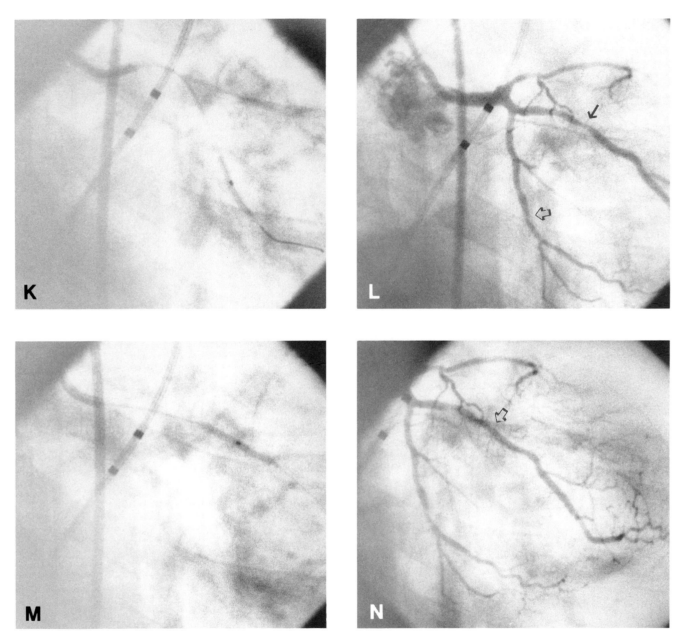

Case 12 K: Left coronary artery, LAO projection. Two millimeter balloon inflated in lesion. **L:** Left coronary artery, RAO projection. Circumflex, postangioplasty (open arrow). Severe lesion in obtuse marginal circumflex branch (solid arrow). **M:** Left coronary artery, RAO projection. Balloon inflated in obtuse marginal circumflex. **N:** Left coronary artery, RAO projection. Obtuse marginal circumflex postangioplasty (arrow).

CASE NUMBER 13

Clinical   55-year-old man admitted with unstable angina and anterior ST and T wave changes; enzymes were normal, and he was sent for angiography

Angiography   RCA: "dominant" mild to moderate irregularities in right main trunk; no collaterals back to left system
LMain: normal
LAD: totally obstructed in proximal third; faint antegrade collateralization of distal vessel
LCX: severe distal disease
LV: apical hypokinesia

Equipment

Guide	Dilatation Catheter	Wire
8.3 F 3 inch medium brachial	2 mm ACX; 2.5 mm ACX	0.014 silicone-coated FS

Strategy and Procedure

The patient was clinically unstable and was shown to have a total obstruction of the LAD (A–D). There also appeared to be moderate disease in the circumflex system involving the bifurcation of the OM branch (B). Because of his clinical syndrome, it was decided to treat the totally occluded LAD and deal with the circumflex at a later date. A short stump of the occluded LAD was best seen in the 15° RAO, 30° cranial view (D), and the spider view was also helpful in wiring the total obstruction (E). The wire was eventually passed across the total obstruction, and attempts to get the 2 mm balloon to cross the lesion with the guide in the standard position were not successful. Therefore, a power position of the brachial guide was used (F). The guide was withdrawn into the more normal position (G) following balloon passage across the lesion. Balloon inflations were carried out at up to 10 atm for as long as 1 min. This produced a patent vessel but an inadequate lumen, and the wire was extended and exchanged for a 2.5 mm ACX balloon, which was positioned at the lesion, and inflations carried out. During the procedure, the midzone of the diagonal branch showed some slow flow, and either spasm or embolic debris was considered. The patient was stable, and nothing was done with that vessel, which eventually cleared. A widely patent vessel was achieved with excellent flow into the distal LAD. The patient has done well clinically and has had a thallium treadmill test that did not show any reversibility in the distribution of the circumflex; he continues to be treated medically.

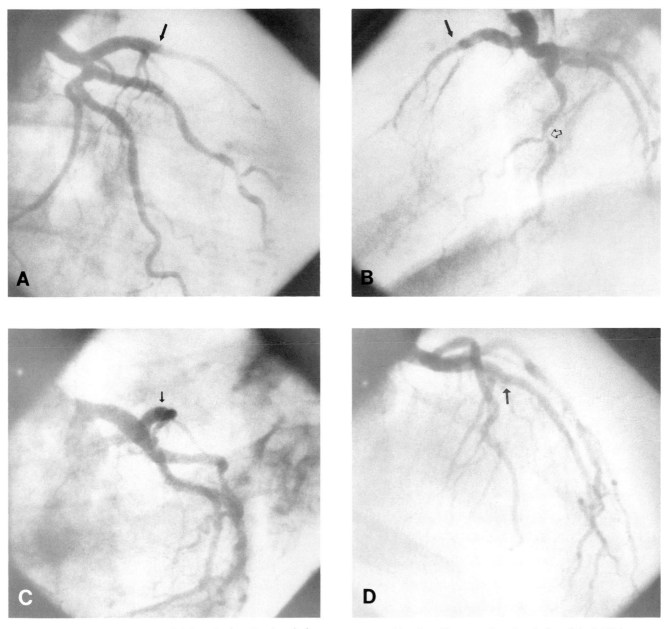

Case 13. A: Left coronary artery, RAO projection. Total occlusion of left anterior descending coronary artery is seen with filling of the diagonal branch just beyond the area of total obstruction (arrow). **B:** Left coronary artery, steep LAO projection. Total occlusion of the LAD is seen at the solid arrow, and the open arrow points out a severe lesion in the high obtuse marginal circumflex branch. **C:** Left coronary artery, spider view. The area of total occlusion of the LAD is seen at the arrow. The acute angle into the LAD from the left main trunk is well evidenced in this view. **D:** Left coronary artery, RAO 15°, cranial 30° projection. A short stump of the totally occluded LAD is seen (arrow).

See following pages for continuation of figures.

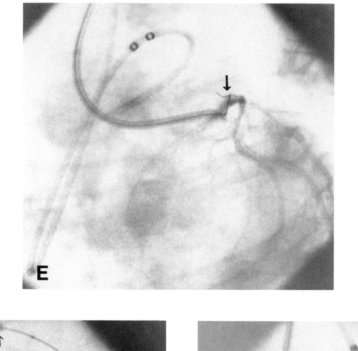

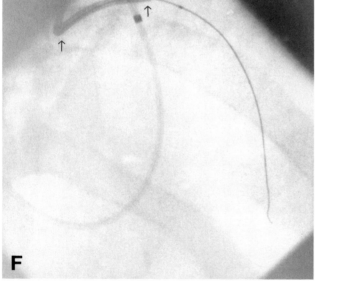

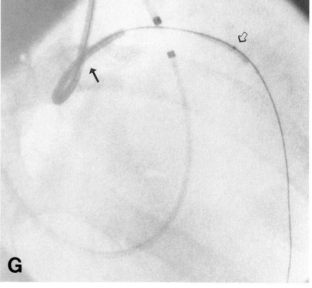

Case 13. E: Left coronary artery, spider projection. This demonstrates the brachial guide seated in the left main trunk and the wire across the total occlusion and traversing the usual area of LAD (arrow). **F:** Left coronary artery, RAO projection. The wire has completely traversed the lesion. The balloon is forced across the lesion by a power position of the brachial guide (arrows). **G:** Left coronary artery, RAO projection. The brachial guide is in its usual position (solid arrow). The balloon is inflated at the site of total occlusion (open arrow).

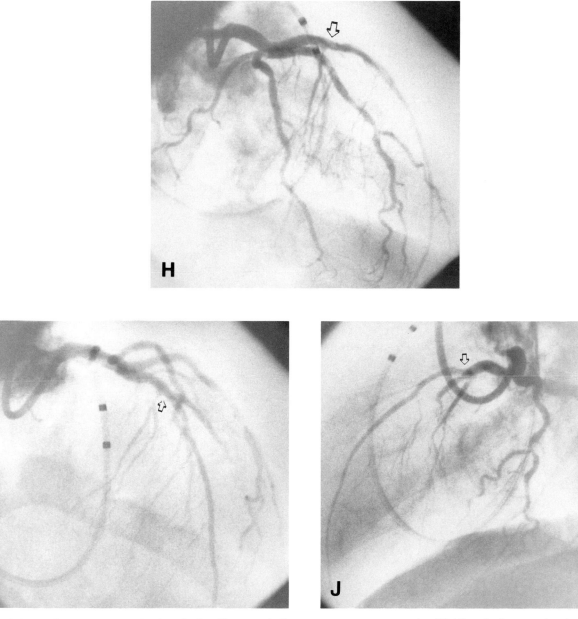

Case 13. H: Left coronary artery, RAO projection. The arrow indicates the previous area of total obstruction, and there is antegrade flow in the LAD with probable diffuse spasm of the distal vessel. **I:** Left coronary artery, angulated RAO projection, postnitroglycerin. Arrow indicates the site of previous total occlusion. **J:** Left coronary artery, left lateral projection. See I.

CASE NUMBER 14

Clinical 42-year-old man first seen at age 38 in 1986 for a total occlusion of the circumflex, successfully treated with angioplasty; returned in 1990 with recurrent chest pain and unstable angina

Angiography

	1986	1990
RCA:	minor disease	total occlusion
LMain:	normal	normal
LAD:	normal	normal
LCX:	totally occluded	normal
LV:	posterior hypokinesia	inferolateral hypokinesia

Equipment

Guide	Dilatation Catheter		Wire	
	1986	1990	1986	1990
JL4/JR4	2.5 mm low profile	2.5 mm ACX; 3.0 mm ACX	0.014 FS	0.014 HTF; 0.014 intermediate

Strategy and Procedure When the patient was first seen in 1986, he presented with an acute syndrome and a total occlusion of the LCX, with no significant disease in the other arteries. This had an abrupt cutoff, suggesting thrombus (A). The 0.014 FS wire buckled at the total occlusion (C), and by advancing the balloon tip over the mandril, this stiffened it enough to cross the total occlusion and provide for balloon inflations (D). The balloon was inflated to 9 atm for as long as 50 sec several times, and an excellent angiographic result was achieved (E). The patient returned with angina in 1990. Diagnostic angiography showed continued excellent patency of the LCX (F) and a new total occlusion of the RCA (G). Intracoronary nitroglycerin provided better distal flow so that the route of the wire could be identified (H,I). An FR4 guide was selected and seated well. The 0.014 HTF wire would not cross the total occlusion, but a 0.014 intermediate wire popped across the area of total occlusion into the distal vessel. The 2.5 mm balloon was positioned at the lesion, and inflations carried out at 8 atm with full balloon inflation at 4 atm (J). Injections then showed reflex distal spasm (K), which cleared with intracoronary nitroglycerin (L). There was a distal lesion that was dilated with a 2.5 mm balloon (M). The wire was extended, and a 3.0 mm balloon positioned at the proximal area of total occlusion and 2 min inflations at 5 atm carried out twice (N). Injections then showed excellent flow and patency and a widely patent artery (O). He has continued to do well 6 months postprocedure.

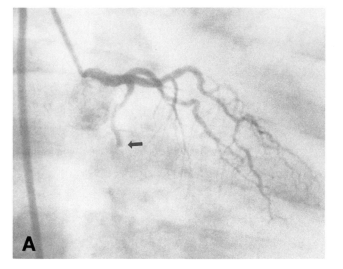

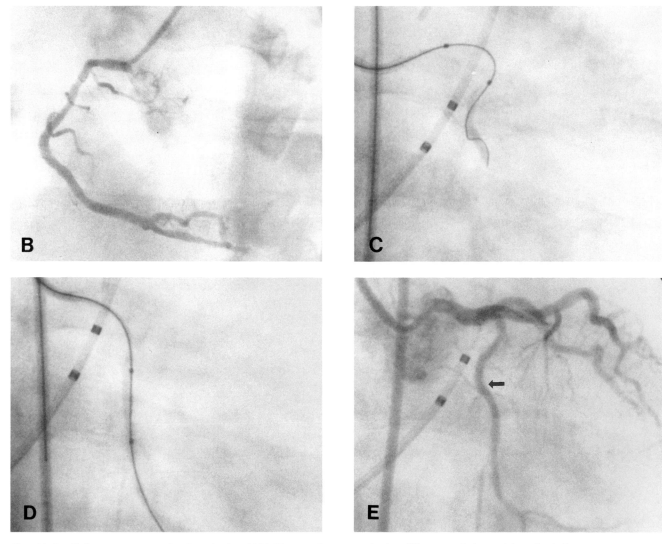

Case 14. A: Left coronary artery, RAO projection, 1986. Blunt total occlusion of circumflex suggesting thrombus (arrow). **B:** Right coronary artery, LAO projection, 1986. **C:** Left coronary artery, RAO projection. Wire tip at total occlusion. **D:** Left coronary artery, RAO projection. Wire across lesion and into distal circumflex with balloon inflated. **E:** Left coronary artery, RAO projection. Postangioplasty. Arrow denotes level of previous total occlusion.

See following pages for continuation of figures.

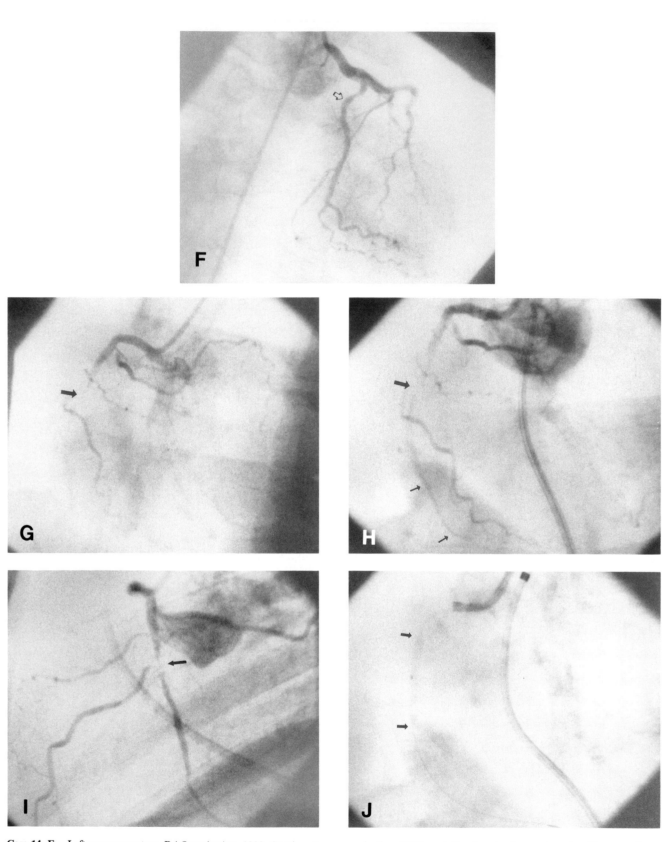

Case 14. F: Left coronary artery, RAO projection, 1990. Continued patency of circumflex (arrow). **G:** Right coronary artery, LAO projection, 1990. Total proximal occlusion of right coronary artery that had previously had minor disease (arrow). **H:** Right coronary artery, LAO projection, 1990, postnitroglycerin. Severe stenosis still present (large arrow), but some improvement in antegrade flow (small arrows). **I:** Right coronary artery, left lateral projection. **J:** Right coronary artery, LAO projection. Balloon inflated at site of total occlusion.

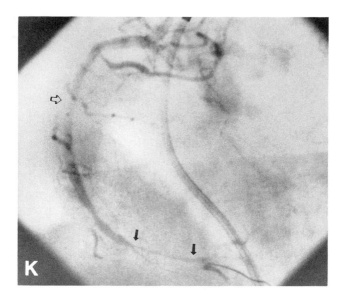

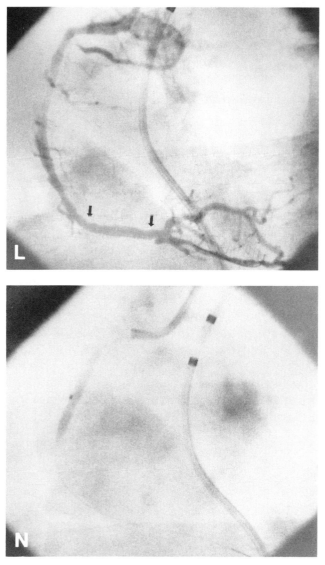

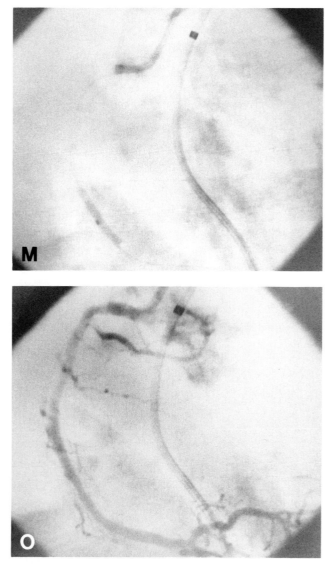

Case 14. K: Right coronary artery, LAO projection. Patent lumen at previous total occlusion (open arrow), and severe distal reflex spasm in distal vessel (solid arrows). **L:** Right coronary artery, LAO projection, postintracoronary nitroglycerin. The distal spasm has been re-lieved (arrows). **M:** Right coronary artery, LAO projection. Balloon inflated at site of distal narrowing. **N:** Right coronary artery, LAO projection. Balloon inflated at site of previous total occlusion. **O:** Right coronary artery, LAO projection. Postangioplasty.

CASE NUMBER 15

Clinical

46-year-old man with admission for inferior myocardial infarction; diagnostic studies showed total occlusion of the right coronary artery with collateralization from the left (A–C) and an inferior scar; a thallium treadmill test showed reversible inferior ischemia, and the patient continued to have angina-type pain with exertion in spite of maximal medical therapy

Angiography

RCA: total occlusion, midzone
LMain: normal
LAD: normal
LCX: normal
LV: inferior scar

Equipment

Guide	Dilatation Catheter	Wire
JR4	2.0 mm ACX; 2.5 mm ACX	0.014 HTF
0.014 intermediate

Strategy and Procedure

The proximal RCA appeared to be diffusely diseased proximal to the total occlusion, and there was good collateral filling of the distal vessel from the left coronary system (A–C). A JR4 guide seated nicely. Attempts to get the 0.014 HTF wire to cross the total occlusion were not successful, even with stiffening of the wire by the balloon catheter. The balloon catheter would not advance through the area of proximal disease. The wire was therefore exchanged for a 0.014 intermediate wire, and this successfully traversed the total occlusion and entered the distal vessel. Balloon inflations were then carried out at the proximal lesion first, and then throughout the area of long disease in the vessel (D–H). Injections then showed an excellent lumen (I), but a small dissection in the proximal third of the vessel. It was decided to mold that area with a slightly larger balloon, and the wire was extended and the balloon exchanged for a 2.5 mm ACX. Overlapping inflations were then made throughout the area of total occlusion at 4 atm and then in the proximal area where the crack had appeared at 10 atm for 3 min each time. Good flow resulted, and an adequate lumen was achieved throughout the right main trunk (K, L).

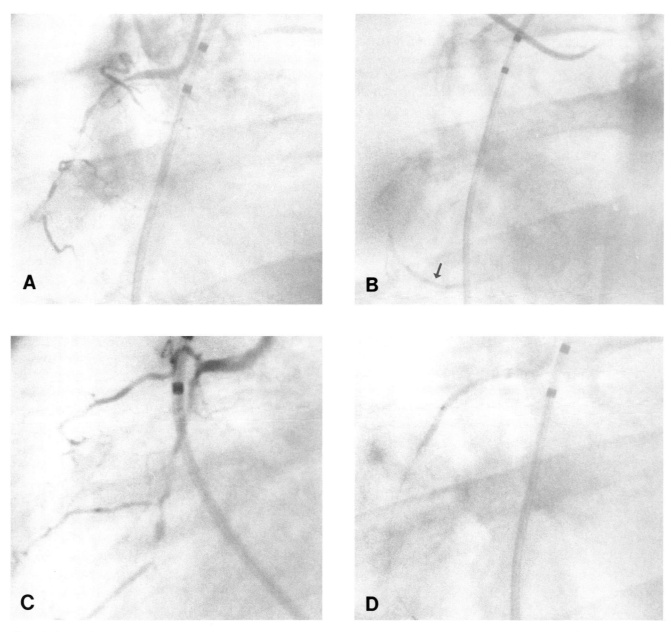

Case 15. A: Right coronary artery, LAO projection. Severe diffuse proximal disease with total obstruction in midzone. **B:** Left coronary artery, LAO projection. Late phase of injection showing collateral filling in distal right coronary artery (arrow). **C:** Right coronary artery, left lateral projection. **D:** Right coronary artery, LAO projection. Two millimeter balloon inflated in proximal area to provide distal access.

See following pages for continuation of figures.

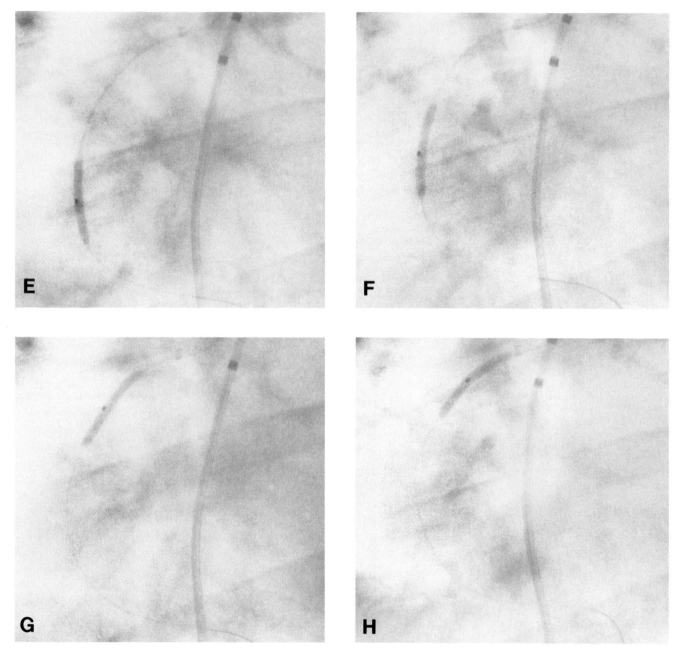

Case 15. E: Right coronary artery, LAO projection. **F:** Right coronary artery, LAO projection. **G:** Right coronary artery, LAO projection. **H:** Right coronary artery, LAO projection.

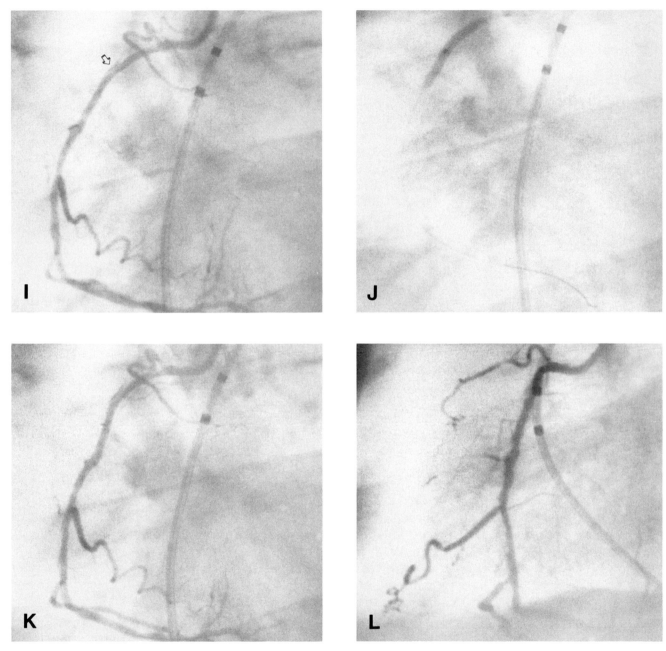

Case 15. I: Right coronary artery, LAO projection. Antegrade flow reestablished through the area of severe disease and total obstruction of the right coronary artery with good distal filling. A small linear dissection in proximal vessel (arrow). **J:** Right coronary artery, LAO projection. Molding inflation. **K:** Right coronary artery, LAO projection. Postangioplasty. **L:** Right coronary artery, left lateral projection. Postangioplasty.

CASE NUMBER 16

Clinical
80-year-old man with previous bypass surgery in 1981; returned in 1990 with unstable angina

Angiography

RCA:	totally occluded
Graft to PDA:	normal
Graft to PL:	90% narrowing in distal third
LMain:	normal
LAD:	totally occluded
Graft to LAD:	patent
LCX:	totally occluded
Graft to LCX:	patent
LV:	normal

Equipment

Guide	Dilatation Catheter	Wire
8 F multipurpose	2.5 mm ACX; 3.0 mm ACX	0.014 modified Veriflex; 0.014 HTF; 0.014 intermediate

Strategy and Procedure

The straight takeoff of the graft allowed excellent seating of the multipurpose tip. To pass through the proximal portion of the 10-year-old graft with decreased likelihood of digging up the lining, a 0.014 Veriflex wire was modified into a "U" shape and passed to the area just proximal to the lesion (B). The deflated balloon was then passed over the modified wire, and the wire removed and replaced with a 0.014 HTF wire, which was believed to be more appropriate to cross the lesion (C,D). There was some buckling at the lesion, and it was necessary to use a 0.014 intermediate wire to cross that area of stenosis. The distal vessel was adequately wired, and balloon inflations with a 2.5 mm balloon carried out at 8 and 10 atm for as long as 1 min, and then an exchange was done for a 3.0 mm balloon and two 60 sec inflations at 8 atm were carried out. Injections then showed good flow and patency, and the postangioplasty angiograms demonstrated an excellent lumen (F). He continues to do well 6 months following the procedure with no recurrence of symptoms.

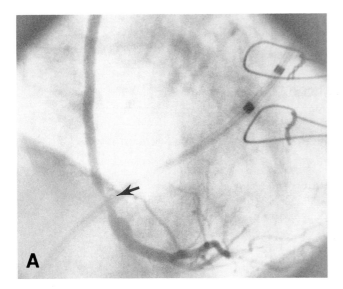

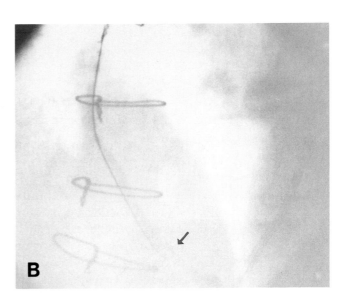

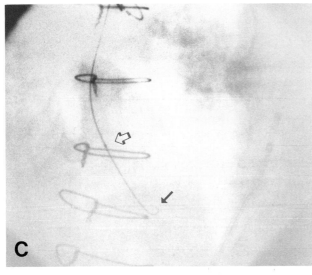

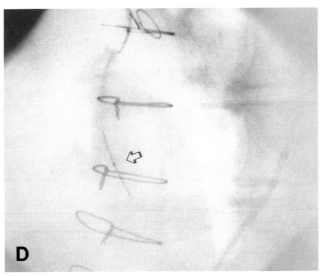

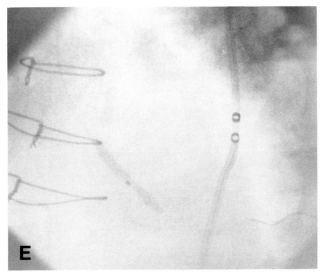

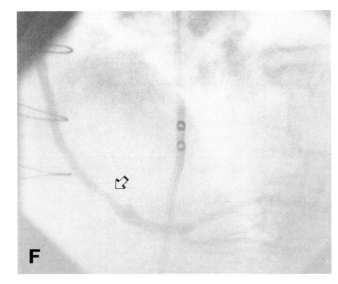

Case 16. A: RCA bypass, LAO projection. Severe lesion in distal third of graft (arrow). **B:** RCA bypass, LAO projection. "U"-shaped leading wire passed to just proximal obstruction (arrow). **C:** RCA bypass, LAO projection. "U" wire proximal to obstruction (solid arrow), and balloon advanced over wire to midgraft (open arrow). **D:** RCA graft, LAO projection. Wire exchange (arrow). See text. **E:** RCA graft, LAO projection. Balloon inflation. **F:** RCA graft, LAO projection. Postangioplasty (arrow).

CASE NUMBER 17

Clinical   70-year-old man with Class IV angina and history of five previous bypasses

Angiography

RCA:	occluded
LMain:	normal
LAD:	occluded
LCX:	occluded
CABG-RCA:	patent
CABG-LADD:	occluded
CABG-LCX OM:	occluded
CABG-LAD:	severe stenosis
CABG-LCX:	patent

Equipment

Guide	Dilatation Catheter	Wire
JR4 SH	3.0 mm skinny; 3.5 mm Stack	0.0.14 HTF

Strategy and Procedure

The patient's lesion in the graft to the LAD appeared to be discrete, but the entire LAD graft is diffusely irregular (A). The wire was passed easily across the stenosis and into the distal LAD. Good backup was achieved from the guide. The 3 mm balloon was inflated to 9 atm several times for as long as 2 min (B). A reasonable result was initially achieved (C). The patient then had the onset of chest pain, and injections showed filling in of the area of dilatation and poor distal flow (D). Further inflations were carried out with a 3 mm balloon that reestablished adequate flow (E,F). There did appear to be dissection or thrombus in the area of dilatation (F). An increase in chest pain occurred with demonstrated nearly absent flow in the distal graft and vessel (G). A 3.5 mm Stack balloon was then inserted and positioned at the lesion (H). Proximal injections with the balloon inflated showed good flow through the inflated balloon into the distal vessel (I). A 10 min inflation at 6 atm showed resolution of the filling defect in the area of original dilatation, but a new lesion 2 cm distal to the original (J). This was dilated for 7 min at 6 atm (K). A good ultimate result was achieved (L).

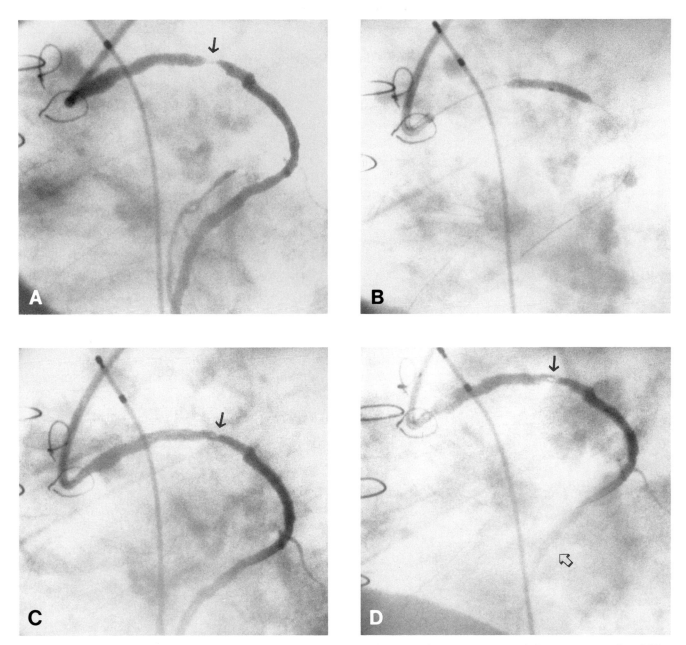

Case 17. A: LAD graft, LAO projection. Severe stenosis in midzone of graft (arrow), with good flow to distal vessel. **B:** LAD graft, LAO projection. Three millimeter balloon inflated in body of graft. **C:** LAD graft, LAO projection. Improvement in lumen, but suggestion of filling defect (arrow). **D:** LAD graft, LAO projection. Worsening of filling defect (solid arrow) and slow flow in distal graft (open arrow).

See following pages for continuation of figures.

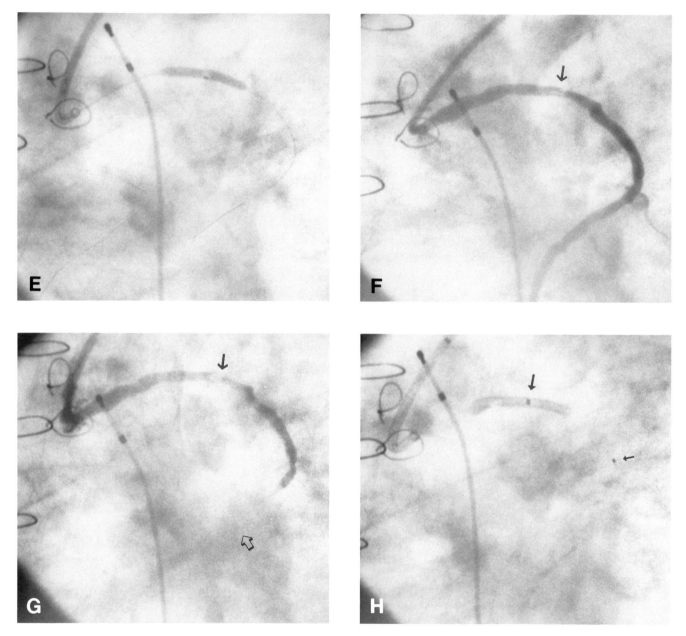

Case 17. E: LAD graft, LAO projection. Repeat molding balloon inflation. **F:** LAD graft, LAO projection. Persistent filling defect in graft (arrow). **G:** LAD graft, LAO projection. Near total occlusion of graft by thrombus/dissection (solid arrow) and virtually no flow in distal graft (open arrow). **H:** 3.5 mm Stack balloon catheter in position (arrows).

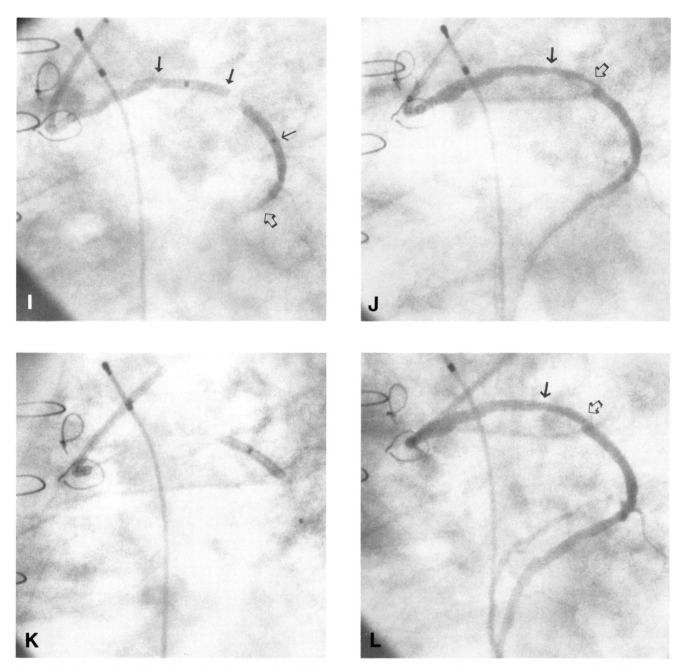

Case 17. I: LAD graft, LAO projection. Stack balloon inflated (solid arrows), and proximal injection demonstrates antegrade flow through the catheter with balloon inflated (open arrow). **J:** LAD graft, LAO projection. Improvement in lumen at original lesion site (solid arrow) and apparent new lesion downstream (open arrow). **K:** LAD graft, LAO projection. Stack balloon inflated at distal lesion. **L:** LAD graft, LAO projection. Postangioplasty results of original lesion (solid arrow) and secondary lesion (open arrow).

CASE NUMBER 18

Clinical
66-year-old woman with bypass surgery in 1984, returned with angina in 1988

Angiography

RCA:	mild disease, left
LMain:	normal
LAD:	total occlusion
LCX:	total occlusion
SVG to LAD:	moderate disease
SVG to LCX:	severe midzone stenosis

Equipment

Guide	Dilatation Catheter	Wire
JL4	3 mm ACX; 3.5 mm SULP	0.014 HTF

Strategy and Procedure

The patient had developed a severe lesion in the midzone of a bypass graft that was nearly 5 years old. The wire was carefully passed across the lesion and into the distal circumflex vessel. Balloon inflations with a 3 mm ACX balloon were carried out to 8 atm for as long as 1 min. A better lumen was achieved, but significant haziness and a suggestion of a dissection was present (B,C). A 3.5 mm balloon was inserted and inflations carried out to 7 atm for as long as 1 min $\times$ 3. This molded an adequate lumen, but haziness in the area of dilatation continued with a suggestion of irregular flaplike material, with no hang-up of contrast in that area (E,F). It was elected to maintain the patient on heparin and return her to the laboratory in several days to assess the healing of the graft. This was done 4 days later, and the graft appeared to be less irregular in the area of dilatation (G,H). The patient had some recurrent chest pain and in a repeat study 3 months later, the lumen of the bypass appeared to have healed perfectly (I,J). She was maintained on antiplatelet agents during that period of time and has been continued on dipyridamole.

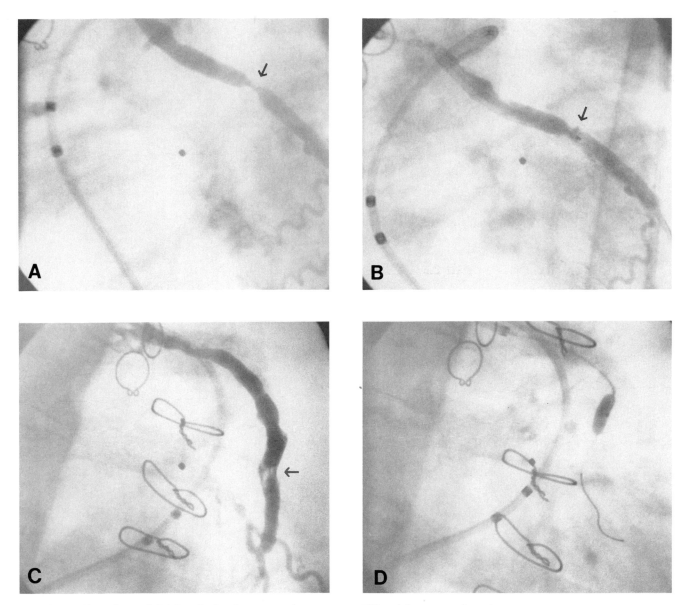

Case 18. A: Circumflex graft, LAO projection. Severe stenosis preangioplasty (arrow). B: Circumflex graft, LAO projection. Postangioplasty (arrow). C: Circumflex graft, RAO projection. Postangioplasty. Filling defect present (arrow). D: Circumflex graft, RAO projection. Molding inflation of balloon.

See following pages for continuation of figures.

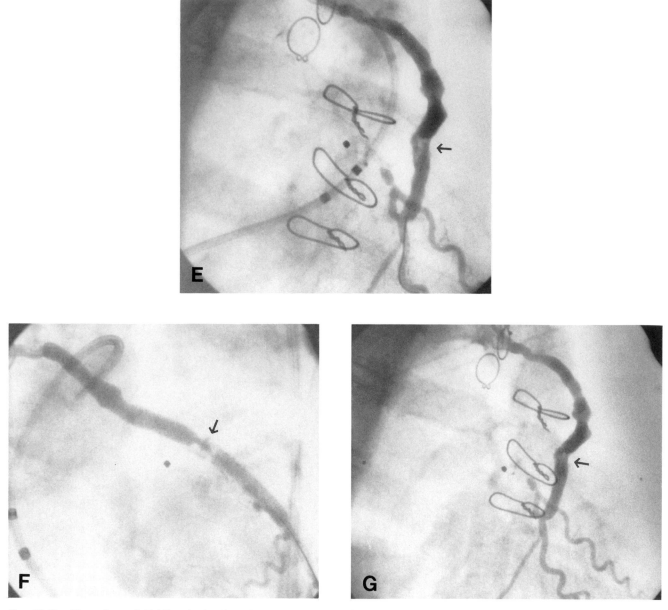

Case 18. E: Circumflex graft, RAO projection. Some improvement in area of filling defect (arrow). **F:** Circumflex graft, LAO projection. Postangioplasty (arrow). **G:** Circumflex graft, RAO projection. Four days postangioplasty (arrow).

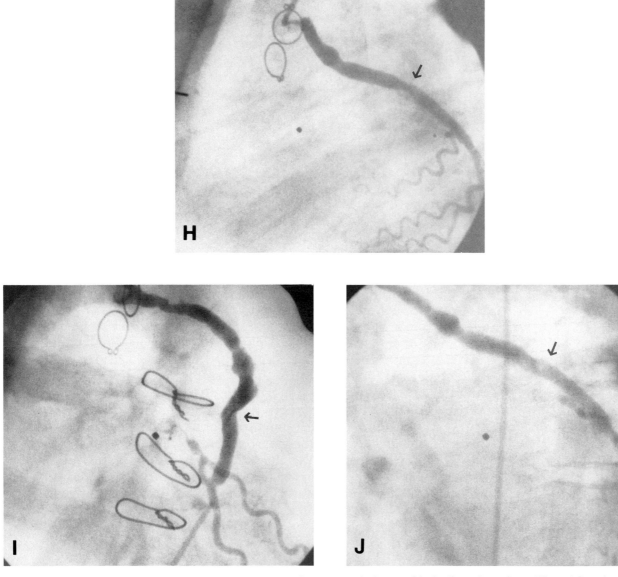

Case 18. H: Circumflex graft, LAO projection. Four days postangio-plasty (arrow). **I:** Circumflex graft, RAO projection. Four weeks post-angioplasty, with healing of previous filling defect (arrow). **J:** Circumflex graft, LAO projection. See I.

CASE NUMBER 19

Clinical
75-year-old woman admitted with unstable angina, who began to develop inferior myocardial infarction in hospital; transferred to laboratory for urgent study

Angiography
RCA:	total occlusion, proximal third
LMain:	normal
LAD:	normal
LCX:	normal
LV:	not done

Equipment

Guide	Dilatation Catheter	Wire
JR4	3.0 mm ACX	0.014 FS

Strategy and Procedure
The angioplasty was done as an ad hoc procedure on an emergency basis. The JR4 guide seated coaxially, and the wire passed very easily across the area of total obstruction and into the distal vessel. Balloon inflations were carried out throughout the area of presumed total obstruction (B–D). Guide catheter injections showed patency of the proximal lumen with several areas of smooth narrowing, suggesting spasm in the distal vessel (E). Intracoronary nitroglycerin was given, which resolved distal spasm (F). The proximal lumen looked quite good, but filling defects were apparent on the TV monitors (F–H). Over a 10 min period, the artery appeared to reaccumulate thrombus in the proximal segment (I). Higher pressure (10 atm) balloon inflations throughout that area (J) were carried out with reestablishment of good flow and reappearance of some distal spasm (K). IC nitroglycerin was given, and an adequate lumen was felt to be present (L). The patient was maintained on heparin for several days and was returned to the laboratory 2 weeks later for repeat angiography to assess results. This showed excellent patency of the proximal lumen and no evidence of distal spasm (M,N). She has continued to do well 1 year postprocedure.

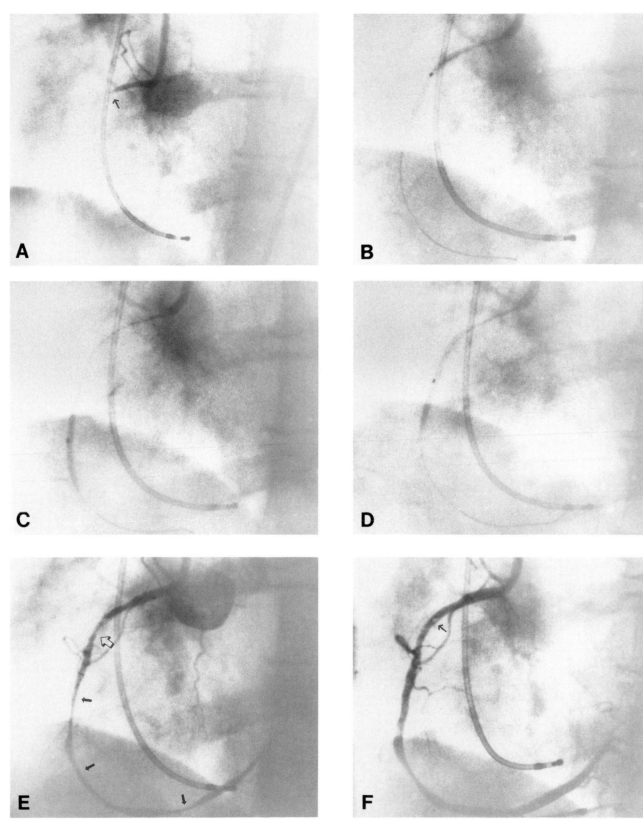

Case 19. A: Right coronary artery, LAO projection. Acute total obstruction of RCA (arrow). **B:** Right coronary artery, LAO projection. Wire across total obstruction and in distal vessel. Balloon inflated at area of total obstruction. **C:** Right coronary artery, LAO projection.

D: Right coronary artery, LAO projection. **E:** Right coronary artery, LAO projection. Patent vessel at level of previous total obstruction (open arrow). Diffuse spasm of distal vessel (solid arrows). **F:** Right coronary artery, LAO projection. Note filling defect (arrow).

See following pages for continuation of figures.

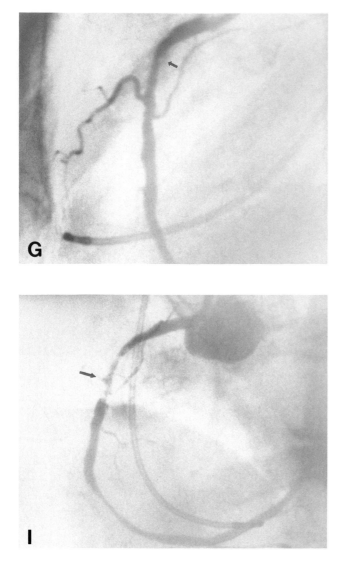

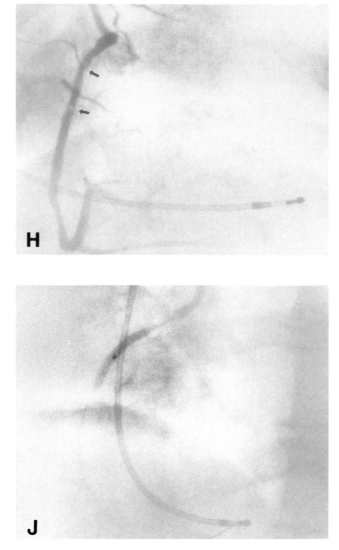

Case 19. G: Right coronary artery, left lateral projection. Note filling defect (arrow). **H:** Right coronary artery, RAO projection. Note filling defects (arrows). **I:** Right coronary artery, LAO projection. Reac- cumulation of thrombotic material in proximal RCA (arrow). **J:** Right coronary artery, LAO projection. Balloon inflated.

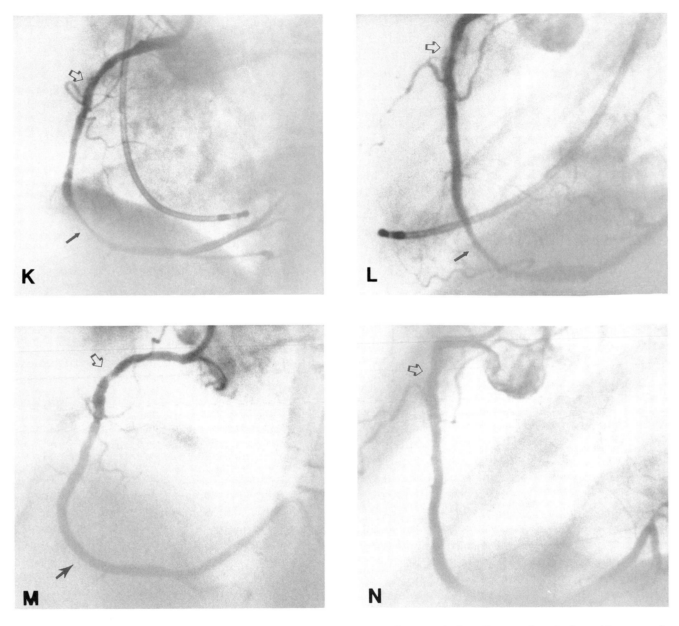

Case 19. K: Right coronary artery, LAO projection. Note patency of vessel in area of previous thrombus (open arrow). Downstream spasm noted (solid arrow). **L:** Right coronary artery, left lateral projection. Postnitroglycerin (see K). **M:** Right coronary artery, LAO projection.

Two weeks postangioplasty. Patency of proximal vessel (open arrow). No evidence of persistent spasm or defects in distal vessel (solid arrow). **N:** Right coronary artery, left lateral projection. Two weeks postangioplasty (arrow).

CASE NUMBER 20

Clinical 54-year-old man with previous pacemaker for intermittent heart block; admitted with changed and abnormal electrocardiogram with inferior and lateral ST segment elevations, suspicious of recent myocardial injury or ischemia

Angiography

RCA:	normal
LMain:	normal
LAD:	90% lesion at origin of first diagonal branch
Main LAD:	normal
LCX:	80% stenosis at origin and long area of 70% disease in midmain LCX
LV:	diffusely hypokinetic

Equipment

Guide	Dilatation Catheter	Wire
JL4	2.0 mm; 2.5 mm; 3.0 mm	0.014 FS

Strategy and Procedure

The diagonal branch of the LAD was first dilated with an excellent result. Balloon inflations at 8 atm for 45 sec ×3. The same wire was then passed across both lesions in the circumflex coronary artery and the balloon advanced across both lesions in the deflated mode. The second lesion was dilated first, with 8 atm for 45 sec ×3, and then the wire was extended and the balloon replaced with a 2.5 mm balloon, which was subsequently inflated at both proximal and midzone lesions at 7 atm for 45 sec ×3 in both areas. An excellent angiographic result was achieved. Three months later, the patient returned with reonset of angina. The study showed recurrence at the origin of the circumflex artery with a partial recurrence in the midzone of the circumflex as well and a good persistent result in the diagonal branch (A). Using a JL4 guide, a 2 mm balloon was passed over a 0.014 flexible steerable wire in the circumflex, and the distal lesion dilated first at 8 atm for 60 sec ×2 (B). The wire was extended, and a 2.5 mm balloon and then a 3 mm balloon were used in the proximal lesion. Maximum pressures with the 3 mm balloon were 7 atm (C). The angiographic results are seen in D. Ten hours later, the patient had the sudden onset of chest pain and ischemic EKG changes and was returned to the laboratory and found to have a total closure of the entire circumflex system (E). The total obstruction was wired and a 2.5 mm balloon positioned at the lesion and inflated to a maximum of 7 atm with reestablishment of flow in the artery (F,G). The lumen was not judged adequate, so the wire was extended and a 3 mm balloon inflated at the proximal lesion (H) with an apparent good result achieved (I). The patient was observed in the laboratory for 45 min with repeated injections and continued patency assured with the wire still across the lesions. Postangiographic results appeared excellent (J), and the patient was restudied 18 months later with continued normalization of all areas dilated.

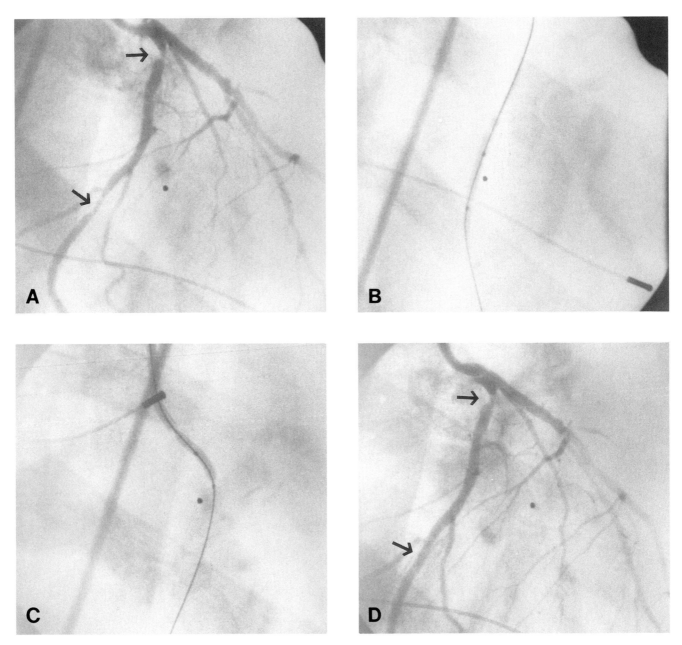

Case 20. A: Left coronary artery, RAO projection. Severe lesion just distal to origin of circumflex (top arrow) and long lesion in midzone of main circumflex artery (bottom arrow). **B:** Left coronary artery, RAO projection. Balloon inflated at distal lesion. **C:** Left coronary artery, RAO projection. Balloon inflated at proximal lesion. **D:** Left coronary artery, RAO projection. Postangioplasty (arrows).

See following pages for continuation of figures.

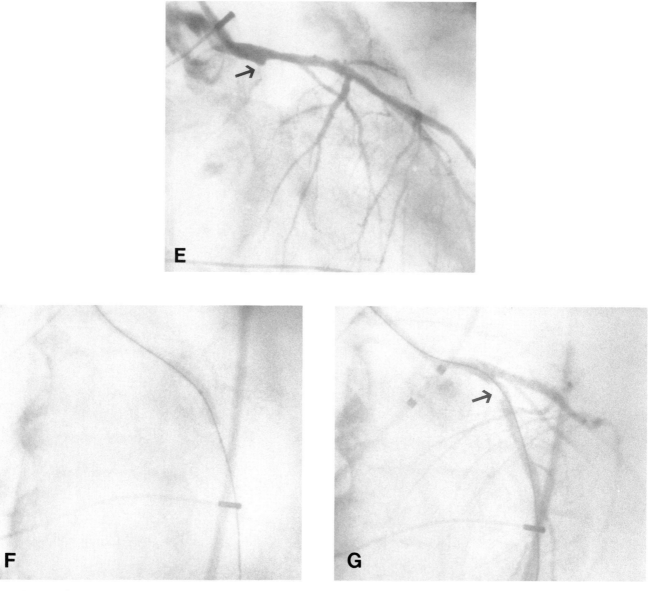

Case 20. E: Left coronary artery, RAO projection. Acute total closure of circumflex artery at site of proximal dilatation 10 hours postangioplasty (arrow). **F:** Left coronary artery, RAO projection. Total occlusion wired and balloon inflated. **G:** Left coronary artery, RAO projection. Flow reestablished through circumflex coronary artery, but obviously compromised lumen (arrow).

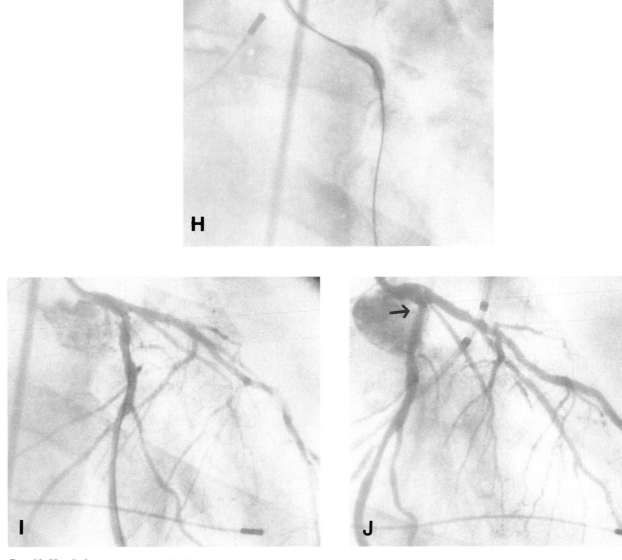

Case 20. H: Left coronary artery, RAO projection. Molding balloon inflation. **I:** Left coronary artery, RAO projection. Contrast injection through guide with wire still across lesion showing better appearance of lumen. **J:** Left coronary artery, RAO projection. Widely patent lumen 1 hour postreopening (arrow).

CASE NUMBER 21

Clinical

75-year-old man with abdominal aortic aneurysm and history of increasing angina; angiography recommended to assess extent of coronary disease prior to major abdominal surgery

Angiography

RCA: dominant with minimal irregularities
LMain: normal
LAD: large tortuous vessel with ectasia and an area of 80–90% narrowing in proximal third
LCX: 90% narrowing at origin of small first obtuse marginal branch, and total occlusion distal to this vessel, with antegrade and retrograde collateral filling of distal circumflex
LV: mild posterior hypokinesia

Equipment

Guide	Dilatation Catheter	Wire
JL4 8	3.0 mm SULP	0.014 flexible "J"

Strategy and Procedure

The LAD is believed to be the most important ischemia-producing lesion and is recognized to carry a higher risk of dissection because of the ectasia and tortuosity surrounding the severe stenosis (A,B). The guide seated coaxially, and the flexible wire was passed across the eccentric lesion, confirming the route of the wire in several projections. Balloon inflations conformed to the tortuosity of the lesion and adjacent vessel (C). Guide injections showed the wire to be in the superior aspect of the artery and suggested dissection (D,E). Molding inflations at 8 atm were carried out for 45 sec ×2 (F). Guide injections then confirmed a significant dissection at the site of dilatation with very slow flow into the distal vessel (G). A decision was quickly made to take the patient to bypass surgery with the wire across the area of dissection to maintain flow in the distal vessel. Patient was taken to surgery in stable condition with this hardware in place (G).

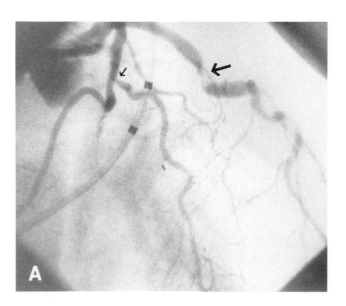

Case 21. A: Left coronary artery, RAO projection. Large arrow shows severe lesion in proximal LAD. Note ectatic appearance of LAD, both proximal and distal to the lesion. Small arrow demonstrates severe narrowing at origin of obtuse marginal branch.

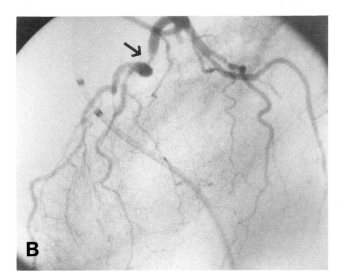

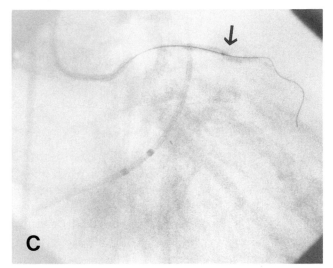

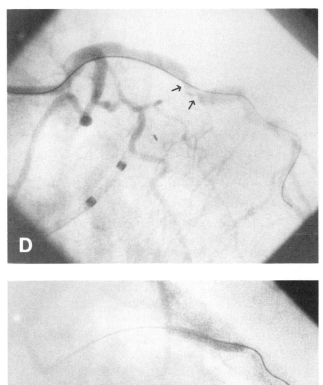

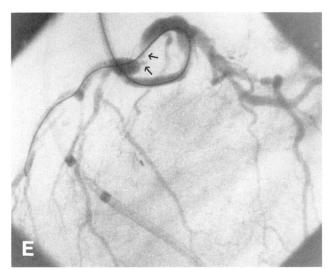

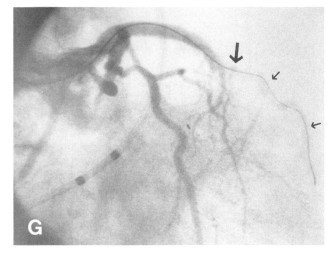

Case 21. B: Left coronary artery, LAO projection. Severe localized lesion at arrow. **C:** Left coronary artery, RAO projection. Balloon inflation at lesion with wire in distal vessel. **D:** Left coronary artery, RAO projection. Injection through guide shows good distal flow. The wire appears to be at the top of the lumen achieved. **E:** Left coronary artery, LAO projection. Injection through guiding catheter with wire still across lesion. Suggestion of dissection demonstrated by small arrows. **F:** Repeat dilatation in area of lesion. **G:** Left coronary artery, RAO projection. Markedly attenuated flow through area of original lesion (large arrow), with slow antegrade flow in distal vessel (small arrows). Patient taken to surgery with hardware in this position and was clinically stable.

CASE NUMBER 22

Clinical 58-year-old man with abrupt onset of unstable angina; hospitalized on IV nitroglycerin with continuing intermittent pain

Angiography

RCA: "dominant" minor proximal irregularities with total occlusion in midzone and collateral filling from LAD and LCX
LMain: minor disease
LAD: 90–95% stenosis proximal third
LCX: mild proximal disease
LV: mild anterior hypokinesia

Equipment

Guide	Dilatation Catheter	Wire
JL4	2.5 mm SULP; 3.0 mm SULP	0.014 FS

Strategy and Procedure

This was done as an ad hoc angioplasty. The soft-tipped guide seated very coaxially, and the wire was passed carefully across the eccentricity of the lesion in the lateral projection (B). With the wire in the distal vessel, inflations of the 2.5 mm balloon were carried out to 7 atm for 60 sec ×4. It was believed that the lumen achieved was not adequate, and the wire was extended and the 2.5 mm balloon replaced with a 3.0 mm SULP balloon, with which two further dilatations at 5 atm were done for 60 sec each. Repeat angiography with the dilatation equipment out showed an apparent excellent result (F–H). Approximately 16 hr later, the patient had the abrupt onset of pain and ST changes, indicating an anterior infarction. He was returned to the laboratory, and a total occlusion of the LAD was apparent from guiding catheter injections (H,I). A 0.016 wire was used, and the total occlusion cannulated with moderate difficulty. A 3.0 mm balloon was positioned at the region of total occlusion, and three dilatations at 6 atm for 60 sec each were performed. An apparent excellent angiographic result was again achieved (L–N). At his 6 month follow-up, he reported 2 weeks of intermittent exertional angina and was restudied. This showed a severe restenosis in the area of previous total obstruction (O,P). Repeat angioplasty was performed with a 3 mm SULP balloon over a 0.014 FS wire, and balloon inflations were carried out at 8 atm for as long as 45 sec ×5. An apparent good lumen with some haziness was achieved (R,S). When seen in follow-up 1 month later, he again complained of some mild, though indistinct chest pains and was restudied with excellent persistent patency of the lumen in the LAD (T,U). With this reassurance, he has continued to do well clinically and has a normal thallium stress EKG 1 year postprocedure.

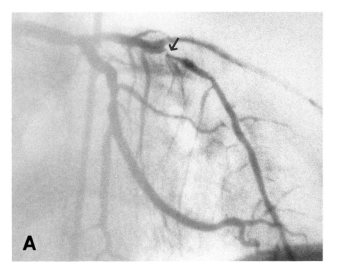

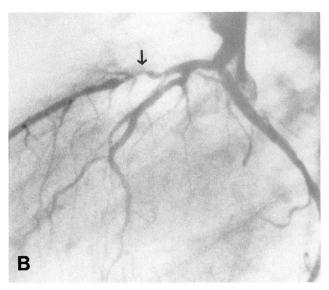

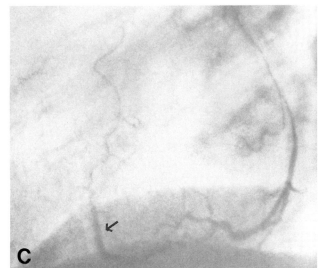

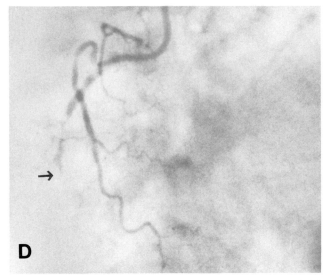

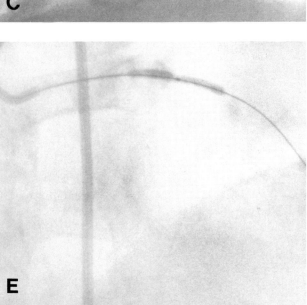

Case 22. A: Left coronary artery, RAO projection. Severe proximal lesion in LAD (arrow). **B:** Left coronary artery, left lateral projection. Preangioplasty (arrow). **C:** Left coronary artery, left lateral projection. Late stage of injection. Collateral filling of distal RCA (arrow). **D:** Right coronary artery, LAO projection. Total obstruction of RCA in midzone (arrow). **E:** Left coronary artery, RAO projection. Balloon inflation in LAD.

See following pages for continuation of figures.

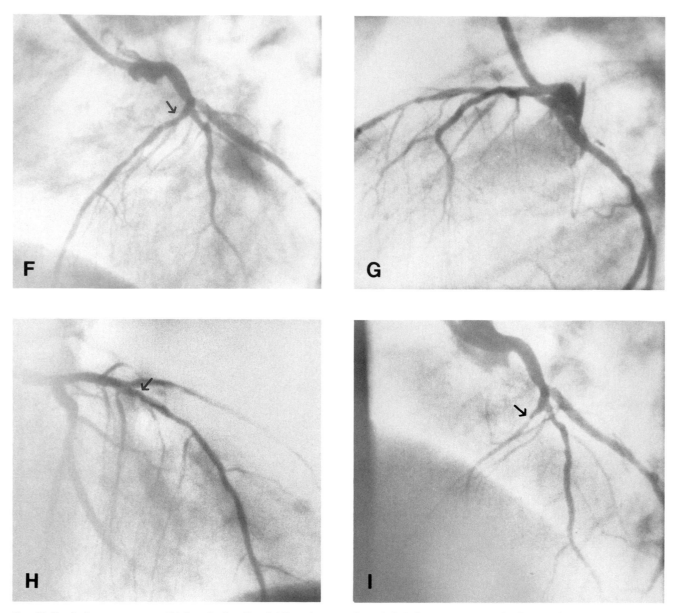

Case 22. F: Left coronary artery, RAO projection. Post-LAD angioplasty (arrow). G: Left coronary artery, left lateral projection. Postangioplasty. H: Left coronary artery, RAO projection. Postangioplasty (arrow). I: Left coronary artery, LAO projection. Sixteen hours postangioplasty, with abrupt reclosure (arrow).

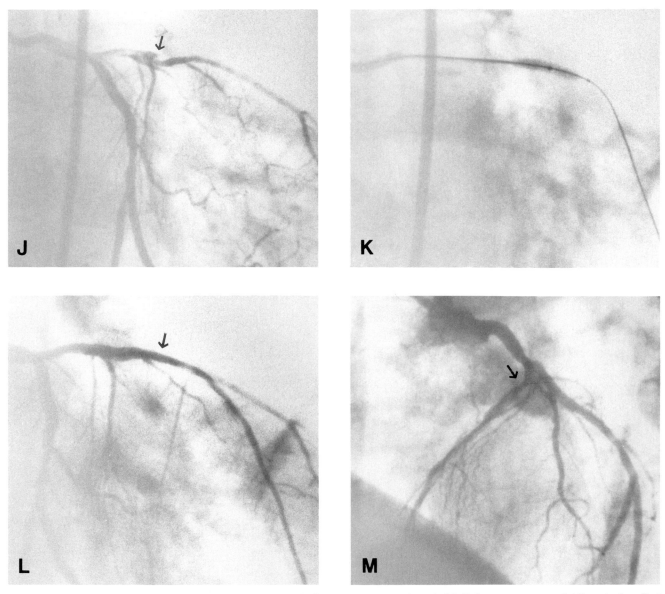

Case 22. J: Left coronary artery, RAO projection. See I. **K:** Left coronary artery, RAO projection. Wire across abrupt reclosure and balloon inflated. **L:** Left coronary artery, RAO projection. Post second angioplasty (arrow). **M:** Left coronary artery, LAO projection. Post second angioplasty (arrow).

See following pages for continuation of figures.

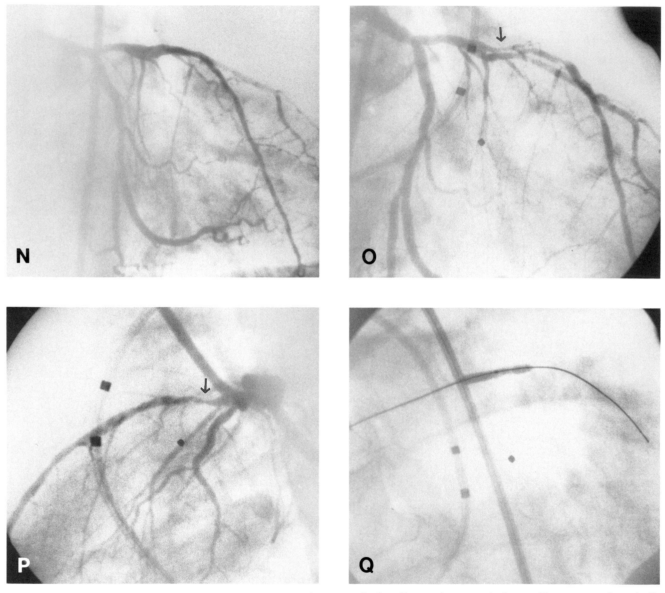

Case 22. N: Left coronary artery, RAO projection. Post second angioplasty. **O:** Left coronary artery, RAO projection. Recurrence 6 months postangioplasty (arrow). **P:** Left coronary artery, left lateral projection. Six months postangioplasty, with recurrence (arrow). **Q:** Left coronary artery, RAO projection. Balloon inflation.

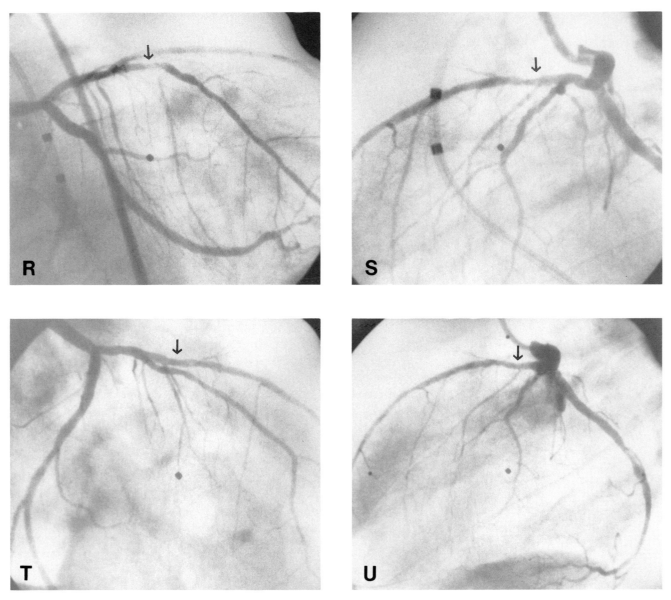

Case 22. R: Left coronary artery, RAO projection. Post repeat angioplasty (arrow). **S:** Left coronary artery, left lateral projection. Post repeat angioplasty (arrow). **T:** Left coronary artery, RAO projection. One month post repeat angioplasty (arrow). **U:** Left coronary artery, left lateral projection. One month post repeat angioplasty (arrow).

CASE NUMBER 23

Clinical

60-year-old man with abrupt onset of small inferior myocardial infarction and postinfarct pain

Angiography

RCA: diffuse hazy severe stenosis distal third (probable thrombus)
LMain: normal
LAD: normal
LCX: normal
LV: normal

Equipment

Guide	Dilatation Catheter	Wire
FL4 SH	2.5 mm ACX	0.014 HTF; 0.014 FS

Strategy and Procedure

The initial diagnostic study suggested the presence of thrombus in the distal RCA (B). While preparing a balloon catheter, the patient had some pain, and an injection showed retarded flow in the distal vessel on a spontaneous nature (C). The wire was passed quickly across the lesion and into the distal vessel, and balloon inflations were carried out at 10 atm for as long as 60 sec. Injections then showed slow flow in the distal vessel, suggesting that a shower of emboli had occurred from the thrombus in the area of stenosis, and he was then given 250,000 units of urokinase. This improved the flow, and an adequate lumen appeared to have been achieved (E). Thirty minutes later, however, he redeveloped pain and ST segment elevation, and the artery was shown to be totally occluded. It was quickly rewired, and the same 2.5 mm balloon used (F,G). This produced complete resolution of the pain and EKG changes, and the lumen achieved appeared to be excellent, but there was still some haziness in the area of dilatation (H). Postangioplasty angiography demonstrated an adequate lumen (I), and he has continued to do well clinically 1 year postprocedure.

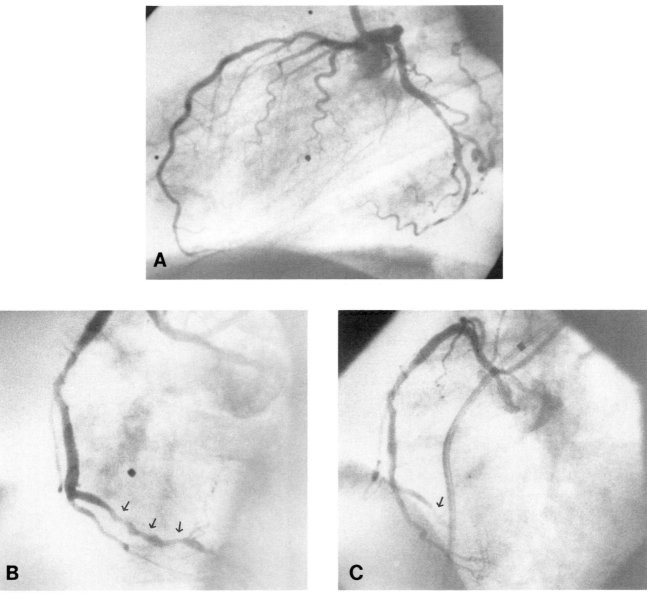

Case 23. A: Left coronary artery, left lateral projection. **B:** Right coronary artery, LAO projection. Area of diffuse disease in distal vessel (arrows). **C:** Right coronary artery, LAO projection. Spontaneous slow distal flow (arrow).

See following pages for continuation of figures.

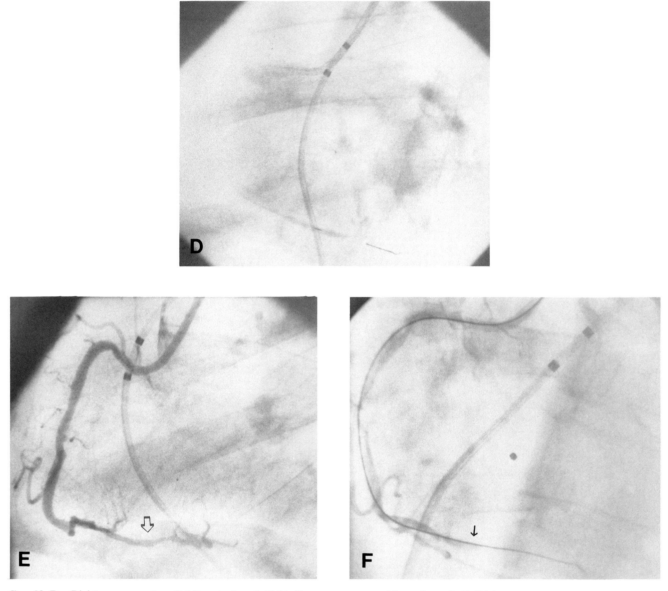

Case 23. D: Right coronary artery, LAO projection. Initial balloon inflation. **E:** Right coronary artery, LAO projection. Postangioplasty, post-urokinase (arrow). **F:** Right coronary artery, LAO projection. Wire in place following abrupt reclosure (arrow).

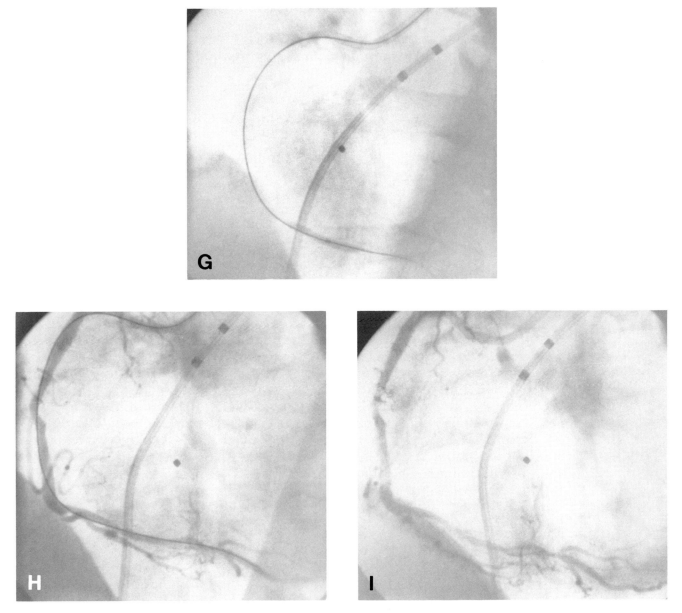

Case 23. G: Right coronary artery, LAO projection. Balloon inflation. **H:** Right coronary artery, LAO projection. Postangioplasty. **I:** Right coronary artery, left lateral projection. Postangioplasty.

CASE NUMBER 24

Clinical

49-year-old man with inferior myocardial infarction 7 years ago; no angina until 2 weeks prior to angiogram; positive treadmill test inferolaterally

Angiography

RCA: total occlusion, midzone
LMain: normal
LAD: no significant disease
LCX: long area of 70–90% stenosis distal to origin of major OM branch
LV: inferior hypokinesia

Equipment

Guide	Dilatation Catheter	Wire
RCA: JR4 SH	2.5 mm SULP	0.014 intermediate
LCX: JL4	2.5 mm SULP	0.014 HTF; 0.014 FS

Strategy and Procedure

Even though RCA occlusion was presumed to be 7 years old, it was decided to try that first. Unable to get intermediate wire to cross area of total obstruction (C). LCX was then approached with 2.5 mm balloon. Inflations (D) yielded initial good lumen (E). Inflations carried out to 7 atm for 40 sec several times. When the balloon and wire were removed, angiography demonstrated an area of dissection and poor distal flow (G). The area was rewired (F) and further balloon inflations done with a 2.5 mm balloon. Within 5 min, the area of dissection was obviously reclosing, and decision was made to take the patient to bypass surgery with the wire across the lesion to maintain flow in the distal vessel (I). It is important to pull the guiding catheter back from the left main for transport (I). The patient was taken to surgery in stable condition and did well at surgery.

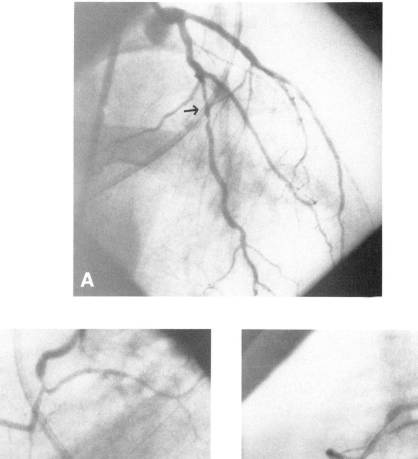

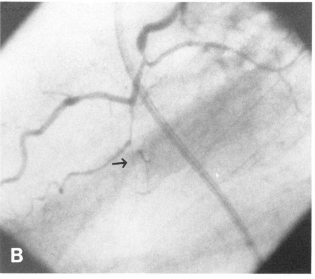

Case 24. A: Left coronary artery, RAO projection. Severe diffuse disease in LCX (arrow). **B:** Right coronary artery, left lateral projection. Total occlusion of RCA (arrow). **C:** Right coronary artery, LAO projection. Unsuccessful attempt to advance wire across total obstruction in RCA (arrow).

See following pages for continuation of figures.

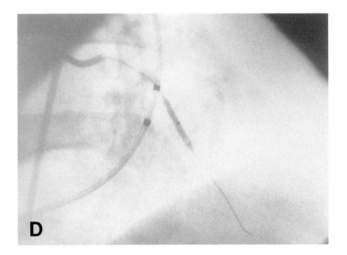

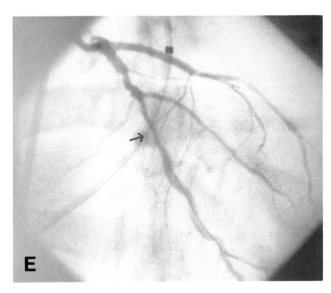

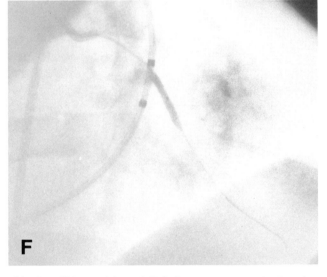

Case 24. D: Left coronary artery, RAO projection. Balloon inflation in LCX. **E:** Left coronary artery, RAO projection. Postangioplasty with wire still in vessel (arrow). **F:** Left coronary artery, RAO projection. Balloon inflation in LCX.

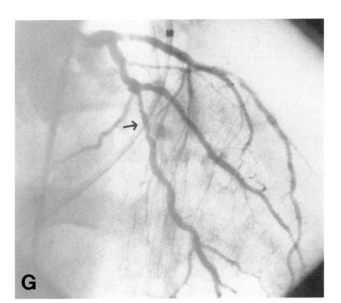

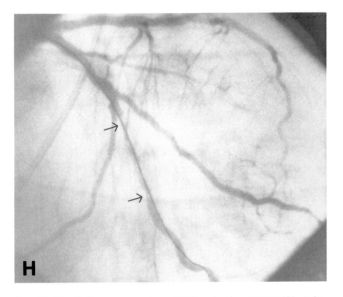

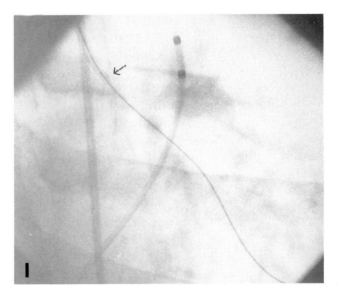

Case 24. G: Left coronary artery, RAO projection. Post-LCX angioplasty (arrow). **H:** Left coronary artery, RAO projection. Rewired LCX with long area of diffuse stenosis (arrows). **I:** Left coronary artery, RAO projection. Wire across lesion and guide tip withdrawn (arrow).

CASE NUMBER 25

Clinical

68-year-old woman with acute inferolateral myocardial infarction, treated with TPA, and subsequent small enzyme rise; continued chest pain led to angiography

Angiography

RCA: "dominant" normal
LMain: normal
LAD: normal
LCX: 90% narrowing with apparent thrombus
LV: not done

Equipment

Guide	Dilatation Catheter	Wire
JL4	2.5 mm ACX; 3.0 mm ACX	0.014 FS

Strategy and Procedure

The patient arrived at the catheterization laboratory having continuing chest pain not responsive to IV nitroglycerin. A left ventriculogram was not done because of her acute clinical syndrome. It was decided to proceed with an ad hoc angioplasty of the LCX lesion. Angiographically, the lesion appeared to have thrombus present (A,B). The 2.5 mm balloon passed easily across the severe stenosis, and balloon inflations were carried out at up to 8 atm for as long as 45 sec. Initial postangioplasty injections showed good flow and patency (D), but intermittent filling of the obtuse marginal branch was obvious (E,F). The patient continued to have pain, and further injections showed deterioration and probable dissection in the main LCX with no flow in the OM (G). The area was recrossed with the 0.014 FS wire, and inflations made with both a 2.5 mm and 3.0 mm ACX balloon (H). Repeated inflations at 5–6 atm for as long as 90 sec with the 3 mm balloon reestablished good antegrade flow in the main circumflex (I), and slow flow again appeared in the obtuse marginal branch. Following long observation, it was believed that the lumen achieved could be trusted (J,K), and the patient was returned to the cardiac unit for continued heparinization. Approximately 20 hr later, she had the reonset of severe chest pain, was restarted on her nitroglycerin drip, and returned to the laboratory. The sheaths, which were still in place, were changed under sterile conditions, and injections through the FL4 guide showed a total occlusion with slow flow in the main circumflex and good flow in the obtuse marginal branch (L). Attempts to recross the lesion with a 0.014 FS and a 0.014 intermediate wire were not successful. The patient and her family elected to allow the infarction to continue and not have bypass surgery. She had approximately 2 more hr of chest pain and has done very well clinically following her hospitalization.

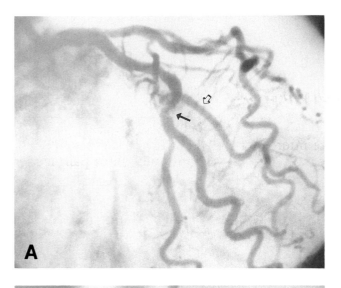

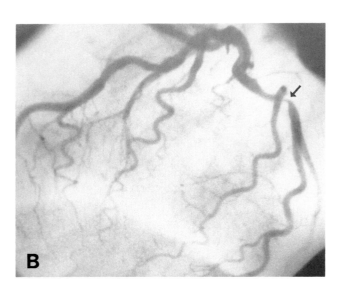

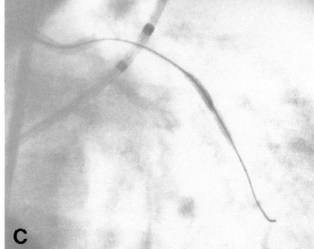

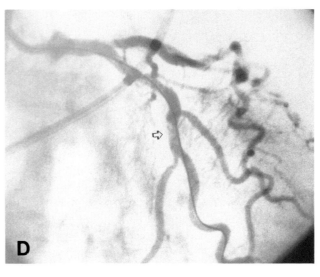

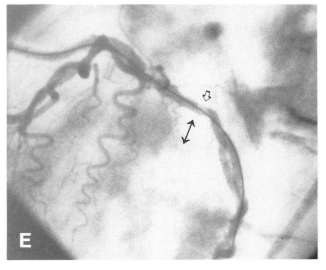

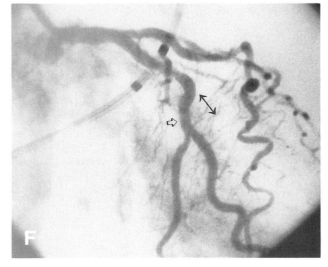

Case 25. A: Left coronary artery, RAO projection. Severe lesion on curve in main circumflex (solid arrow). Note obtuse marginal branch (open arrow). **B:** Left coronary artery, left lateral projection. Preangioplasty (arrow). **C:** Left coronary artery, RAO projection. Balloon inflation on curve. **D:** Left coronary artery, RAO projection. Postangioplasty. Note adequate filling of OM branch (arrow). **E:** Left coronary artery, LAO projection. Postangioplasty (open arrow). Note absence of filling of OM branch (double arrow). **F:** Left coronary artery, RAO projection. See E.

See following pages for continuation of figures.

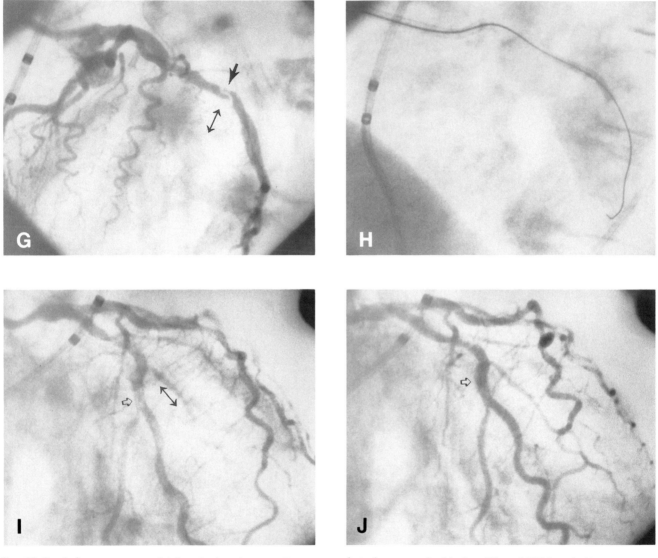

Case 25. G: Left coronary artery, LAO projection. Apparent dissection in area of dilatation (single arrow) and absence of filling of OM branch (double arrow). **H:** Left coronary artery, LAO projection. Balloon inflation. **I:** Left coronary artery, RAO projection. Postangio-plasty (open arrow) with slow filling of OM branch (double arrow). **J:** Left coronary artery, RAO projection. Thirty minutes postangio-plasty (arrow).

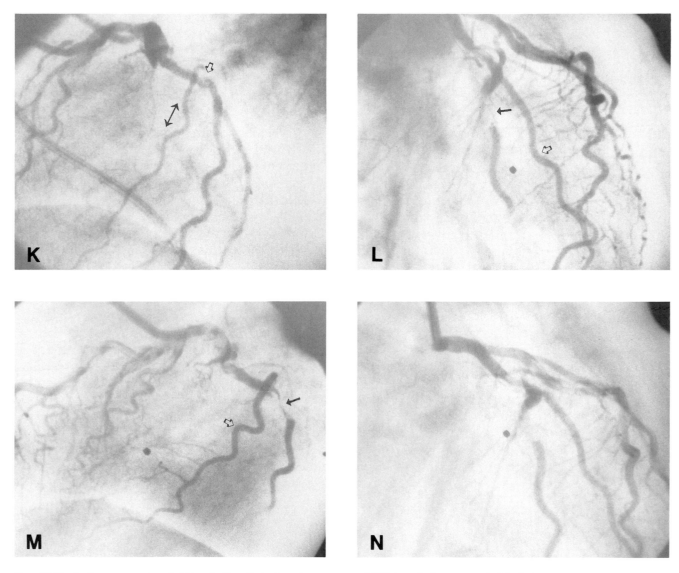

Case 25. K: Left coronary artery, LAO projection. Forty-five minutes postangioplasty (arrow). Note filling of OM branch (double arrow). **L:** Left coronary artery, RAO projection. Twenty-four hours postangioplasty. Abrupt closure of dilated segment (solid arrow). Note patency of OM branch (open arrow). **M:** Left coronary artery, left lateral projection. Twenty-four hours postangioplasty. See L. **N:** Left coronary artery, RAO projection.

CASE NUMBER 26

Clinical 45-year-old man with severe diabetes and lower extremity amputation with unstable angina

Angiography

RCA:	total occlusion	LAD:	total occlusion proximal third
LMain:	normal	LCX:	severe proximal lesion

Equipment

Guide	Dilatation Catheter	Wire
8.3 F 3 inch medium brachial	2.5 mm SULP; 3.0 mm SULP	0.014 FS

Strategy and Procedure

The patient presented with left ventricular dysfunction and congestive heart failure. Angiography showed total occlusions of the right coronary artery and left anterior descending coronary artery and a severe lesion in the proximal circumflex affecting his remaining viable myocardium. His severe diabetic arteriosclerotic disease and chronic hepatic disease secondary to congestive heart failure made him a very poor surgical candidate. It was decided to attempt angioplasty of the artery supplying his only remaining myocardium with the patient on cardiopulmonary support. CPS was instituted through the left femoral artery and vein, and the venous cannula can be seen in A. The severe lesion in the LCX is seen in B, as is the total occlusion of the ectatic LAD. With the patient on cardiopulmonary bypass with a flow of 4 liters/min, the wire was passed easily across the lesion and a 2.5 mm balloon positioned at the stenosis. Inflations were carried out at 5 atm for as long as 1 min, with the patient completely stable during the balloon inflations. The wire was extended and the balloon removed and replaced with a 3 mm SULP balloon catheter. This was positioned at the lesion, and the balloon was dumbbelled to 11 atm when it fully opened, and other molding inflations at 7 atm were taken for 60 sec each with the patient extremely stable on CPS. Postangioplasty angiography showed a good result in the proximal circumflex, and an elective repeat study 4 months later showed a persistent good lumen in the vessel (F,G).

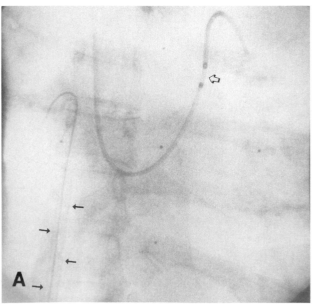

Case 26. A: AP projection. Multipurpose pacing wire in place (open arrow). Venous cannula of CPS device led to right atrium by "J" wire (solid arrows).

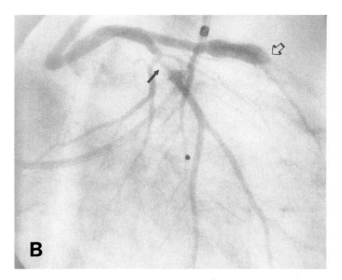

B

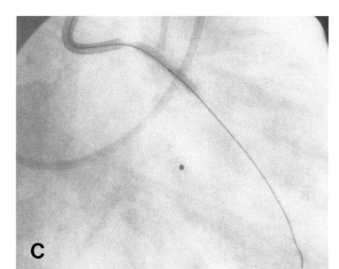

C

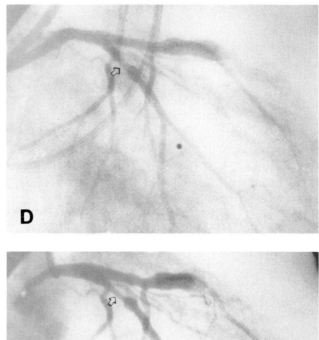

D

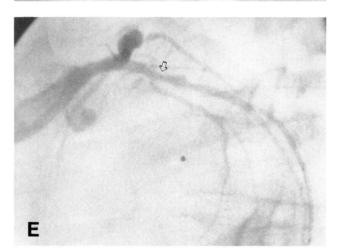

E

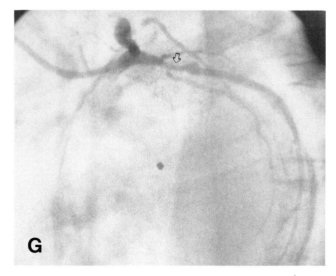

F

G

Case 26. B: Left coronary artery, RAO projection. Note total obstruction of aneurysmal LAD (open arrow). Severe lesion in main circumflex demonstrated (solid arrow). **C:** Left coronary artery, RAO projection. Balloon inflation in proximal circumflex with some indentation in midballoon. **D:** Left coronary artery, RAO projection. Postangi-

oplasty (arrow). **E:** Left coronary artery, LAO projection. Postangioplasty (arrow). **F:** Left coronary artery, RAO projection. Four months postangioplasty (arrow). **G:** Left coronary artery, LAO projection. Four months postangioplasty (arrow).

CASE NUMBER 27

Clinical

76-year-old man first treated in 1987 with angioplasty of the ramus intermedius branch and a normal dominant circumflex artery; previous total occlusion of the LAD and nondominant right coronary artery; returned in 1990 with severe angina and angiography demonstrated as below

Angiography

RCA:	"nondominant" diffusely diseased
LMain:	normal
LAD:	totally occluded
Ramus:	minor irregularities
LCX:	"dominant" 90% proximal narrowing
LV:	diffuse hypokinesia with 3+ mitral regurgitation

Equipment

Guide	Dilatation Catheter	Wire
JL4	3 mm ACX; 3.5 mm ACX	0.014 FS

Strategy and Procedure

The patient had a striking progression of disease over a 3-year period in his dominant circumflex artery. He had a previous anterior myocardial infarction and has a nondominant right coronary artery. He also has diffusely poor left ventricular function with mitral regurgitation and was believed to be a poor surgical candidate on that basis. It was decided to proceed with angioplasty using cardiopulmonary support. The CPS system was inserted from the right femoral approach and functioned well prior to procedure (B). The angioplasty was straightforward with no difficulty wiring the lesion, and balloon inflations were carried out with the 3 mm balloon to 10 atm for as long as 45 sec. Each time the balloon was inflated, the patient's pressure dropped. He had PVCs and was put on 4 liters/min of cardiopulmonary support. This stabilized him, and the wire was extended, the balloon replaced with a 3.5 mm ACX, and inflations carried out for 1 and 1½ min at 7 atm. An excellent angiographic result was achieved (D), and the use of CPS allowed for a stable procedure with adequate balloon inflations.

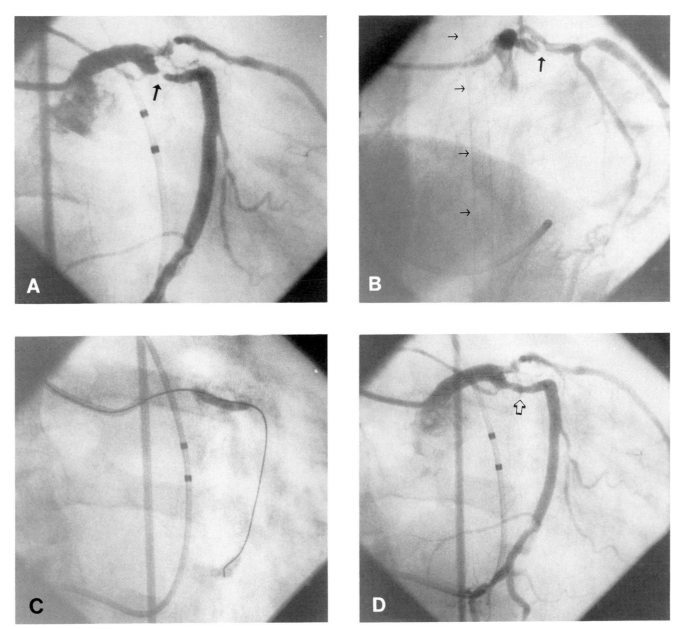

Case 27. A: Left coronary artery, RAO projection. Severe proximal LCX lesion (arrow). **B:** Left coronary artery, LAO projection. Severe LCX lesion (large arrow). Note CPS venous cannula (small arrows).

C: Left coronary artery, RAO projection. Balloon inflation. **D:** Left coronary artery, RAO projection. Postangioplasty (open arrow).

CASE NUMBER 28

Clinical
65-year-old man first studied in 1985 with no significant disease; returned with unstable angina

Angiography

	1985	1989
RCA:	nondominant	nondominant
LMain:	normal	normal
LAD:	normal	normal
LCX:	anomalous origin from right cusp with minor irregularities in midzone and no significant obstructive disease	severe irregular lesion in main trunk
LV:	normal	normal

Equipment

Guide	Dilatation Catheter	Wire
N/A	N/A	N/A

Strategy and Procedure
When the patient was first studied in 1985, he had no significant disease in his large circumflex, which originated from an anomalous position in the right cusp. In 1989, this large circumflex had a very diffuse irregular lesion (D), which was believed to present increased risk at angioplasty because of the apparent ulcer and irregularity of the lesion. The distal circumflex supplied through this vessel was extensive in distribution, and it was believed that the patient should have bypass surgery rather than angioplasty.

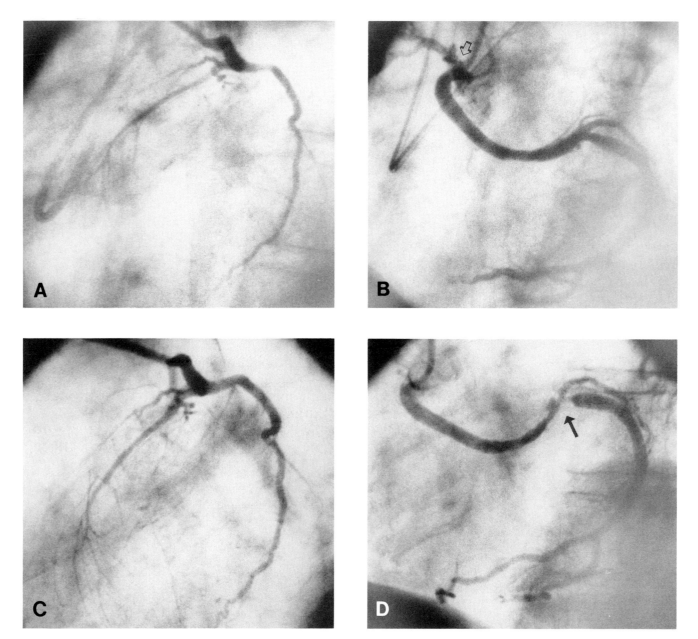

Case 28. A: Left coronary artery, LAO projection, 1985. **B:** Right coronary artery, LAO projection, 1985. Anomalous origin of large dominant circumflex artery from right coronary cusp (arrow). **C:** Left coronary artery, LAO projection, 1990. **D:** Right coronary artery, LAO projection, 1990. This demonstrates a new grossly irregular lesion (arrow) in the large dominant circumflex artery, which originates from the right coronary sinus.

CASE NUMBER 29

Clinical   58-year-old man with 3-month history of exertional angina and reversible anterior thallium defect

Angiography   RCA: "dominant" 30–40% proximal lesion
                      LMain: normal
                      LAD: total occlusion with retrograde collaterals from right
                      LCX: normal
                      LV: mild anterior hypokinesia

Equipment

Guide	Dilatation Catheter	Wire
JL4	3.0 mm LPS	0.014 FS

Strategy and Procedure

Done as ad hoc angioplasty. The stump of the LAD is quite nicely seen in both RAO and lateral views (B,C). The JL4 guide seated coaxially, and the 0.014 FS wire was traversed quite easily. The 3 mm balloon crossed the lesion, and a 40 mm pressure gradient was measured. Balloon inflations to 8 atm for as long as 60 sec throughout the area of total occlusion produced no pain, presumably due to collaterals. The pressure gradient was reduced to 8 mmHg, and postangioplasty angiography showed an excellent lumen with rapid antegrade flow in the distal vessel (D). The patient did well clinically for 4 years and then returned with angina. Repeat angiography showed a persistent excellent result in the LAD treated with angioplasty (E), but a new lesion in the LMain and progression of disease in the LCX and RCA (E,F). Because of the left main lesion, the patient was referred for bypass surgery with bypasses placed to the LCX, RCA, and LAD.

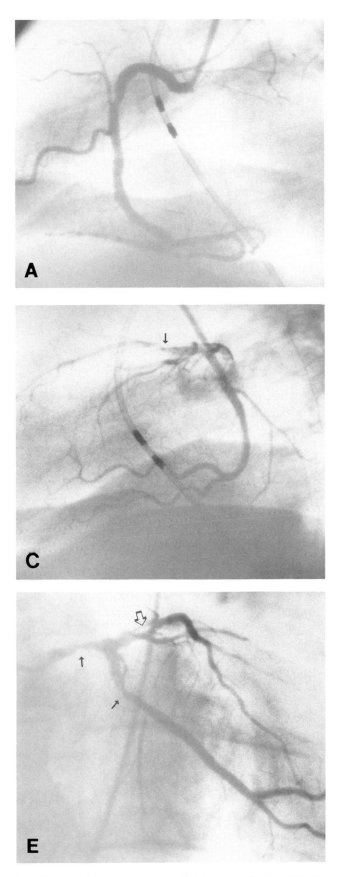

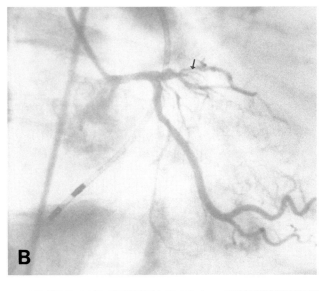

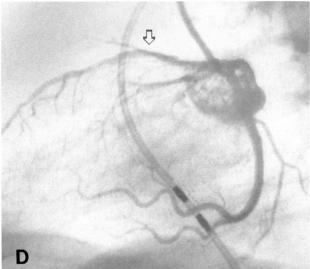

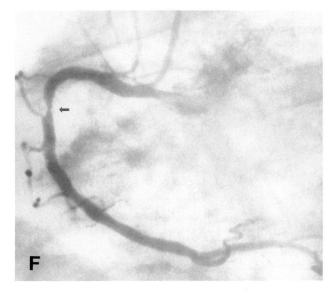

Case 29. A: Right coronary artery, left lateral projection, 1985. **B:** Left coronary artery, RAO projection, 1985. Total obstruction of LAD (arrow). **C:** Left coronary artery, left lateral projection, 1985. See B. **D:** Left coronary artery, left lateral projection, 1985. Postangioplasty (arrow). **E:** Left coronary artery, RAO projection, 1989. Persistent patency of LAD (open arrow). New lesions in left main and LCX (solid arrows). **F:** Right coronary artery, left lateral projection, 1989. New lesion in proximal RCA (arrow).

CASE NUMBER 30

Clinical   59-year-old woman with recent onset of unstable angina, admitted to hospital, and the night prior to angiography showed extreme elevation of ST segments in the inferior leads, associated with pain and responsive to nitroglycerin

Angiography

RCA:	subtotal occlusion in proximal third
LMain:	normal
LAD:	normal
LCX:	moderate disease
LV:	normal

Equipment

Guide	Dilatation Catheter	Wire
N/A	N/A	N/A

Strategy and Procedure   The patient had an episode of apparent Printzmetal angina. The diagnostic angiography showed a subtotal occlusion in the proximal RCA at a time when the patient was not having pain and had no EKG changes. There were no collaterals from the left coronary system (A,B). While a balloon was being prepared, intracoronary nitroglycerin was given, which resulted in opening of the vessel (C). There appeared to be some diffuse proximal spasm as well as distal spasm in the vessel, and repeated injections with intracoronary nitroglycerin achieved a widely patent lumen. Observation in the cath lab showed repeated episodes of proximal spasm (E–H), which responded transiently to intracoronary nitroglycerin, but which recurred. The patient was then given sublingual nifedipine, and persistence of a perfect lumen over 1 hr's observation in the laboratory was documented (I). It was therefore decided to treat the patient with high doses of calcium blockers and not perform balloon angioplasty in this setting.

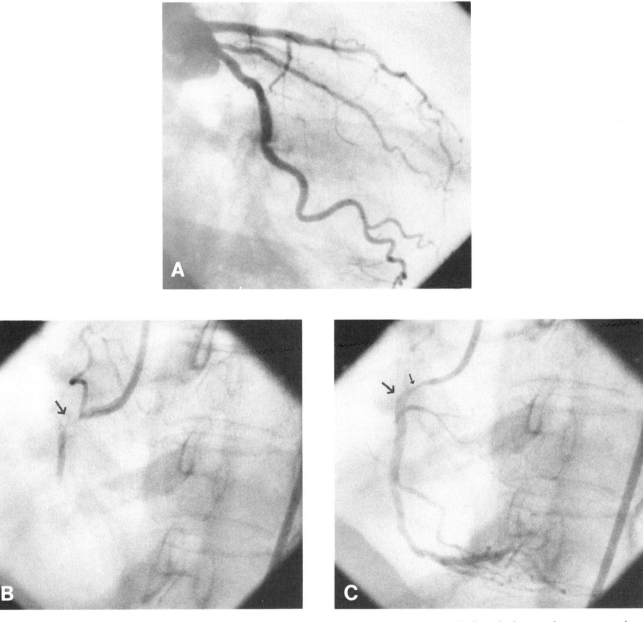

Case 30. A: Left coronary artery, RAO projection. No significant disease is seen in the left coronary system. **B:** Right coronary artery, LAO projection. Initial injection of contrast shows subtotal stenosis in the proximal third (arrow) with minimal flow into the distal vessel.

C: Right coronary artery, LAO projection, postintracoronary nitroglycerin. Demonstrates quite full patency at site of previous stenosis (large arrow) and some proximal apparent spasm (small arrow).

See following pages for continuation of figures.

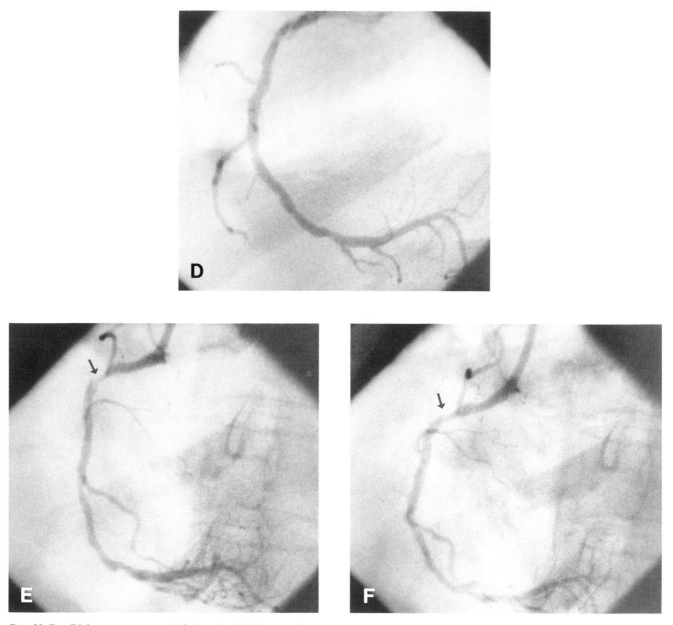

Case 30. D: Right coronary artery, left lateral projection, postnitroglycerin. Apparent relief of proximal spasm with diffuse irregularity throughout the artery. **E:** Right coronary artery, LAO projection. Spontaneous reonset of angina and ST changes correspond to signifi-

cant renarrowing of the proximal vessel (arrow). **F:** Right coronary artery, LAO projection. Reestablishment of antegrade flow and relief of spasm (arrow) following intracoronary nitroglycerin.

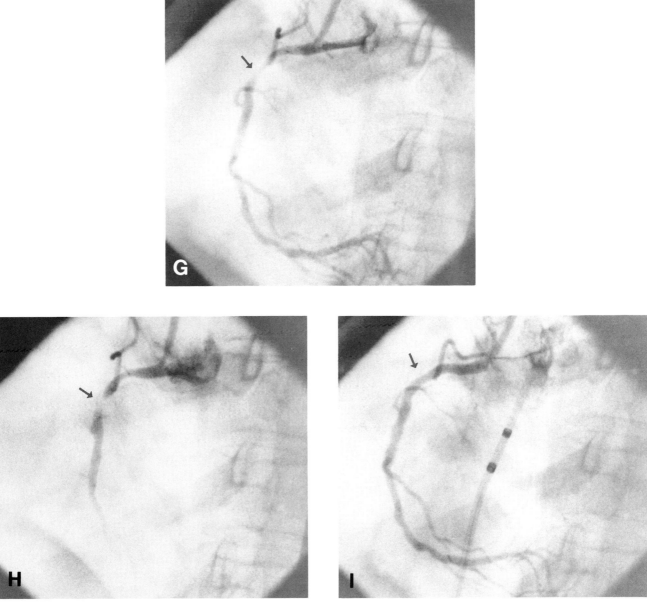

Case 30. G: Right coronary artery, LAO projection. Spontaneous return of spasm (arrow). **H:** Right coronary artery, LAO projection. Worsening of spasm (arrow) with slow antegrade flow. **I:** Right coronary artery, LAO projection, 30 min postsublingual nifedipine, with good persistent patency of area of proximal spasm (arrow).

CASE NUMBER 31

Clinical

Young man first seen at age 33 for unstable angina in 1987; dilatation of tandem circumflex lesions done at that time; repeat angina in 1989 with new circumflex lesion and diffuse disease in RCA, treated with Rotablator angioplasty

Angiography

	1987	1989
RCA:	small diffusely irregular	diffuse severe disease
	without obstruction	in midzone on tortuous segment
LMain:	normal	normal
LAD:	normal	normal
LCX:	tandem proximal lesions	new lesion distal to previous angioplasty
LV:	normal	normal

Equipment

Guide		Dilatation Catheter		Wire	
1987	1989	1987	1989	1987	1989
JL4	LCX: JL4	3.0 mm LPS	2.5 mm SULP	0.014 FS	0.014 HTF
	RCA: 9 F JR4		2.0 mm Rotablator		Rotablator

Strategy and Procedure

In 1987, the only significant lesions were in the circumflex coronary artery (A–D). A JL4 guide was used and seated nicely in the left main trunk. A 3 mm LPS balloon catheter system was positioned over a 0.014 FS wire, and a pressure gradient of 8 mmHg was measured. Balloon inflations were carried out to 7 atm for as long as 60 sec, and the pressure gradient was obliterated. A good angiographic result was obtained (E,F). The patient did well clinically until 1989 when he returned with angina. Angiograms then showed a good persistent result in the circumflex, but a new lesion downstream from the original dilatation (G). This was dilated using a JL4 guide and a 2.5 mm SULP balloon catheter, inflated to 8 atm for as long as 1 min several times. A good result was obtained (H). Diffuse disease had developed in the RCA (I,J). It was decided to treat the long lesion on the tortuous segment of the artery with a Rotablator rather than with conventional balloon angioplasty. A 2 mm Rotablator dilatation system was then used throughout the right coronary artery (K–M), and an excellent lumen was achieved (N,O). The patient refused follow-up study, but did return in 1990, 1 year later, with recurrent angina. An angiogram at that time showed a good persistent result in the circumflex (P) and a good result in the area treated with Rotablator angioplasty in the right coronary artery (Q). A new lesion had, however, developed in the distal RCA (Q), and this was treated with balloon angioplasty (R) with a good result (S). He continues to do well 6 months post his last procedure.

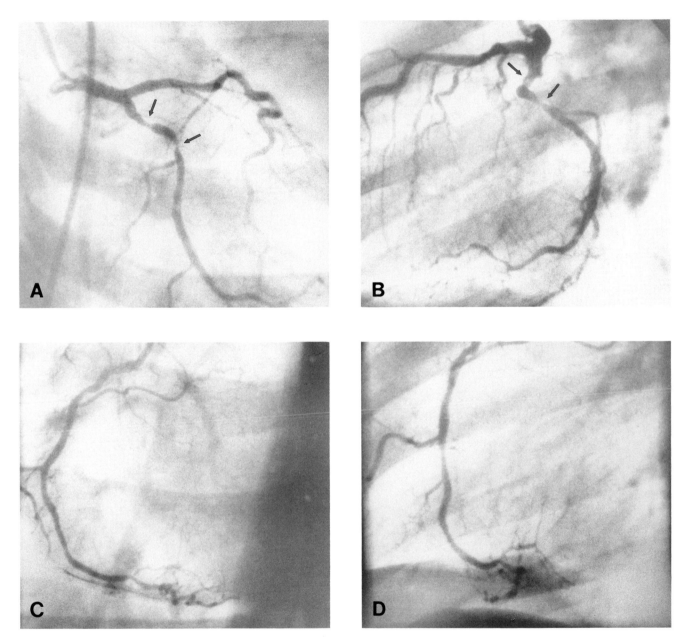

Case 31. A: Left coronary artery, RAO projection, 1987. Tandem lesions in proximal circumflex demonstrated (arrows). **B:** Left coronary artery, left lateral projection, 1987. See A. **C:** Right coronary artery, LAO projection, 1987. **D:** Right coronary artery, left lateral projection, 1987.

See following pages for continuation of figures.

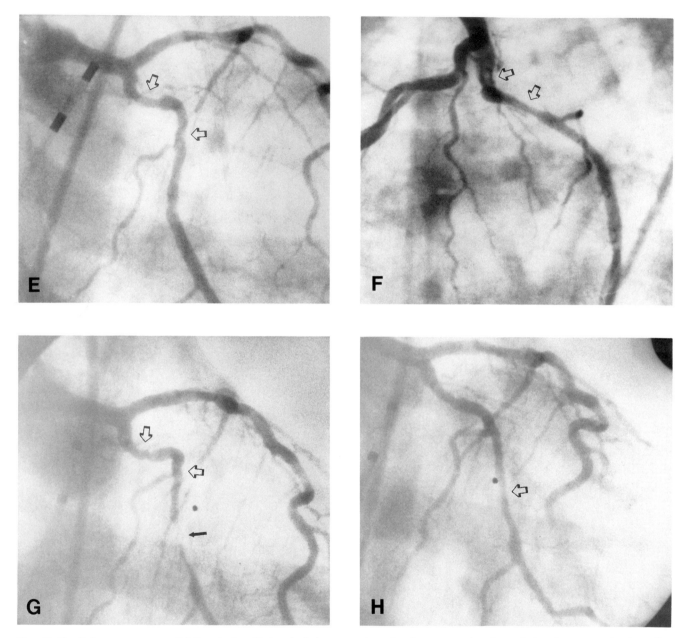

Case 31. E: Left coronary artery, RAO projection. Postangioplasty, 1987 (arrows). **F:** Left coronary artery, LAO projection. Postangioplasty, 1987 (arrows). **G:** Left coronary artery, RAO projection, 1989. Persistent good results from angioplasty of proximal tandem lesions in circumflex (open arrows) and new lesion downstream in circumflex (solid arrow). **H:** Left coronary artery, RAO projection, 1989. Postangioplasty (arrow).

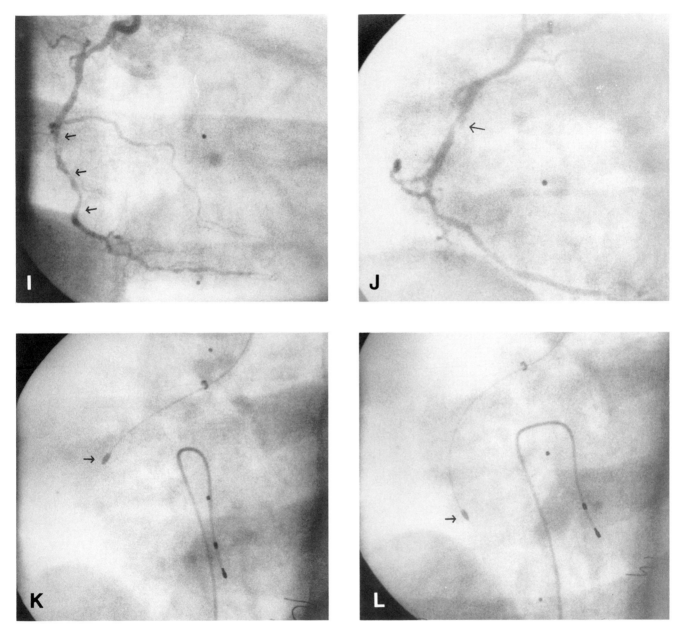

Case 31. I: Right coronary artery, RAO projection, 1989. New diffuse disease in distal third of right main trunk (arrows). **J:** Right coronary artery, LAO projection, 1989. Cleftlike lesion preangioplasty (arrow). **K:** Right coronary artery, LAO projection. Two millimeter Rotablator burr in RCA (arrow). **L:** Right coronary artery, LAO projection. See K.

See following pages for continuation of figures.

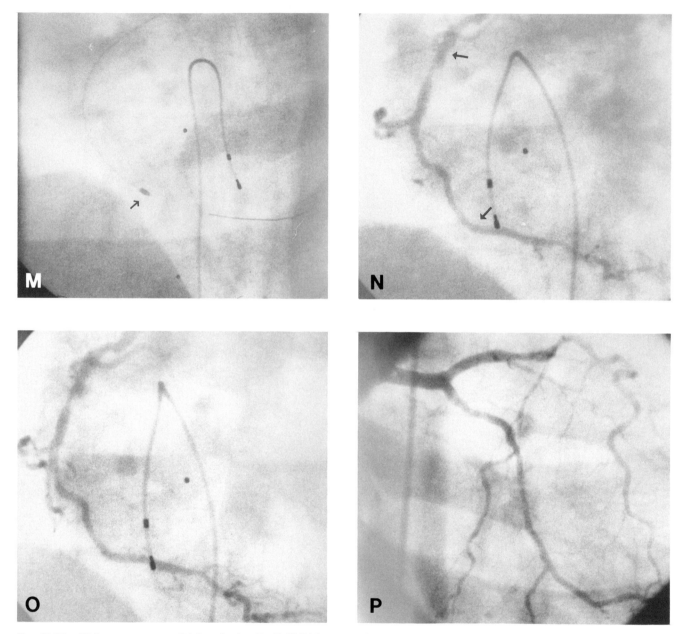

Case 31. M: Right coronary artery, LAO projection. See K. **N:** Right coronary artery, LAO projection. Results of Rotablator angioplasty between arrows. **O:** Right coronary artery, LAO projection. Thirty minutes post-Rotablator angioplasty. **P:** Left coronary artery, RAO projection, 1990. Persistent good results in circumflex.

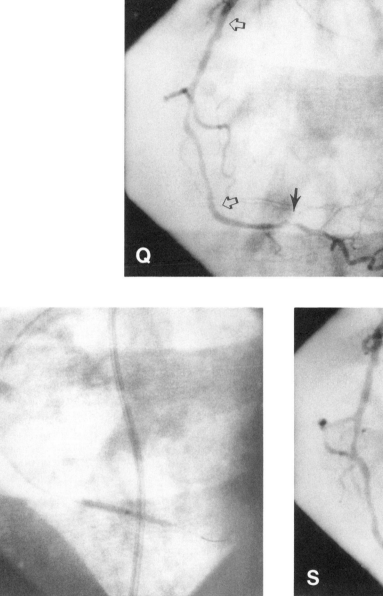

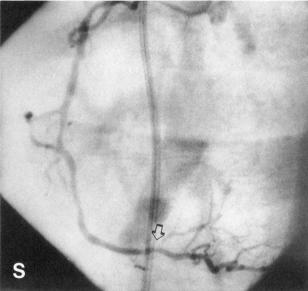

Case 31. Q: Right coronary artery, LAO projection. Persistent good results from Rotablator angioplasty between open arrows and new distal lesion in right coronary artery (solid arrow). **R:** Right coronary artery, LAO projection. Balloon inflated at distal lesion. **S:** Right coronary artery, LAO projection. Postangioplasty (arrow).

CASE NUMBER 32

Clinical

51-year-old man first seen in January 1990 with unstable angina; several recurrences and eventual stent placement

Angiography

RCA:	normal
LMain:	normal
LAD:	severe proximal lesion
LCX:	normal
LV:	normal

Equipment

Guide	Dilatation Catheter			Wire		
	1/90	3/90	6/90	1/90	3/90	6/90
JL4	2.5 mm ACX	3.0 mm ACX	3.0 mm ACX	0.014 FS	0.014 FS	0.016 Hyperflex

Strategy and Procedure

When the patient was first seen with a severe proximal lesion, it appeared ideal for angioplasty. The lesion was easily crossed, and a 2.5 mm ACX balloon initially used, with inflations to 10 atm for as long as 1 min. The lumen was judged not adequate, and the wire extended and balloon exchanged for a 3.0 mm ACX that was positioned at the lesion, and inflations of 10 atm for as long as 1 min were carried out. This produced a good lumen (C). In 3/90, he had a recurrence (D) that was redilated with a good result (E), utilizing a 3.0 mm ACX at 12 atm for 90 sec intervals ×3. In 6/90, he had return of symptoms, and angiography demonstrated another recurrence. He was most reluctant to undergo surgery, which was suggested to him, and he chose the alternative of a stent placement. Using a 0.016 Hyperflex guide wire, the lesion was easily crossed and a 3 mm ACX balloon positioned at the area of stenosis with dilatations to 10 atm (G), with a good result (H). A 3 mm Gianturco-Roubin stent was then delivered to the area of stenosis over a 3 mm Profile Plus balloon catheter (I). Two balloon inflations were carried out to seat the stent, and then the balloon was removed and replaced with the ACX 3 mm balloon and further inflations within the stent carried out to 7 atm for as long as 1 min to anchor the stent (J). Injections with the wire still across the lesion showed good flow and patency, including in the side branches (K). The final result showed an excellent lumen, and the patient continues to do well 6 months post stent placement.

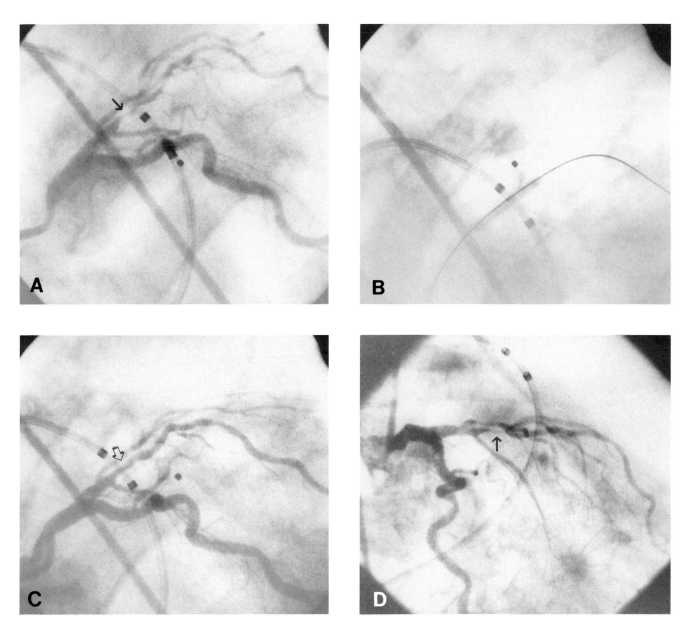

Case 32. A: Left coronary artery, angulated LAO projection, 1/90. Pre-PTCA (arrow). B: Left coronary artery, angulated RAO projection, 1/90. Balloon inflations. C: Left coronary artery, angulated RAO projection, 1/90. Post-PTCA (arrow). D: Left coronary artery, RAO projection, 3/90. Recurrent lesion, pre-PTCA (arrow).

See following pages for continuation of figures.

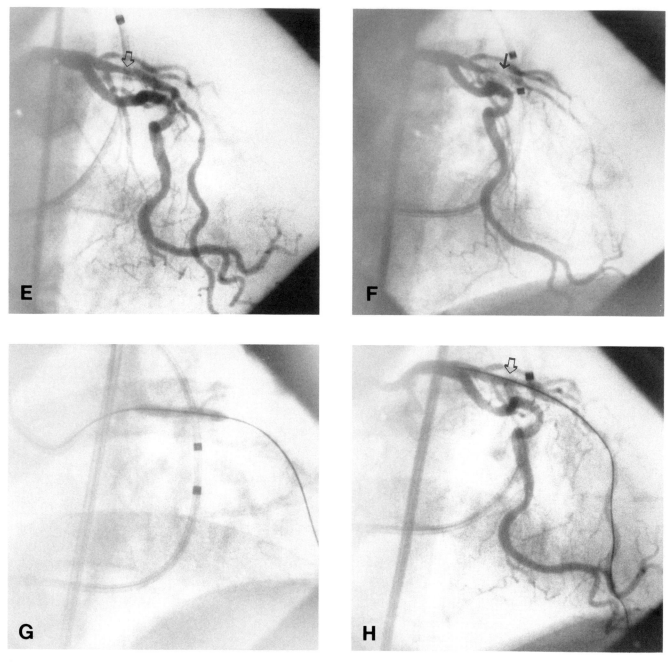

Case 32. E: Left coronary artery, RAO projection, 3/90. Post-PTCA (arrow). **F:** Left coronary artery, RAO projection, 6/90. Recurrent lesion in proximal LAD (arrow). **G:** Left coronary artery, RAO projec- tion, 6/90. Balloon angioplasty. **H:** Left coronary artery, RAO projec- tion, 6/90. Post-POBA (arrow).

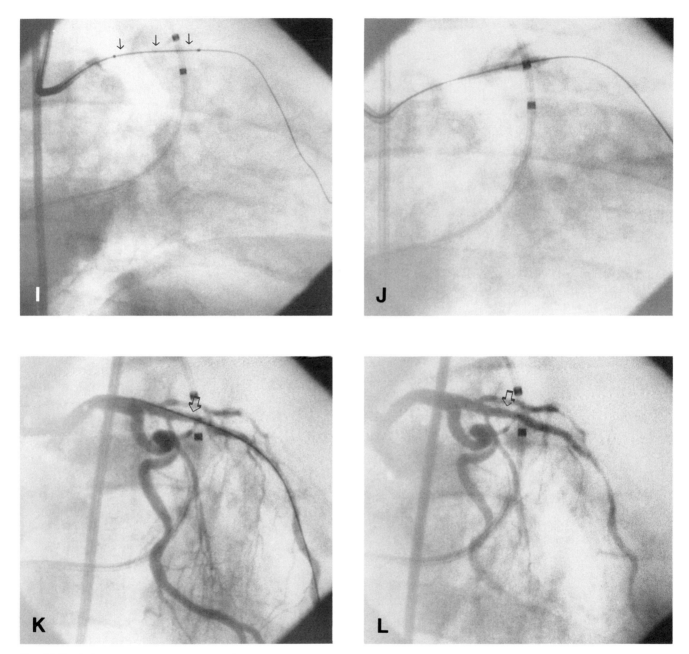

Case 32. **I:** Left coronary artery, RAO projection, 6/90. Stent delivery (arrows). **J:** Left coronary artery, RAO projection, 6/90. Stent molding inflation. **K:** Left coronary artery, RAO projection, 6/90. Post stent placement with wire across lesion (arrow). **L:** Left coronary artery, RAO projection, 6/90. Stent in place (arrow).

APPENDIX *II:* PROTOCOLS

A. CONSENT TO PARTICIPATE IN PERCUTANEOUS TRANSLUMINAL CORONARY ANGIOPLASTY

You are being invited to participate in a study to determine the effectiveness of a nonoperative procedure which has been designed to open up the narrowed portion (plaques) of the blood vessels (coronary arteries) which feed the heart muscle. The technique, which has been named "percutaneous transluminal coronary angioplasty" (PTCA), has been used for many years in the blood vessels (arteries) of the leg. In the last ten years, technical advancements have allowed its use in the coronary arteries.

We are learning which patients are most likely to benefit from the procedure, how effective it is in improving blood flow to the heart, and how long this improvement will last. You were selected because your coronary arteriogram and symptoms suggest that you are a good candidate for this procedure.

If you elect this form of treatment, the procedure will be performed using techniques very similar to those used to perform your coronary arteriogram. The essential difference is that in addition to injecting dye into the coronary arteries, a small, flexible, balloon-tipped catheter will be placed in the narrow region of the coronary artery. When inflated, the balloon compresses the plaque against the blood vessel wall itself—thus enlarging the opening (lumen) in the coronary artery.

It is estimated that the procedure will take about one to two hours and that the discomfort should not be appreciably different from that of a coronary arteriogram.

The occurrence of complications in an individual case is difficult to predict. The types of possible complications are likely to be similar to coronary arteriography and may include pain or discomfort due to leakage from the blood vessels in the leg or arm after the study. Occasionally a clot may form in these peripheral vessels and may require surgical removal. It is possible that more serious complications could occur requiring heart surgery, or result in a heart attack or death. These latter complications are rare with coronary arteriography.

In the past few years, especially due to the effort of pioneer investigators, some statistics are available on the incidence of serious complications. These may include abrupt reclosure of the "dilated" segment of the coronary arteries requiring emergency heart surgery (3%), heart attack (5%), or death (a fraction of 1%).

At the present time, the incidence of complications from percutaneous transluminal coronary angioplasty is approximately that of coronary bypass surgery.

Also, during the course of percutaneous transluminal coronary angioplasty certain medications may be utilized such as drugs from the nitroglycerin family and/or medications to relieve or prevent coronary spasm such as the calcium channel blockers (for example, nifedipine). These medications are designed to diminish the likelihood of coronary spasm which may occur in association with PTCA. In addition, suppression of one of the clotting mechanisms (platelets) will be necessary during and after coronary angioplasty. These medications may include aspirin and dipyridamole initially and for several months thereafter.

Your acceptance or rejection of our recommendation to undergo PTCA will not prejudice us for or against your medical care. If you decide to participate you are free to withdraw your consent and discontinue participation at any time without prejudice or effect on your medical care. If you have any questions, we expect you to ask us. If you have any additional questions later, Dr. _____ (phone: _____) will be happy to answer them.

YOUR SIGNATURE INDICATES THAT YOU HAVE READ AND UNDERSTAND THE FOREGOING INFORMATION, THAT YOU HAVE DISCUSSED THE PROPOSED TREATMENT AND THE THERAPEUTIC ALTERNATIVES WITH A PRINCIPAL OPERATOR AND HIS/HER STAFF, AND THAT YOU HAVE DECIDED TO SELECT PTCA BASED UPON THE INFORMATION PROVIDED.

_____
Signature of Patient

_____
Date

_____
Signature of Witness

_____
Date

_____
Signature of Physician

_____
Date

B. DYE REACTION PROTOCOL

I.   Evening prior to PTCA
    A. Prednisone 60 mg po q 12 hr
    B. Cimetidine 300 mg po q 6 hr
    C. Benadryl 50 mg po q 6 hr
II. On call to catheterization laboratory
    A. Be certain of excellent peripheral IV
    B. Hydrocortisone 100 mg IV
    C. Cimetidine 300 mg po
    D. Benadryl 50 mg IM
III. During PTCA procedure
    A. Right heart catheter with large central lumen and pacemaker capability in place
    B. Epinephrine, vasopressors, atropine on table
    C. Use nonionic contrast medium
    D. Limit amount of contrast used
    E. If anaphylaxis occurs
        1. Epinepherrine 0.2 mg IV q 1–2 min as necessary
        2. Hydrocortisone 100 mg IV
        3. Rapid infusion of normal saline IV to maintain filling pressure
        4. Availability of anesthesia/intubation
IV. After PTCA procedure
    A. Prednisone 60 mg po q 12 hr $\times$ 2 doses
    B. Cimetidine 300 mg po q 6 hr $\times$ 4 doses

C. PRE-PTCA ORDERS

Date & Time	Doctor's Orders

These orders supersede all previous orders

ADMITTING

  1. Admit to heart center

HISTORY

  2. Old hospital record to floor
  3. Diagnosis:
  4. Allergies:
  5. Date of PTCA:

CONSENTS

  6. A. Permit for cardiac catheterization
      B. Consent for percutaneous transluminal coronary angioplasty
      C. Operative permit for possible coronary artery bypass grafts

VITAL SIGNS

  7. TPR, tid

DIET

  8. Prudent heart diet. NPO after midnight the day of exam
     Weight: on admission and day of exam on electric scale

INPUT AND OUTPUT

  9. D5W TKO in left arm with #18- or #20-gauge angiocath

RESP CARE/MONITOR

  10. No smoking
  11. EKG

MEDICATIONS

  12. Pre-med: Valium 5 mg po and Benedryl 50 mg IM on call to Cath Lab

(continued)

C. PRE-PTCA ORDERS (continued)

Date & Time	Doctor's Orders

X-RAY

    13. PA and lateral chest X-ray

LAB WORK

    14. CBC, platelet count, PT, PTT, UA, electrolytes, BUN, creatinine, A-1 panel, EKG, type and screen, CPK totals and isoenzymes

OTHER   Prep: Both groins and right antecubital

    15. Have patient void before leaving ward. Send patient in hospital gown, with dentures in and glasses (if present), with chart, on surgilift to Cardiac Cath Lab on call at:

_____   _____

Physician's Signature   Date

D. POST-PTCA ORDERS

Date & Time	Doctor's Orders

These orders supplement all previous orders

VITAL SIGNS

    1. q 15 min $\times$4 or until stable, then q 30 min $\times$2, then every 1 hr $\times$4
    2. Check "cath site" for signs of bleeding, color, temperature, and pulse q 30 min $\times$ 4, then q 1 hr $\times$4

ACTIVITY

    3. Remove sandbag after 4 hr
    4. Bed rest for _____

DIET

    5. Dietician to see patient tomorrow for instruction of prescribed diet
    6. NPO until _____

INPUT AND OUTPUT

    7. IV ( )_____ml/hr for _____hr (total: _____ml), then heparin lock

MEDICATIONS

    8. Analgesic (for "cath" site):
    Nitroglycerin 1/150 gr sublingual q 2 hr $\times$4 doses, then PRN for angina Hold if BP less than 90 systolic
    Isordil 10 mg po qid. Hold if BP less than 90 systolic
    Nifedipine 20 mg po qid. Hold if BP less than 90 systolic
    ASA-enteric coated 325 mg po qd
    Persantine 75 mg po bid
    DC inderal (if on)

EKG

    9. EKG at _____ and _____ today and at 8:00 A.M. tomorrow

LABORATORY

    10. H + H and CPK-MB at 4:00 P.M. today and at 8:00 A.M. tomorrow

_____   _____

Physician's Signature   Date

E. BALLOON CATHETER SPECIFICATIONS

	Deflated balloon profiles (inches)										Length (mm)	Pressure		Wire[c]	Shaft (French)[d]	Contrast[e]	Marker[f]
	1.5 mm	2.0 mm	2.25 mm	2.5 mm	2.75 mm	3.0 mm	3.25 mm	3.5 mm	3.75 mm	4.0 mm		Max[a]	Nom[b]				
ACS (*polyethylene*)																	
ACS Mini (*1.3 mm*)	.025	—	—	—	—	—	—	—	—	—	20	8	6	NA	2.9	No	M
Delta	—	.044	—	.050	—	.054	—	.062	—	.062	20	10	6	.018	4.3	Yes	P, D
Simpson Robert	—	.045	—	.050	—	.055	—	.062	—	.063	20	10	6	.018	4.3–4.7	Yes	P, D
Hartzler Micro II	.033	.035	—	.042	—	.045	—	.050	—	—	20	10	6	NA	3.7	No	M
Hartzler LPS	.031	.032	—	.041	—	.042	—	.046	—	.053	20	10	6	NA	2.9–4.3	No	M
Simpson Ultra Low	—	.040	—	.046	—	.049	—	.059	—	.059	20	10	6	.014	4.3–4.7	Yes	M, D
Simpson Ultra Low II	—	.037	—	.044	—	.047	—	.051	—	.054	20	10	6	.014	3.7	Yes	M
Hartzler ACX	—	.031	—	.032	—	.035	—	.037	—	.038	20	10	6	.014	3.7	No	M
ACS RX	—	.040	—	.044	—	.046	—	.049	—	.053	20	10	6	.018	4.5	Yes	M
Stack perfusion	—	—	—	.064	—	.065	—	.067	—	—	20	10	6	.018	4.5	Yes	M, D
Angled balloon	—	.047	—	.056	—	.060	—	—	—	—	25	10	6	.018	4.3	Yes	P, D
CORDIS (*polyester*)																	
Atlas LP	—	.041	—	.043	—	.046	—	.052	—	—	20	12		.018	4.0	Yes	M
MANSFIELD (*polyethylene*)																	
Glider	—	.032	—	.035	—	.040	—	.044	—	.046	20	10	6	.014	4.0	No	P
Pro Act	—	.038	—	.040	—	.042	—	.050	—	.053	20	10	8.6	.014	4.0	No	M
Heart Trak III	—	.040	—	.046	—	.051	—	.053	—	.059	20, 25	10	8.6	.018	4.5	Yes	P, D
Max Trak	—	.040	—	.046	—	.051	—	.053	—	.059	20, 25	10	8.6	.018	4.5	Yes	P, D
MEDTRONIC (*polyethylene,*																	
ThruFlex	—	.034	—	.038	—	.042	—	.046	—	—	20	10	6	.016[h]	3.5	Yes	M, D
Omniflex	—	.034	—	.038	—	.042	—	.046	—	—	20	10	6	NA	2.9	No	M
Prime	—	.040	—	.044	—	.049	—	.053	—	.056	25	10	6	.018[i]	4.3	Yes	M
SCHNEIDER-SHILEY (*polyethylene terephthalate*)																	
Microsoftrac	.033	.034	—	.036	—	.038	—	.042	—	.044	20	16	10	.014	4.3/3.2	No	M
Monorail	.032	.034	—	.036	—	.040	—	.042	—	.044	20	16	10	.014	3.0	No	M

E. BALLOON CATHETER SPECIFICATIONS (continued)

	Deflated balloon profiles (inches)										Length (mm)	Pressure		Wire[c]	Shaft (French)[d]	Contrast[e]	Marker[f]
	1.5 mm	2.0 mm	2.25 mm	2.5 mm	2.75 mm	3.0 mm	3.25 mm	3.5 mm	3.75 mm	4.0 mm		Max[a]	Nom[b]				
SCI-MED (*polyolefin copolymer*)																	
Dilating guide wire	.017	—	—	—	—	—	—	—	—	—				NA	1.8	No	None
ACE	—	.022	—	.030	—	.032	—	.036	—	—	20	10	7	NA	1.8	No	P
Skinny	.027	.031	—	.033	—	.037	—	.040	—	.042	20	12	8	.014	3.5/3.0	No	M
Long Skinny	—	.031	—	.034	—	.038	—	.040	—	.044	20	12	8	.014	3.5/3.0	No	M
Strong	—	.036	—	.038	—	.043	—	—	—	—	30	14	8	.014	4.3	No	M
Trak Plus	—	.040	—	.046	—	.049	—	—	—	—	20	14	8	.018	4.3	Yes	M
USCI (*polyethylene terephthalate*)																	
Probe	—	.020	—	.025	—	.030	—	—	—	—	20,15	10	5	NA	1.7	No	P
Mini-Profile	—	.031	—	.033	—	.035	—	.037	—	—	20	10	5	.018	3.5	No	M
Simplus PE/t	—	.034	—	.034	—	.036	—	.037	—	.042	20	10	5	.018	4.3	No	M
Profile Plus	—	.033	.038	.038	.039	.039	.040	.040	.041	.041	20	10	5	.018[g,i]	4.3	Yes	M, D
(*polyvinyl*)																	
LPS	—	.039	—	.047	—	.050	—	.051	—	.053	25	10	7	.018[g,h]	4.3	Yes	P, D
LPS II	—	.036	—	.047	—	.050	—	.051	—	.053	20	10	7	.018[g,i]	4.3	Yes	M
LPS II Short	—	.036	—	.047	—	.050	—	—	—	—	12	10	7	.018[g,i]	4.3	Yes	M

All specifications are per manufacturer's product information, unless otherwise indicated.

From: Avedissian MG, Killeavy ES, Garcia JM, Dear WE: Percutaneous transluminal coronary angioplasty: A review of current balloon dilitation systems. Cathet Cardiovasc Diagn 18:263–275, 1989.

[a]Maximum pressure, in bar, per *Texas Heart Institute experience*. (Note: Balloons ≥ 3.0 mm tolerate 1–3 bar less than the maximum pressure listed.)

[b]Nominal pressure, in bar: pressure at which balloon reaches indicated size.

[c]Maximum allowable wire size; NA = not applicable.

[d]Shaft diameter, French.

[e]Ability of distal contrast injection.

[f]Marker positions: P, proximal; M, mid; D, distal.

[g].018 wire = no pressure or dye injection.

[h]Except 2.0 mm balloon, which uses maximum wire size of .014.

[i]Except 2.0 mm balloon, which uses maximum wire size of .016.

F. GUIDING CATHETER SPECIFICATIONS

	Length (cm)	I.D.[a] (inches)	Tip marker	Flexible tip	Deformable tip	Side hole available	Curve styles available
ACS							
ET Hi-Flow 8F/7.5F tip	100	.076	Yes	Yes	No	Yes	Judkins, Amplatz, IMA
CORDIS							
Brite-tip 8F	100	.074	Yes	Yes	Yes	Yes	Judkins, Amplatz, Arani, El Gamal, Multipurpose, Bypass, IMA
INTERVENTIONAL MEDICAL							
IMI 8F	100	.076	Yes	Yes	No	Yes	Judkins, Amplatz, Arani, El Gamal, Multipurpose, Bypass, IMA, Out-of-plane Judkins
IMI 9F	100	.088	Yes	Yes	No	Yes	Judkins, Amplatz, Arani, El Gamal, Multipurpose, Bypass, IMA, out-of-plane Judkins
MALLINCKRODT							
Softtouch 8F	100	.079	No	Yes	No	Yes	Judkins, Amplatz
SCHNEIDER-SHILEY							
Softtip 7F	80, 100	.063	No	Yes	Yes	Yes	Judkins (short and regular tip), Amplatz, Arani, El Gamal, Multipurpose, Bypass, IMA, Out-of-plane Judkins
Softtip 8F	80, 100	.076	No	Yes	Yes	Yes	Judkins (short and regular tip), Amplatz, Arani, El Gamal, Multipurpose, Bypass, IMA, out-of-plane Judkins, Brachial[b]
Softtip 9F	80, 100	.080	No	Yes	Yes	Yes	Judkins (short and regular tip), Amplatz, Arani, El Gamal, Multipurpose, Bypass, IMA, Out-of-plane Judkins
USCI							
Standard 8F	100	.068	No	No	No	Yes	Judkins, Amplatz, Arani, El Gamal, Multipurpose, Out-of-plane Judkins
Standard 9F	100	.072	No	No	No	Yes	Judkins, Amplatz, El Gamal, Multipurpose, Out-of-plane Judkins
Large Lumen 8F	100	.072	Yes	Yes	Yes	Yes	Judkins, Amplatz, Arani, El Gamal, multipurpose, bypass, IMA, Out-of-plane Judkins, Brachial IMA,[c] Diagnostic curve ("Dx" series), Block RCA, Williams RCA
Finesse Large Lumen 8F	100	.072	Yes	Yes	Yes	Yes	Judkins, Amplatz, Arani, Out-of-plane Judkins, Diagnostic curve ("Dx" series)
Stertzer Brachial 8.3F	90, 105	.068	No	Yes	No	Yes	Multipurpose and Bent Tip with variable curve size and tip length

All specifications are per manufacturer's product information, unless otherwise indicated.
From: Avedissian MG, Killeavy ES, Garcia JM, Dear WE: Percutaneous transluminal coronary angioplasty: A review of current balloon dilation systems. Cathet Cardiovasc Diagn 18:263–275, 1989.
[a]I.D. = inner diameter.
[b]80 cm length.
[c]70 cm length.

G. GUIDE WIRE SPECIFICATIONS

	Diameter (inches)	Tip style	Tip construction (cm)[a]	Torqueability[b]	Flexibility[b]	Malleability[b]	Length (cm)	Radiopaque portion (cm)
ACS								
Hi Torque Standard	0.014	Straight and "J"	—	3+	2+	3+	175	2
	0.018	Straight	2	4+	1+	4+	175	2
Hi Torque Intermediate	0.014	Straight and "J"	2	3+	3+	3+	175	3
	0.018	Straight	2	4+	3	3+	175	3
Hi Torque Floppy	0.018	Straight	2	4+	4+	2+	175	2
Hi Torque Floppy II	0.014	Straight and "J"	2	3+	4+	3+	175	2
PDT	0.014	Straight	1	2+	3+	2+	175	1
Exchange (HTF type)	0.014	Straight	2	1+	4+	1+	300	NA
	0.018	Straight	2	1+	4+	1+	300	NA
Doc Wire	0.014	NA	NA	NA	NA	NA	145	NA
Extension	0.018	NA	NA	NA	NA	NA	145	NA
USCI								
Standard	0.014	"J" only	—	3+	2+	3+	175	25
	0.016	"J" only	—	4+	1+	4+	175	25
Flex	0.014	Straight and "J"	2	3+	3+	1+	175	25
	0.016	Straight and "J"	2	4+	3+	1+	175	25
Veriflex	0.014	Straight and "J"	3	3+	4+	1+	175	25
Hi Per Flex	0.014	"J" only	3	4+	3+	3+	180	25
	0.016	"J" only	3	4+	3+	3+	180	25
Exchange (FLEX type)[c]	0.014–0.016	Straight	2	2+	3+	2+	300	25
Stertzer-Myler Extension	0.016	NA	NA	NA	NA	NA	122	NA
Linx Extension	0.014	NA	NA	NA	NA	NA	122	NA

NA, not applicable. *All specifications are per manufacturer's product information, unless otherwise indicated.*
From: Avedissian MG, Killeavy ES, Garcia JM, Dear WE: Percutaneous transluminal coronary angioplasty: A review of current balloon dilitation systems. Cathet Cardiovasc Diagn 18:263–275, 1989. Used with permission from author.
[a]See text for discussion of "tip construction."
[b]Subjectively evaluated, scale: 0+ = minimum, 4+ = maximum.
[c]Distal 125 cm are .014 diameter; proximal 175 cm are .016 diameter.

BIBLIOGRAPHY and SUGGESTED READINGS

CHAPTER 1. A HISTORY OF CARDIAC CATHETERIZATION

1. Forssman W: "Experiments on Myself. Memoirs of a Surgeon in Germany." New York: Saint Martin's Press, 1974, p 81

2. Grmek MD: "Catalogue des Manuscrits de Claude Bernard." Paris: Masson et Cie, 1967.

3. Harvey W: "De Motu Cordis." Translated by Chauncey Leake, Tercentenary Edition. Springfield, IL: Charles C. Thomas, 1928.

4. Chaveau A, Marey EJ: Appareils et experiences cardiographiques. In "Memoirs de l'Academie Imperiale de Medicien, Paris, Vol. 26." 1863, p 268.

5. Forssman W: Die Sondierung des rechten Herzens. Klin Wochenschr 8:2085–2087, 1929.

6. Bleichoder, Ungar, Loeb: Three short articles. Klin Wochenschr 49:1503, 1912.

7. Forssman W: Addendum to manuscript. Klin Wochenschr 8:2287, 1929.

8. Forssman W: Uber Kontrasrdarstellung de Hohlen des lebenden rechten Herzens und der Lungenschagader. Munchen Med Wochenschr 78:489, 1931.

9. Liljestrand G: In: "Le Prix Nobel cn 1956." Stockholm: Nobel Foundation, 1957.

10. Klein O: Zur Bestimmung des zirkulatorischen minutens Volumen nach den Fickschen Prinzip (Gewinnung des gemischten venosen Blutes mittels Herzsondierung). Munchen Med Wochenschr 77:1311, 1930.

11. Padilla, Cossio, Berconsky: Dondeo del Corazon; technia. Semana Med 21:79, 1932.

12. Cournand A, Ranges HA: Catheterization of the right auricle in man. Proc Soc Exp Biol Med 46:462, 1941.

13. Cournand A: Cardiac catheterization. Development of the technique, its contribution to experimental medicine, and its initial applications in man. Acta Med Scand 579[Suppl]:4–32, 1975.

14. Bradley SE, Curry JJ: Catheterization of the renal vein. In Goldring W, Chasis H (eds): "Hypertension and Hypertensive Disease." New York: Commonwealth Fund, 1944.

15. Bradley SE, Ingelfinger FJ, Bradley GP, Curry JJ: The estimation of hepatic blood flow in man. J Clin Invest 24:390–397, 1945.

16. Brannon ES, Weens HS, Warren JV: Atrial septal defect. Study of hemodynamics by the technique of right heart catheterization. Am J Med Sci 210:480, 1945.

17. Baldwin E deF, Moore LV, Noble RP: The demonstration of ventricular septal defect by means of right heart catheterization. Am Heart J 32:152, 1944.

18. McMichael J, Sharpey-Schafer EP: The action of intravenous digoxin in man. 13:1123, 1944.

19. Sturzbecher H: Cholers, Dieffenbach and the catheterization of the heart, 1831. Deutch Med J 22:470–471, 1971.

20. Reboul H, Racine M: Ventriculographie cardiaque experimentale. Presse Med 37:763–767, 1933.

21. Nuvoli U: Arteriografia dell'aorta toracica mediante puncture dell'aorta ascendente o del ventriculos. Policlinico 43:227–230,233–234,237, 1936.

22. Ponsdomenech ER, Nunez VB: Heart puncture in man for diodrast visualization of the ventricular chambers and great vessels. Am Heart J 41:643, 1951.

23. Smith PW, Wilson CW, Cregg HA, Klassen KP: Cardioangiography. J Thorac Surg 28:273–280, 1954.

24. Cregg HA, Smith PW, Wilson CW, Bull JW: Cardioangiography. Radiology 65:368–372, 1955.

25. Lehman JS, Mussler BG, Lykens HP: Cardiac ventriculography. Am J Roentgenol 77:207–234, 1957.

26. Brock R, Milstein BB, Ross DN: Percutaneous left ventricular puncture in the assessment of aortic stenosis. Thorax 11:163, 1956.

27. Fleming P, Gibson R: Percutaneous left ventricular puncture in the assessment of aortic stenosis. Thorax 12:37–49, 1957.

28. Yu PN, Lovejoy FW Jr, Schreiner BF, Leahy RH, Stanfield CA, Walther H: Direct left ventricular puncture in the evaluation of aortic and mitral stenosis. Am Heart J 55:926–940, 1958.

29. Ross DN: Percutaneous left ventricular puncture in the assessment of the obstructed left ventricule. Guy's Hosp Rep 108:159–162, 1959.

30. Radner S: Suprasternal puncture of the left atrium for flow studies. Acta Med Scand 148:57–61, 1954.

31. Hansen AT, Fabricius J, Pedersen A, Sandoe E: Suprasternal puncture of the left atrium and great vessels. Experience from 500 punctures. Am Heart J 63:443–450, 1953.

32. Lemmon WM, Lehman JS, Boyer RA: Suprasternal transaortic coronary arteriography. Circulation 19:47–54, 1959.

33. Facquet JM, Alhomme P, Lemoine JM: Colvez and Lagadur: La pression auriculaire gauche recieillie por voie transbroncheque, dans le cardiopathies mitrales. Arch Mal Coeur 47:136, 1954.

274 Bibliography and Suggested Readings

34. Allison PR, Linden RJ: The bronchoscopic measurement of left auricular pressure. Circulation 7:669, 1953.

35. Morrow AG, Braunwald E, Haller JA, Sharp EH: Left atrial pressure pulse in mitral valve disease. Circulation 16:399, 1957.

36. Davila JC, Rivera PC, Voci C: Combined catheterization of the heart utilizing a modified transbronchial technique, percutaneous left ventricular puncture and venous and arterial catheterization. Am Heart J 57:415, 1959.

37. Bjork VO, Malmstrom G, Uggla LG: Left auricular pressure measurements in man. Ann Surg 138:718–723, 1953.

38. Fischer DL, McCaffrey MH: Right and left atrium puncture for simultaneous right and left heart catheterization. Circulation 14:935, 1956.

39. Wood EH, Sutter W, Swan HJC, Helmholtz HF: The technical special instrumentation problems associated with catheterization of the left side of the heart. Proc Staff Meet, Mayo Clin 31:108, 1956.

40. Blakemore W.S., Schnable TG, Kuo PT, Conn HL, Langfield SB, Heiman DD, Woske H: Diagnostic and physiologic measurements using left heart catheterization. J Thorac Surg 34:436, 1957.

41. Litwack RS, Samet P, Bernstein WH, Silverman LM, Turkewitz H, Lesser ME: The effect of exercise upon the mean diastolic left atrial-left ventricular gradient in mitral stenosis. J Thorac Surg 34:449, 1957.

42. Ross J Jr: Catheterization of the left heart through the interatrial septum: A new technique and its experimental evaluation. Surg Forum 9:297, 1959.

43. Cope C: Technique for transseptal catheterization of the left atrium: Preliminary report. J Thorac Surg 37:482–486, 1959.

44. Brockenbrough EC, Braunwald E: A new technic of left ventricular angiocardiography and transseptal left heart catheterization. Am J Cardiol 6:1062–1064, 1960.

45. Bevegard S, Carlens E, Jonsson B, Karlof I: A technique for transseptal left heart catheterization via the right external jugular vein. Thorax 15:299–302, 1960.

46. Rashkind WJ, Miller WN: Creation of an atrial septal defect without thoracotomy: Palliative approach to complete transposition of the great arteries. JAMA 196:991–992, 1966.

47. Park SC, Zuberbuhler JR, Neches WH, Lenox CC, Zoltun RA: A new atrial septostomy technique. Cathet Cardiovasc Diagn 1:195–202, 1975.

48. Mullins CE: New catheter and technique for transseptal left heart catheterization in infants and children. Circulation 59/60[Suppl II]:II-251, 1979.

49. Lock JE, Khalilullah M, Shrivastava S, Bahl V, Keane JF: Percutaneous catheter commissurotomy in rheumatic mitral stenosis. N Engl J Med 313:1515–1518, 1985.

50. Castellanos A, Pereiras R: Counter-part aortography. Rev Cuban Cardial 2:187, 1940.

51. Radner S: An attempt at the roentgenologic visualization of the coronary blood vessels in man. Acta Radiol 26:497–502, 1945.

52. Radner S: Thoracic aortography by catheterization from the radial artery. Acta Radiol 29:178–180, 1948.

53. Zimmerman HA: Presentation at the Twenty-Second Annual Scientific Session of the American Heart Association, Atlantic City, NJ, June 4, 1949.

54. Zimmerman HA, Scott RW, Becker NO: Catheterization of the left side of the heart in man. Circulation 1:357–359, 1950.

55. Wiggers CJ: "Physiology in Health and Disease, ed 4." Philadelphia: Lea and Febiger, 1944.

56. Limon Lason, R Bouchard A: El cateterismo intracardico: Cateterizacion de las cavidades izquierdas en el hombre. Registro simultaneo de presion y electrocardiograma intracavatarios. Arch Inst Cardiol Mexico 21:271, 1950.

57. Pierce EC: Percutaneous femoral artery catheterization in man with special reference to aortography. J Surg Gynecol Obstet 93:56–74, 1951.

58. Seldinger SI: Catheter replacement of the needle in percutaneous arteriography. A new technic. Acta Radiol 39:368–376, 1953.

59. Prioton JB, Thevenet A, Pellissier M, Puech P, Latour H., Pourquier J: Cardiographie ventriculaire gauche par cathétérisme retrograde percutane femoral. Presse Med 65:1948–1951, 1957.

60. Ingraham FD, Alexander E, Matson DD: Polyethylene. New synthetic plastic for use in surgery; experimental applications in neurosurgery. JAMA 135:82–87, 1947.

61. Odman P: Radiopaque polyethylene catheter. Acta Radiol 45:117–124, 1956.

62. Olin T: EKG-styrd Kontrastinjektion vid angiografi. Twenty-Second Congress of Nordisk for. For Medicinsky Radiologi, at Abo, 1958.

63. Littman D, Starobin OE, Hall JH, Matthews RJ, Williams JA: A new method of left ventricular catheterization. Circulation 21:1150–1155, 1960.

64. Bellman S, Frank HA, Lambert P, Littman D, Williams JA: Coronary arteriography. I. Differential opacification of the aortic stream by catheters of special design-experimental development. N Engl J Med 262:325–328, 1960.

65. Williams JA, Littman D, Hall J, Bellman S, Lambert P, Frank H: New principle for coronary arteriography. II. Clinical experience with loop end catheter. N Engl J Med 262:328–332, 1960.

66. Dotter CT: Left ventricular and systemic arterial catheterization: A simple percutaneous method using a spring guide. Am Roentgenol Radium Ther Nucl Med 83:969–984, 1960.

67. Dotter CT, Gensini GG: Percutaneous retrograde catheterization of the left ventricle and systemic arteries of man. Radiology 75:171–184, 1960.

68. Sones FM Jr: Cine coronary arteriography. Circulation 20:773, 1959 (abstr).

69. Judkins MP: Percutaneous transfemoral selective coronary arteriography. Radiol Clin North Am 6:467, 1968.

70. Swan HJC, Ganz W, Forrester JS, Marcus H, Diamond G, Chonette D: Catheterization of the heart in man with use of a flow directed balloon-tipped catheter. N Engl J Med 28:3447, 1970.

71. Gruentzig A, Hopff H: Perkutane Rekanalisation chronischer arterieller Verschlusse mit einem neuen Dilatationskatheter. Deutsche Med Wochenschr 99:2502, 1974.

72. Sanchez-Perez JM, Carter RA: Time factors in cerebral angiography and an automatic seriograph. Am J Roentgenol 62:509–518, 1949.

73. Dotter CT, Steinberg I, Temple HJ: Automatic roentgenray roll film magazine for angiocardiography and cerebral angiography. Am J Roentgenol 62:355, 1949.

74. Scott WG, Moore S: Rapid serialization of X-ray exposures by radiography, utilizing rollfilm nine and one-half inches wide. Radiology 53:846, 1949.

75. Gidlund AS: New apparatus for direct cineroentgenography. Acta Radiol 32:81, 1949.

76. Sturm RE, Morgan RH: Screen intensification systems and their limitations. Am J Roentgenol 62:617, 1949.

77. Moon RJ: Amplifying and intensifying fluoroscopic images by means of scanning X-ray tube. Science 112:339, 1950.

78. Janker R: "Roentgenotogische Funktionsdiagnostic Wupper." Elberfeld: Garandit, 1954.

79. Sones FM Jr: Cinecardioangiography. Pediatr Clin North Am 5:945, 1958.

80. Rousthoi P: Uber Angiokardiographie. Vorlautige Mitteilung. Acta Radiol 14:419, 1933.

81. Radner S: An attempt at the roentgenographic visualization of the coronary blood vessels in man. Acta Radiol 26:497, 1945.

82. Manses-Hoyos J, Gomez del Campo C: Angiography of the thoracic aorta and coronary vessels with direct injection of an opaque solution into the aorta. Radiology 50:211, 1948.

83. Jonsson G: Visualization of the coronary arteries: Preliminary report. Acta Radiol 29:536, 1948.

84. DiGuglielmo L, Guttadauro MA: A roentgenologic study of the coronary arteries in the living. Acta Radiol [Suppl 97]:1–82, 1952.

85. Dotter CT, Frische LH: Visualization of the coronary circulation by occlusive aortography: A practical method. Radiology 76:502, 1958.

86. Ricketts HJ, Abrams HA: Percutaneous selective coronary cinearteriography. JAMA 181:620, 1962.

87. Ferris LP, Spence PW, King BG, Williams HB: Electric engineering 55:498, 1936.

88. Wiggers CJ: Am Heart J 20:399, 1940.

89. Zoll PM, Linenthal AJ, Phelps MD Jr: Termination of refractory tachycardia by external electric countershock. Circulation 24:1078, 1961.

90. Lown B, Neuman J, Amarasingham R, Berkovitz BV: Comparison of alternating current with direct current countershock across the closed chest. Am J Cardiol 10:223, 1962.

91. Kouwenhoven WB, Jude JR, Knickerbocker GG: Closed chest cardiac massage. JAMA 173:1064, 1960.

92. Jude JR, Kouwenhoven WB, Knickerbocker GG: Cardiac arrest: Report of application of external cardiac massage on 118 patients. JAMA 178:1063, 1961.

93. Dotter CT, Judkins MP: Transluminal treatment of arteriosclerotic obstruction. Description of a technique and a preliminary report of its application. Circulation 30:654, 1964.

94. Gruentzig AR, Turina MI, Schneider JA: Experimental percutaneous dilation of coronary artery stenosis. Circulation 53–54 [Suppl II]:II-81, 1976 (abstr).

95. Gruentzig AR, Myler RK, Hanna ES, Turina MI: Coronary transluminal angioplasty. Circulation 55–56[Suppl III]:III-84, 1977 (abstr).

CHAPTER 2. CORONARY ANGIOPLASTY EQUIPMENT

Abele JE: Balloon catheters and transluminal dilatation technical considerations. Am J Roentgenol 135:901–906, 1980.

Arani DT: A new catheter for angioplasty of the right coronary artery and aorto-coronary bypass grafts. Cathet Cardiovasc Diagn 11:647–653, 1985.

Arani DT, Bunnell IL, Visco JP, Conley JG: Double loop guiding catheter: A primary catheter for angioplasty of the right coronary artery. Cathet Cardiovasc Diagn 15:-125–131, 1988.

Athanasopoulis CA: Percutaneous transluminal coronary angioplasty: General principles. Am J Roentenol 135:893–900, 1980.

Avedissian MG, Killeavy ES, Garcia JM, Dear WE: Percutaneous transluminal coronary angioplasty: A review of current balloon dilatation systems. Cathet Cardiovasc Diagn 18:263–275, 1989.

Carr ML: The use of the guiding catheter in coronary angioplasty: The technique of manipulating catheters to obtain the necessary power to cross tight coronary stenoses. Cathet Cardiovasc Diagn 12:189–197, 1986.

Dorros G, Lewin RF: The brachial artery method to transluminal internal mammary artery angioplasty. Cathet Cardiovasc Diagn 12:341–346, 1986.

Dorros G, Lewin RF: The probe exchange catheter. Cathet Cardiovasc Diagn 16:263–266, 1989.

Dorros G, Lewin RF, Mathiak L: Probe, a balloon wire: Initial experience. Cathet Cardiovasc Diagn 14:286–288, 1988.

El Gamal MI, Bonnier JJ, Michels HR, van Gelder LM: Improved success rate of percutaneous transluminal graft and coronary angioplasty with the El Gamal guiding catheter. Cathet Cardiovasc Diagn 11:89–96, 1985

Encasteneda-Zuniga WR: "Addition Transluminal Angioplasty." New York: Thieme-Stratton, 1983.

Gerlok AJ Jr, Regen DM, Shaft MI: An examination of the physical characteristics leading to angioplasty balloon rupture. Radiology 144:421–422, 1982.

Hartz WH, McLean GK: Current technology of angioplasty catheters and accessories. In Jang GD (ed): "Angioplasty." New York: McGraw-Hill, 1986, pp 156–169.

Heibig J, Angelini P, Leachman DR, Beall MM, Beall AC: Use of mechanical devices for distal hemoperfusion during balloon catheter coronary angioplasty. Cathet Cardiovascular Diagn 15:143–149, 1988.

Jang DJ (ed): "Angioplasty." New York: McGraw-Hill, 1986.

Kamada RO, Fergusson DJG, Itagaki RK: Percutaneous entry of the brachial artery for transluminal coronary angioplasty. Cathet Cardiovasc Diagn 15:132–133, 1988.

Krajcer Z, Boskovic D, Angelini P, Leatherman LL, Springer A, Leachman RD: Transluminal coronary angioplasty of right coronary artery: Brachial countdown approach. Cathet Cardiovasc Diagn 8:553–564, 1982.

Levin DC, Harrington DP, Bettmann, MA, Garnek JD, Torman H, Murray T, Boxt LM, Geller SC: Equipment choices, technical aspects and pitfalls of percutaneous transluminal angioplasty. Cardiovasc Intervent Radiol 7:1–10.

Myler RK, Boucher RA, Cumberland DC, Stertzer SH: Guiding catheter selection for right coronary artery angioplasty. Cathet Cardiovasc Diagn 19:58–67, 1990.

Myler RK, Mooney MR, Stertzer SH, Clark DA, Hidalgo BO, Fishman J: The balloon on a wire device: A new ultra-low-profile coronary angioplasty system/concept. Cathet Cardiovasc Diagn 14:135–140, 1988.

Nicholas AB, Smith R, Berke AD, Shlofmitz RA, Powers ER: Importance of balloon size in coronary angioplasty. J Am Coll Cardiol 13:1094–1100, 1989.

Oesterle SN: Angioplasty techniques for stenoses involving coronary artery bifurcations. Am J Cardiol 61:29G–32G, 1988.

Phillips WJ: Extendable probe. Cathet Cardiovasc Diagn 18:262, 1989.

Pinkerton CA, Slack JD, Orr CM, VanTassel JW: Percutaneous transluminal angioplasty involving internal mammary artery bypass grafts: A femoral approach. Cathet Cardiovasc Diagn 13:414–418, 1987.

Quigley PJ, Hinohara T, Phillips HR, Peter RH, Behar VS, Kong Y, Simonton CA, Perez JA, Stack RS: Myocardial protection during coronary angioplasty with an autoperfusion balloon catheter in humans. Circulation 78:1128–1134, 1988.

Salinger MH, Kern MJ: First use of a 5 French diagnostic catheter as a guiding catheter for percutaneous transluminal coronary angioplasty: Preliminary report. Cathet Cardiovasc Diagn 18:276–278, 1989.

Spaccavento LJ, Breisblatt WM: Use of femoral artery guiding catheters via the left brachial artery for transluminal coronary angioplasty. Cathet Cardiovasc Diagn 20:182–184, 1990.

Thomas ES, Williams DO: Simultaneous double balloon coronary angioplasty through a single guiding catheter for bifurcation lesions. Cathet Cardiovasc Diagn 15:260–264, 1988.

USCI: Clinical Update PTCA Factors in Guiding Catheter Selection.

CHAPTER 3. SELECTION OF PATIENTS FOR PTCA

Alfonso F, Macaya C, Iniguez A, et al.: Percutaneous transluminal coronary angioplasty after non-Q-wave acute myocardial infarction. Am J Cardiol 65:835–839, 1990.

Brundage BH: Because we can, should we? J Am Coll Cardiol 15:544–545, 1990.

Clark DA: "Coronary Angioplasty." New York: Alan R. Liss, Inc., 1987.

Diver DJ, McGabe CH, McKay RG, et al.: Coronary angioplasty of a "culprit" lesion in patients with multivessel coronary disease. J Am Coll Cardiol 9:16A, 1987 (abstr).

Kahn JK, Rutherford BD, McConahay DR, Johnson WL, Giorgi LV, Hartzler GO: Supported "high risk" coronary angioplasty using intraaortic balloon pump counterpulsation. J Am Coll Cardiol 15:1151–1155, 1990.

Kahn JK, Rutherford BD, McConahay DR, et al.: Short- and long-term outcome of percutaneous transluminal coronary angioplasty in chronic dialysis patients. Am Heart J 119:484–489, 1990.

O'Keefe JH Jr, Hartzler GO, Rutherford BD, et al.: Left main coronary angioplasty: Early and late results of 127 acute and elective procedures. Am J Cardiol 64:144–147, 1989.

San Francisco Heart Institute, San Francisco-Peninsula Cardiovascular Medical Corporation, Inc., and then-associated member doctors; slides, charts, data, statistics, computer databases, files and tapes, illustrations and other materials, 1984–1988.

Shawl FA, Domanski MJ, Hernandez TJ, et al.: Emergency percutaneous cardiopulmonary bypass support in cardiogenic shock from acute myocardial infarction. Am J Cardiol 64:967–970, 1989.

Teirstein P, Giorgi L, Johnson W, et al.: PTCA of the left coronary artery when the right coronary artery is chronically occluded. Am Heart J 119:479–483, 1990.

Tuzcu M, Nisanci Y, Simpfendorfer C, Dorosti K, Franco I, Hollman J, Whitlow P: Percutaneous transluminal coronary angioplasty in silent ischemia. Am Heart J 119:797–801, 1990.

Tuzcu M, Simpfendorfer C, Dorosti K, Franco I, Golding L, Hollman J, Whitlow P: Long-term outcome of unsuccessful percutaneous transluminal coronary angioplasty. Am Heart J 119:791–796, 1990.

Vogel RA, Shawl F, Tommaso C, et al.: Initial report of the National Registry of Elective Cardiopulmonary Bypass Supported Coronary Angioplasty. J Am Coll Cardiol 15:23–29, 1990.

CHAPTER 4. PTCA STRATEGY

Arora RR, Raymond RE, Dimas AP, et al.: Side branch occlusion during coronary angioplasty: Incidence, angiographic characteristics, and outcome. Cathet Cardiovasc Diagn 18:210–212, 1989.

Clark DA: "Coronary Angioplasty." New York: Alan R. Liss, Inc., 1987.

Clark DA: Elective angioplasty at the time of angiography can benefit the patient. Intervent Cardiol 3:4–5, 1989.

Cowley MJ, Snow FR, DiSciascio G, et al.: Perfluorochemical perfusion during coronary angioplasty in unstable and high-risk patients. Circulation 81 [Suppl IV]:27–34 1990.

Ellis SG, Roubin GS, King SB, et al.: Antiographic and clinical predictors of acute closure after native vessel coronary angioplasty. Circulation 77(2):372–379, 1988.

Fischell T: Coronary artery spasm after percutaneous transluminal coronary angioplasty: Pathophysiology and clinical consequences. Cathet Cardiovasc Diagn 19:1–3, 1990.

Kruskal JB, Commerford PJ, Franks JJ, Kirsch RE: Fibrin and fibrinogen-related antigens in patients with stable and unstable coronary artery disease. N Engl J Med 317(22):1361–1365, 1987.

Meier B, Gruentzig AR, King SB, et al.: Risk of side branch occlusion during coronary angioplasty. Am J Cardiol 53:10, 1986.

Ogilby JD, Kopelman HA, Klein LW, Agarwal JB: Adequate heparinization during PTCA: Assessment using activated clotting times. Cathet Cardiovasc Diagn 18:206–209, 1989.

San Francisco Heart Institute, San Francisco-Peninsula Cardiovascular Medical Corporation, Inc., and then-associated member doctors; slides, charts, data, statistics, computer databases, files and tapes, illustrations and other materials, 1984–1988.

Spaccavento LJ, Tomlinson GC, Grassman ED: Hugging balloon coronary angioplasty of a large left circumflex coronary artery. Cathet Cardiovasc Diagn 19:190–194, 1990.

Voudris V, Marco J, Morice MC, et al.: "High-risk" percutaneous transluminal coronary angioplasty with preventive intraaortic balloon counterpulsation. Cathet Cardiovasc Diagn 19:160–164, 1990.

Warren SG, Barnett JC: Guiding catheter exchange during coronary angioplasty. Preliminary report. Cathet Cardiovasc Diagn 20:212–215, 1990.

CHAPTER 5. COMPLEX PTCA I: MULTIPLE-VESSEL DISEASE AND LONG SEGMENTAL STENOSES

Alcan KE, Stertzer SH, Wallsh E, DePasquale NP, Bruno MS: The role of intra-aortic balloon counterpulsation in patients undergoing percutaneous transluminal angioplasty. Am Heart J 105:527–530, 1983.

Clark DA: "Coronary Angioplasty." New York: Alan R. Liss, Inc., 1987.

Crowley MJ, Dorros G, Kelsey SF, VanRaden M, Detre KM: Acute coronary events associated with percutaneous transluminal coronary angioplasty. Am J Cardiol 53:12C–16C, 1984.

Cowley MJ, Vetrovec GW, Disciascio G, Lewis SA, Hirsh PD, Wolfgang TC: Coronary angioplasty of multiple vessels: Short-term outcome and long-term results. Circulation 6:1314–1320, 1985.

Dangoisse V, Gutieras VP, David PR, Lesperance J, Crepeau J, Dydra I, Bourassa MG: Recurrence of stenosis after successful percutaneous transluminal coronary angioplasty (PTCA). Circulation 66[Suppl II]:II-331, 1982 (abstr).

de Frijtner P, Wijns W, Simoons ML, Reiber JHC: Is single vessel angioplasty of the ischemia related vessel in unstable angina and multivessel disease an efficacious treatment? Circulation 70[Suppl II]:II-108, 1984 (abstr).

Dorros G, Stertzer SH, Cowley MJ, Myler RK: Complex coronary angioplasty: Multiple coronary dilatations. Am J Cardiol 53:126C–130C, 1984.

Duprat G, David PR, Lesperance J, Val PG, Fines P, Robert P, Bourassa MG: An optimal size of balloon catheter is critical to angiographic success early after PTCA. Circulation 70[Suppl II]:II-295, 1984 (abstr).

George B, Myler RK, Stertzer SH, Clark DA, Cote GF, Shaw RE, Fishman-Rosen J, Murphy MC: Balloon angioplasty of coronary bifurcation lesions—The kissing balloon technique. Cathet Cardiovasc Diagr 12:124–138, 1986.

Gruentzig AR, Hollman J: Improved primary success rate in transluminal coronary angioplasty using a steerable guidance system. Circulation 66[Suppl II]:II-330, 1982 (abstr).

Hall RJ, Virendra M, Massumi A, Garcia E, Fighali S: Percutaneous transluminal coronary angioplasty update. Texas Heart Inst J 11:10–16, 1984.

Hartzler GO: Percutaneous coronary angioplasty in patients with multivessel disease. In Jang GD (ed): "Angioplasty." New York: McGraw-Hill, 1986, pp. 321–336.

Kaltenbach M, Beyer J, Walter S, Klepzig H, Schmidts L: Prolonged application of pressure in transluminal coronary angioplasty. Cathet Cardiovasc Diagn 10:213–219, 1984.

Kelsey SF, Mullin SM, Detre KM, Mitchell H, Cowley MJ, Gruentzig AR, Kent KM: Effect of investigator experience on percutaneous transluminal coronary angioplasty. Am J Cardiol 53:56C–64C, 1984.

Knudtson ML, Hansen JL, Manyari DE, Roth DL, Flintoft VF: The role of incomplete revascularization by PTCA in patients with multivessel coronary artery disease. Circulation 70 [Suppl II]:II-108, 1984 (abstr).

Leimgruber PP, Roubin GS, Anderson V, Bredlau CE, Whitworth HB, Douglas JS, King SB, Gruentzig AR: Influence of intimal dissection on restenosis after successful coronary angioplasty. Circulation 72:530–535, 1985.

Leimgruber PP, Roubin GS, Hollman J, Cotsonis GA, Meier B, Douglas JS, King SB, Gruentzig AR: Restenosis after successful coronary angioplasty in patients with single-vessel disease. Circulation 73:710–717, 1986.

Levine S, Ewels CJ, Rosing DR, Kent KM: Coronary angioplasty: Clinical and angiographic follow-up. Am J Cardiol 55:673–676, 1985.

Mabin TA, Holmes DR Jr, Smith HC, Vlietstra RE, Reeder GS, Bresnahan JF, Bove AA, Hammes LN, Elveback LR, Orszulak TA: Follow-up clinical results in patients undergoing percutaneous transluminal coronary angioplasty. Circulation 71:754–760, 1985.

Margolis JR, Krieger R, Glemser E: Coronary angioplasty: Increased restenosis rate in insulin dependent diabetics. Circulation 70[Suppl II]:II-175, 1984 (abstr).

Mata LA, Bosch X, David PR, Rapold HJ, Corcos T, Bourassa MG: Clinical and angiographic assessment 6 months after double vessel percutaneous coronary angioplasty. J Am Coll Cardiol 6:1239–1244, 1985.

Meier B, Gruentzig AR, King SB III, Douglas JS, Hollman J, Ischinger T, Galan K: Higher balloon dilatation pressures in coronary angioplasty. Am Heart J 107:619–622, 1984.

Mock MB, Reeder GS, Schaff HV, Holmes DR, Vlietstra RE, Smith HC, Gersh BJ: Percutaneous transluminal coronary angioplasty versus coronary artery bypass. N Engl J Med 312:916–919, 1985.

Myler RK: Transfemoral approach to percutaneous coronary angioplasty. In Jang Gd (ed): "Angioplasty." New York: McGraw-Hill, 1986, pp 198–259.

Roubin GS, Leimgruber PP, Douglas JS Jr, King SP III, Gruentzig AR: Angioplasty in multivessel coronary artery disease: Patient selection and dilatation strategy. J Am Coll Cardiol 5:445, 1985 (abstr).

Roubin G, Redd D, Leimgruber P, Abi-Mansour P, Tate J, Gruentzig AR: Restenosis after multi-lesion and multivessel coronary angioplasty (PTCA). J Am Coll Cardiol 7:22, 1986 (abstr).

San Francisco Heart Institute, San Francisco-Peninsula Cardiovascular Medical Corporation, Inc., and then-associated member doctors; slides, charts, data, statistics, computer databases, files and tapes, illustrations and other materials, 1984–1988.

Schmitz H, Essen R, Meyer J, Effert S: The role of balloon size for acute and late angiographic results in coronary angioplasty. Circulation 70[Suppl II]:II-295, 1984 (abstr).

Thornton MA, Gruentzig AR, Hollman HJ, King SB, Douglas JS: Coumadin and aspirin in prevention of recurrence after transluminal coronary angioplasty: A randomized study. Circulation 69:721–727, 1984.

Vandormael MG, Chaitman BR, Ischinger I, Aker UT, Harper M, Hernandez J, Deligonul U, Kennedy HL: Immediate and short-term benefit of multilesion coronary angioplasty: Influence of degree of revascularization. J Am Coll Cardiol 6:983–991, 1985.

Vlietstra RE, Holmes Dr Jr, Reeder GS, Mock MB, Smith HC, Bove AA, Bresnahan JF: Balloon angioplasty in multivessel coronary artery disease. Mayo Clin Proc 58:563–567, 1983.

Vogel RA: Digital radiographic assessment of coronary flow reserve. In Buda AJ, Delp EJ (eds): "Digital Cardiac Imaging." Boston: Martinus Nijhoff, 1985, pp 106–118.

Whitworth HB, Pilcher GS, Roubin GS, Gruentzig AR: Do proximal lesions involving the origin of the left anterior descending artery (LAD) have a higher restenosis rate after coronary angioplasty (PTCA)? Circulation 72[Suppl III]:III-398, 1985 (abstr).

Zaidi AR, Hollman JL, Galan K: Multivessel angioplasty, procedure, and follow-up trends. Circulation 70[Suppl II]:II-266, 1984 (abstr).

CHAPTER 6. COMPLEX PTCA II: TOTAL OCCLUSIONS

Andreae GE, Myler RK, Clark DA, et al.: Acute complications following coronary angioplasty of totally occluded vessels. Circulation 76[Suppl IV]:IV-400, 1987.

Butman S: Angioplasty of recent total coronary occlusions: Cardiac death can occur in "low-risk" cases. Cathet Cardiovasc Diagn 19:34–38, 1990.

Clark DA: "Coronary Angioplasty." New York: Alan R. Liss, Inc., 1987.

Clark DA, Wexman MP, Murphy MC, Fishman-Rosen J, Shaw RE, Stertzer SH, Myler RK: Factors predicting recurrence in patients who have had angioplasty (PTCA) of totally occluded vessels. J Am Coll Cardiol 7:2, 20A, 1986 (abstr).

de Feyter PF, Serruys P, van den Brand M, et al.: Percutaneous transluminal angioplasty of totally occluded venous bypass graft: A challenge that should be resisted. Am J Cardiol 64:88–90, 1989.

Dervan JP, Baim SA, Chernikes J, Grossman W: Transluminal angioplasty of occluded coronary arteries; use of a movable guide wire system. Circulation 68:776–784, 1983.

Detre K, Holubkov R, Kelsey S, et al.: Percutaneous transluminal coronary angioplasty in 1985–1986 and 1977–1981: The National Heart, Lung and Blood Institute Registry. N Engl J Med 318:265–270, 1988.

DiSciascio G, Cowley MJ, Vetrovec GW, Wolfgang TC: Patterns of recurrence following coronary angioplasty of multiple lesions. Clin Res 32:828A, 1984 (abstr).

DiSciascio G, Vetrovec GW, Cowley MJ, Wolfgang TC: Early and late outcome of percutaneous transluminal coronary angioplasty for subacute and chronic total coronary occlusion. Am Heart J 111:833–839, 1986.

Fergusen DW, Kouba DR, Little MM, Osborne JL, White CW, Kioschos JM: Combined intracoronary streptokinase and percutaneous coronary angioplasty for reperfusion of chronic total coronary occlusion. J Am Coll Cardiol 4:820–824, 1984.

Heyndrickx GR, Serruys PW, Brand M, Bandormael M, Reiber JHC: Transluminal angioplasty after mechanical recanalization in patients with chronic occlusions of coronary artery. Circulation 66[Suppl II]:II-5, 1982 (abstr).

Holmes DR, Vlietstra RE, Reeder GS, et al.: Angioplasty in total coronary artery occlusion. J Am Coll Cardiol 3:845–849, 1984.

Kereiakes DJ, Selmon MR, McAuley BJ, McAuley DB, Sheehan DJ, Simpson JB: Angioplasty in total coronary artery occlusion: Experience in 76 consecutive patients. J Am Coll Cardiol 6:526–533, 1985.

Kipperman RM, Feit AS, Einhorn AM, Co JA: Intracoronary thrombectomy: A new approach to total occlusion. Cathet Cardiovasc Diagn 18:244–248, 1989.

Meier B, Carlier M, Finci L, et al.: Magnum wire for balloon recanalization of chronic total coronary occlusion. Am J Cardiol 64:148–154, 1989.

Saenz CB, Harrell R, Sawyer JA, Hood WP Jr: Acute percutaneous transluminal coronary angioplasty complicated by embolism to a coronary remote from the site of infarction. Cathet Cardiovasc Diagn 13:266–268, 1987.

Safian RD, McCabe CH, Sipperly ME, et al.: Initial success and long-term follow-up of percutaneous transluminal coronary angioplasty in chronic total occlusions versus conventional stenoses. Am J Cardiol 61:23G–28G, 1988.

San Francisco Heart Institute, San Francisco-Peninsula Cardiovascular Medical Corporation, Inc., and then-as-sociated member doctors; slides, charts, data, statistics, computer databases, files and tapes, illustrations and other materials, 1984–1988.

Savage R, Hollman J, Gruentzig AR, King S, Dovelas J, Tankersley R: Can percutaneous transluminal coronary angioplasty be performed in patients with total occlusion? Circulation 66[Suppl II]:II-330, 1982 (abstr).

Stone GW, Rutherford BD, McConahay DR, et al.: Procedural outcome of angioplasty for total coronary artery occlusion: An analysis of 971 lesions in 905 patients. J Am Coll Cardiol 15:849–856, 1990.

Vetrovec GW, Cowley MJ, Wolfgang TC: Non-emergency PTCA for total coronary occlusion: Immediate and late results. Circulation 70:146, 1984 (abstr).

Wexman MP, Clark DA, Murphy MC, Fishman-Rosen J, Shaw RE, Stertzer SH, Myler RK: Patient selection, complications, and predictors of success in PTCA of total occlusion. Circulation 72[Suppl III]:III-179, 1986.

CHAPTER 7. COMPLEX PTCA III: BIFURCATION LESIONS

Clark DA: "Coronary Angioplasty." New York: Alan R. Liss, Inc., 1987.

Cowley MJ, Block PC: Percutaneous transluminal coronary angioplasty. Mod Concepts Cardiovasc Dis 5:25–29, 1981.

George BS, Myler RK, Stertzer SH, Clark DA, Cote G, Shaw RE, Fishman-Rosen J, Murphy M: Balloon angioplasty of coronary bifurcation lesions: The kissing balloon technique. Cathet Cardiovasc Diagn, 12(2):124–138, 1986.

Hall RJ, Virendra M, Massumi A, Garcia E, Fighali S: Percutaneous transluminal angioplasty update. Texas Heart Inst J 11:10–16, 1984.

Leimgruber PP, Modenhauser RT, Libow MA, Douglas JS, Jr, Gruentzig AR: Fate of occluded side branches after coronary angioplasty. Circulation 70[Suppl II]:II-296, 1984 (abstr).

McAuley BJ, Sheehan DJ, Simpson JB: Coronary angioplasty of stenosis at major bifurcations: Simultaneous use of multiple guidewires and dilatation catheters. Circulation 70[Suppl II]:II-108, 1984 (abstr).

Meier B: Kissing balloon angioplasty. Am J Cardiol 53: 918–920, 1984.

Meier B, Gruentzig AR, King SB III, Douglas JS Jr, Hollman J, Ischinger T, Aueron F, Galan K: Risk of side branch occlusion during coronary angioplasty. Am J Cardiol 53:10–14, 1984.

Pinkerton MD, Slack JD, Van Tassel JW, Orr CM: Angioplasty for dilatation of complex coronary artery bifurcation stenoses. Am J Cardiol 55:1626–1628, 1985.

San Francisco Heart Institute, San Francisco-Peninsula Cardiovascular Medical Corporation, Inc., and the-associated member doctors; slides, charts, data, statistics, computer databases, files and tapes, illustrations and other materials, 1984–1988.

Velasquez G, Castaneda-Zuniga W, Formanek A, Zollikofer C, Barreto A, Nikoloff D, Amplatz K, Sullivan A: Nonsurgical angioplasty in Leriche syndrome. Radiology 134:359–360, 1980.

Vertrovec GW, Cowley MJ, Wolfgang TC, Ducey KC: Effects of percutaneous transluminal angioplasty on lesion-associated branches. Am Heart J 109:921–925, 1985.

Zack PM, Ischinger TM: Experience with a technique for coronary angioplasty of bifurcation lesions. Cathet Cardiovasc Diagn 10:433–443, 1984.

CHAPTER 8. COMPLEX PTCA IV: BYPASS GRAFTS

Alcan KE, Stertzer SH, Wallsh E, De Pasquale NP, Bruno MS: The role of intra-aortic balloon counterpulsation in patients undergoing percutaneous transluminal angioplasty. Am Heart J 105:527–530, 1983.

Aueron F, Gruentzig AR: Distal embolization of a coronary artery bypass graft atheroma during percutaneous transluminal coronary angioplasty. Am J Cardiol 53: 953–954, 1984.

Block PC, Cowley MJ, Kaltenbach M, Kent KM, Simpson J: Percutaneous angioplasty of stenoses of bypass grafts or of bypass graft anastomotic sites. Am J Cardiol 53: 666–668, 1984.

Bulkley BH, Hutchins GM: "Accelerated atherosclerosis." A morphologic study of 97 saphenous vein coronary artery bypass grafts. Circulation 55:163–169, 1977.

Campeau L, Enjalbert M, Lesperance J, Bourassa MG, Kwiterovich P, Wacholder S, Sniderman A: The relationship of risk factors to the development of atherosclerosis in saphenous vein grafts and the progression of disease in the native circulation: A study of 10 years after aortocoronary bypass surgery. N Engl J Med 311:1329–1332, 1984.

Clark DA: "Coronary Angioplasty." New York: Alan R. Liss, Inc., 1987.

Corbelli J, Franco I, Hollman J, Simpfendorfer C, Galan K: Percutaneous transluminal coronary angioplasty after previous coronary artery bypass surgery. Am J Cardiol 56:398–403, 1985.

Cowley MJ, Dorros G, Kelsey SF, Van Raden M, Detre KM: Acute coronary event associated with percutaneous transluminal coronary angioplasty. Am J Cardiol 53:12c–16c, 1984.

Dorros G, Johnson WD, Tector AJ, Schmahl TM, Kalush SL, Janke L: Percutaneous transluminal coronary angioplasty in patients with prior coronary artery bypass grafting. J Thorac Cardiovasc Surg 87:17–26, 1984.

Douglas JS Jr, Gruentzig AR, King SB III, Hollman J: Long-term results of percutaneous transluminal angioplasty for aorto-coronary saphenous vein graft stenosis. Circulation 66[Suppl II]:124, 1982 (abstr).

Douglas JS Jr, Gruentzig AR, King SB III, Hollman J, Ischinger T, Meier B, Craver JM, Jones E, Waller JL, Bond DK, Guyton R: Percutaneous transluminal coronary angioplasty in patients with prior coronary bypass surgery. J Am Coll Cardiol 2:745–754, 1983.

El Gamal M, Bunnier H, Michels R, Heijman J, Stassen E: Percutaneous transluminal angioplasty of stenosed aortocoronary bypass grafts. Br Heart J 52:617–628, 1984.

Favaloro RG: Saphenous vein auto graft replacement of severe segmental coronary artery occlusion: Operative technique. Ann Thorac Surg 5:334–339, 1968.

Ford WB, Wholey MH, Zikria EA, Somadani SR, Sullivan ME: Percutaneous transluminal dilatation of aortocoronary saphenous vein bypass grafts. Chest 79:529–535, 1981.

Fuster V, Chesebro JH: Role of platelets and platelet inhibitors in aortocoronary artery vein-graft disease. Circulation 73:227–232, 1986.

Griffith LSC, Bulkley BH, Hutchins GM, Brawley RK: Occlusive changes at the coronary artery-bypass graft anastomosis. Morphologic study of 95 grafts. J Thorac Cardiovasc Surg 73:668–679, 1977.

Guthaner DF, Robert EW, Alderman EL, Wexler L: Long-term serial angiographic studies after coronary artery bypass surgery. Circulation 60:250–259, 1979.

Hamby RI, Aintablian A, Handler M, Voleti C, Weisz D, Garvey JW, Wisoff G: Aorotocoronary saphenous vein bypass grafts. Long-term patency, morphology and blood flow in patients with patent grafts early after surgery. Circulation 60:901–909, 1979.

Hollman J: Percutaneous transluminal angioplasty in patients with failed coronary bypass grafts. In Jang GD (ed): "Angioplasty," New York: McGraw-Hill, 1985, pp 346–356.

Kolessov VI: Mammary artery-coronary artery anastromosis as method of treatment for angina pectoris. J Thorac Cardiovasc Surg 54:535–544, 1967.

Kouchoukos NT, Karp RB, Oberman A, Russel RO Jr, Allison HW, Holt JH Jr: Long-term patency of saphenous veins for coronary bypass grafting. Circulation 58[Suppl I]:96–99, 1979.

Krause AH Jr, Page US, Bigelow JC, Okies JE, Dunlap SF: Reoperation in symptomatic patients after direct coronary artery revascularization. J Thorac Cardiovasc Surg 75:499–504, 1978.

Leimgruber PP, Roubin GS, Hollman J, Cotsonis GA, Meier B, Douglas JS, King SB III, Gruentzig AR: Restenosis after successful coronary angioplasty in patients with single-vessel disease. Circulation 73:710–717, 1986.

Loop FD, Thurer RL, Lytle BW, Cosgrove DM: Reoperation for myocardial revascularization. World J Surg 2:719–729, 1968.

Morrison DA: Coronary angioplasty for medically refractory unstable angina in patients with prior coronary bypass surgery. Cathet Cardiovasc Diagn 20:174–181, 1990.

Norwood WI, Cohn LH, Collins JJ: Results of reoperation for recurrent angina pectoris. Ann Thorac Surg 23:9–13, 1977.

Platko WP, Hollman J, Whitlow PW, Franco I: Percutaneous transluminal angioplasty of saphenous vein graft stenosis: Long-term follow-up. J Am Coll Cardiol 14: 1645–1650, 1989.

Reeder GS, Bresnahan JF, Holmes DR, Mock MB, Orszulak TA, Smith HC, Vlietstra RE: Angioplasty for aortocoronary bypass graft stenosis. Mayo Clin Proc 61:14–19, 1986.

Reul GJ, Cooley DA, Ott DA, Coelho A, Chapa L, Eterovic I: Reoperation for recurrent coronary artery disease. Arch Surg 114:1269–1275, 1979.

San Francisco Heart Institute, San Francisco-Peninsula Cardiovascular Medical Corporation, Inc., and then-associated member doctors; slides, charts, data, statistics, computer databases, files and tapes, illustrations and other materials, 1984–1988.

Seides SF, Borer JS, Kent KM, Rosing DR, McIntosh CL, Epstein SE: Long-term anatomic fate of coronary-artery bypass grafts and functional status of patients five years after operation. N Engl J Med 298:1213–1217, 1978.

Smith SH, Geer JC: Morphology of saphenous vein-coronary artery bypass grafts. Arch Pathol Lab Med 107:13–18, 1983.

Spray TL, Roberts WC: Changes in saphenous veins used as aortocoronary bypass grafts. Am Heart J 94:500–516, 1977.

Vouhe P, Grondin CM: Reoperation for coronary graft failure: Clinical and angiographic results in 43 patients. Ann Thorac Surg 27:328–334, 1979.

Waller BF, Rothbaum DA, Gorfinkel HJ, Ulbright TM, Linnemeier TJ, Berger SM: Morphologic observations after percutaneous transluminal balloon angioplasty of early and late aortocoronary saphenous vein bypass grafts. J Am Coll Cardiol 4:784–792, 1984.

CHAPTER 9. DIRECT PTCA IN ACUTE MYOCARDIAL INFARCTION

1. O'Keefe JH Jr, Rutherford BD, McConahay DR, Ligon RW, Johnson WL, Giorgi LV, Crockett JE, McCallister BD, Conn RD, Gura GM, Good TH, Steinhaus DM, Bateman TM, Shimshak TM, Hartzler GO: Early and late results of coronary angioplasty without antecedent thrombolytic therapy for acute myocardial infarction. Am J Cardiol 64:1221, 1989.

2. Kahn JK, Hartzler GO: Percutaneous thrombus aspiration in acute myocardial infarction. Cathet Cardiovasc Diagn (in press).

3. Althouse R, Maynard C, Olsufka M, Kennedy JW: Incidence of contraindications to thrombolysis in patients with myocardial infarction. Circulation 78:II-211, 1988.

4. Cragg DR, Bonema JD, Jaiyesimi IA, Ramos RG, Timmis GC, O'Neill WW, Schreiber TL: Ineligibility for intravenous thrombolytic therapy predicts high mortality after myocardial infarction. Circulation 80:II-522, 1989.

5. The TIMI Study Group: Comparison of invasive and conservative strategies after treatment with intravenous tissue plasminogen activator in acute myocardial infarction. N Engl J Med 320:618, 1989.

6. Topol EJ et al.: A randomized trial of immediate versus delayed elective angioplasty after intravenous tissue plasminogen activator in acute myocardial infarction. N Engl J Med 317:581, 1987.

7. O'Neill WW, Topol EJ, Pitt B: Reperfusion therapy of acute myocardial infarction. Prog Cardiovasc Dis 30: 235, 1988.

8. Califf RM, Topol EJ, George BS, Kerieakes DJ, Samaha JK, Worley SJ, Anderson J, Sassahara A, Lee K, Stack RS: TAMI 5: A randomized trial of combination thrombolytic therapy and immediate catheterization. Circulation 80:II-418, 1989.

9. Bates ER, Califf RM, Stack RS, Aronson L, George BS, Candela RJ, Kereiakes DJ, Abbottsmith CW, Anderson L, Pitt B, O'Neill WW, Topol EJ: Thrombolysis and angioplasty in myocardial infarction (TAMI 1) Trial: Influence of infarct location on arterial patency, left ventricular function and mortality. J Am Coll Cardiol 13:12, 1989.

10. Brodie BR, Weintraub RA, Stuckey TD, Le Bauer EJ, Katz JD, Kelly TA, Hansen CJ: Direct angioplasty for acute myocardial infarction: Results in candidates and non-candidates for thrombolytic therapy. Circulation 80:II-624, 1989.

11. Rothbaum DA, Linnemeier TJ, Landin RJ, Steinmetz EF, Hillis JS, Hallam CC, Noble RJ, See MR: Emergency percutaneous transluminal coronary angioplasty in acute myocardial infarction: A 3 year experience. J Am Coll Cardiol 10:264, 1987.

12. Kimura T, Nosaka H, Ueno K, Nobuyoshi M: Role of coronary angioplasty in myocardial infarction. Circulation 74:II-22, 1986.

13. Marco J, Caster L, Szatmary LJ, Fajadet J: Emergency percutaneous transluminal coronary angioplasty without thrombolysis as initial therapy in acute myocardial infarction. Int J Cardiol 15:55, 1987.

14. Ellis SG, O'Neill WW, Bates ER, Walton JA, Nabel EG, Werns SW, Topol EJ: Implications for patient triage from survival and left ventricular functional recovery analyses in 500 patients treated with coronary angioplasty for acute myocardial infarction. J Am Coll Cardiol 13:1251, 1989.

15. Kase CS, O'Neal AM, Fisher M, Girgis GN, Ordia JI: Intracranial hemorrhage after use of tissue plasminogen activator for coronary thrombolysis. Ann Intern Med 112:17, 1990.

16. Blankenship JA, Almquist AK: Cardiovascular complications of thrombolytic therapy in patients with a mistaken diagnosis of acute myocardial infarction. J Am Coll Cardiol 14:1579, 1989.

17. Stone G, Rutherford BD, McConahay DR, Johnson WL, Giorgi LV, Ligon RW, Hartzler GO: Direct coronary angioplasty in acute myocardial infarction: Outcome in patients with single vessel disease. J Am Coll Cardiol (in press).

18. Kahn JK, Rutherford BD, McConahay DR, Johnson WL, Giorgi LV, Ligon RW, Hartzler GO: Primary angioplasty for acute myocardial infarction in patients with multivessel coronary artery disease. Circulation 80:II-625, 1989.

19. Kahn JK, Rutherford BD, McConahay DR, Johnson WL, Giorgi LV, Ligon RW, Hartzler GO: Usefulness of angioplasty during acute myocardial infarction in patients with prior coronary artery bypass grafting. Am J Cardiol (in press).

20. Laramee LA, Rutherford BD, Ligon RW, McConahay DR, Hartzler GO: Coronary angioplasty for cardiogenic shock following myocardial infarction. Circulation 78:II-634, 1988.

CHAPTER 10. RECURRENCE FOLLOWING SUCCESSFUL PTCA

Arora RR, Konrad K, Badhwar K, Hollman J: Restenosis after transluminal coronary angioplasty: A risk factor analysis. Cathet Cardiovasc Diagn 19:17–22, 1990.

Block PC: Restenosis after percutaneous transluminal coronary angioplasty—Anatomic and pathophysiological mechanisms: Strategies for prevention. Circulation 81:IV-2–IV-4, 1990.

Block PC, Cowley MJ, Kaltenbach M, Kent KM, Simpson J: Percautaneous angioplasty of stenoses of bypass grafts or of bypass graft anastomotic sites. Am J Cardiol 53:666–668, 1984.

Brown KA, Osbakken M, Boucher CA, Strauss HW, Pohost GM, Okada RD: Positive exercise thallium-201 test responses in patients with less than 50% maximal coronary stenosis: Angiographic and clinical predictors. Am J Cardiol 55:54–57, 1985.

Bruneval P, Guermonprez JL, Perrier P, et al.: Coronary artery restenosis following transluminal coronary angioplasty. Arch Pathol Lab Med 110:1186–1187, 1986.

Cequier A, Bonan R, Crepeau J, et al.: Restenosis postangioplasty and progression of coronary atherosclerosis. Circulation (II) 76:1479, 1987.

Clark DA: "Coronary Angioplasty." New York: Alan R. Liss, Inc., 1987.

Clark DA, Wexman MP, Murphy MC, et al.: Factors predicting recurrence in patients who have had angioplasty (PTCA) of totally occluded vessels. J Am Coll Cardio 7:20A, 1986 (abstr).

Cote G, Myler RK, Stertzer SH, et al.: Percutaneous transluminal angioplastyof stenotic coronary artery bypass grafts: Three years' experience. J Am Coll Cardiol 9:8–17, 1987.

Cowley MJ, Mullin SM, Kelsey SF, et al.: Sex differences in early and long-term results of coronary angioplasty in the NHLBI PTCA Registry. Circulation 71:90–97, 1985.

Dangoisse V, Guiteras Val P, David PR, et al.: Recurrence of stenosis after successful percutaneous transluminal coronary angioplasty (PTCA). Circulation 66[Suppl II]:II-331, 1982 (abstr).

DiSciascio G, Copwley MJ, Vetrovec GW, Wolfgang TC: Angiographic patterns of restenosis after coronary angioplasty of multiple vessels. J Am Coll Cardiol 7:63A, 1986 (abstr).

Dorros G, Johnson WD, Tector AJ, Schmahl TM, Kalush SL, Janke L: Percutaneous transluminal coronary angioplasty in patients with prior coronary artery bypass grafting. J Thorac Cardiovasc Surg 87:17–26, 1984.

Douglas JS, Gruentzig AR, King SB, et al.: Percutaneous transluminal coronary angioplasty in patients with prior coronary bypass surgery. J Am Coll Cardiol 2:745–754, 1983.

Fleiss JL: "Statistical Methods for Rates and Proportions." New York: John Wiley & Sons, 1973, pp 23–34.

Galan KM, Deligonul U, Kern MJ, et al.: Increased frequency of restenosis in patients continuing to smoke cigarettes after percutaneous transluminal coronary angioplasty. Am J Cardiol 61:260–263, 1988.

George B, Myler RK, Stertzer SH, et al.: Balloon angioplasty of coronary bifurcation lesions—The kissing balloon technique. Cathet Cardiovasc Diagn 12:124–138, 1986.

Gould KL, Lipscomb K. Hamilton GW: Physiologic basis for assessing critical coronary stenosis. Am J Cardiol 33:87–94, 1974.

Grigg LE, Kay TWH, Valentine PA, et al.: Determinants of restcnosis and lack of effect of dietary supplementation with eicosapentaenoic acid on the incidence of coronary artery restenosis after angioplasty. J Am Coll Cardiol 13:665–672, 1989.

Gruentzig AR: Transluminal dilatation of coronary artery stenosis. Lancet 1:263–266, 1978.

Gruentzig AR, Myler RK, Hanna EH, Turina MI: Coronary transluminal angioplasty. Circulation 55–56[Suppl III]:III-84, 1977 (abstr).

Gruentzig AR, Myler RK, Stertzer SH, Kaltenbach M, Turina MI: Coronary percutaneous transluminal angioplasty: Preliminary results. Circulation 58[Suppl II]:II-56, 1978 (abstr).

Gruentzig AR, Senning A, Siegenthaler WE: Non-operative dilatation of coronary artery stenosis: Percutaneous transluminal coronary angioplasty. N Engl J Med 301: 61–68, 1979.

Hall DP, Gruentzig AR: Influence of lesion length on initial success and recurrence rates in coronary angioplasty. Circulation 70[Suppl II]:II-176, 1984 (abstr).

Hamm C, Kupper W, Thier W, Mathey DG, Bleifeld W: Factors predicting recurrent stenosis in patients with successful coronary angioplasty. J Am Coll Cardiol 5:518, 1985 (abstr).

Harrison DG, White CW, Hiratska LF, et al.: The value of lesion cross-sectional area determined by quantitative coronary angiography in assessing physiologic significance of proximal left anterior descending coronary arterial stenoses. Circulation 69:1111–1119, 1984.

Hirshfield JW, MacDonald R, Goldberg S, et al.: Patient related variables predictive of restenosis after PTCA—A report from the M-Heart Study. Circulation (II) 76:853, 1987.

Hoffmeister JM, Whitworth HB, Leimgruber PP, Abi-Mansour P, Tate JM, Gruentzig AR: Analysis of anatomic and procedural factors related to restenosis after double lesion coronary angioplasty (PTCA). Circulation 72[Suppl II]:III-398, 1985 (abstr).

Hollman J, Galan K, Franco I, Simpfendorfer C, Fatica K, Beck G: Recurrent stenosis after coronary angioplasty. J Am Coll Cardiol 7:20A, 1986 (abstr).

Holmes DR, Vlietstra RE, Smith HC, et al.: Restenosis after percutaneous transluminal coronary angioplasty (PTCA): A report from the PTCA registry of the National Heart, Lung, and Blood Institute. Am J Cardiol 53:77C–81C, 1984.

Jang GC, Gruentzig AR, Block PC, Myler RK, Stertzer SH: Delayed effect of vessel restenosis on the procedure cost of coronary angioplasty. Circulation 66[Suppl II]:II-330, 1982 (abstr).

Kirkeeide RL, Gould KL, Parsel L: Assessment of coronary stenosis by myocardial perfusion imaging during pharmacologic coronary vasodilation. VII. Validation of coronary flow reserve as a single integrated functional measure of stenosis severity reflecting all its geometric dimensions. J Am Coll Cardiol 7:101–113, 1986.

Knudtson ML, Flintoft VF, Roth DL, et al.: Effect of short-term prostacyclin administration on restenosis after percutaneous transluminal coronary angioplasty. J Am Coll Cardiol 15:691–697, 1990.

Leimgruber PP, Roubin GS, Anderson V, Bredlau CE, Whitworth HB, Douglas HB, King SB, Gruentzig AR: Influence of intimal dissection on restenosis after successful coronary angioplasty. Circulation 72:530–535, 1985.

Leimgruber PP, Roubin GS, Hollman J, et al.: Restenosis after successful coronary angioplasty in patients with single-vessel disease. Circulation 73:710–717, 1986.

Leimbruber PP, Roubin GS, Rice CR, Tate JM, Gruentzig AR: Influence of intimal dissection after coronary angioplasty (PTCA) on restenosis rate. Circulation 70[Suppl II]:II-175, 1984 (abstr).

Marantz T, Williams DO, Reinert S, Gewirtz H, Most AS: Predictors of restenosis after successful coronary angioplasty. Circulation 70[Suppl II]:II-176, 1984 (abstr).

Margolis JR, Kreiger R, Glemser E: Coronary angioplasty: Increased restenosis rate in insulin dependent diabetes. Circulation 70[Suppl II]:II-175, 1984 (abstr).

Mata LA, Bosch X, David PR, Rapold HJ, Corcos T, Bourassa MG: Clinical and angiographic assessment 6 months after double vessel percutaneous coronary angioplasty. J Am Coll Cardiol 6:1239–44, 1985.

McBride W, Lange RA, Hillis LD: Restenosis after successful coronary angioplasty. N Engl J Med 318:1734–1736, 1988.

Meier B, Gruentzig AR, King SB, et al.: Higher balloon dilatation pressure in coronary angioplasty. Am Heart J 107:619–622, 1984.

Milner MR, Gallino RA, Leffingwell A, et al.: Usefulness of fish oil supplements in preventing clinical evidence of restenosis after percutaneous transluminal coronary angioplasty. Am J Cardiol 64:294–299, 1989.

Myler RK: Coronary angioplasty: Widening indications/current state of the art. Paper presented at the American College of Cardiology Conference on Conventional and New Approaches to the Prevention and Treatment of Acute Myocardial Infarction, May 1, 1984.

Myler RK, Shaw RE, Stertzer SH, Clark DA, Fishman-Rosen J, Murphy MC: Recurrence after coronary angioplasty. Cathet Cardiovasc Diagn 13:77–86, 1987.

Myler RK, Topol EJ, Shaw RE, et al.: Multiple vessel coronary angioplasty: Classification, results and patterns of restenosis in 494 consecutive patients. Cathet Cardiovasc Diagn 13:1–15, 1987.

Reis GJ, Boucher TM, Sipperly ME, et al.: Randomized trial of fish oil for prevention of restenosis after coronary angioplasty. Lancet ii:177–181, 1989.

Roubin G, Redd D, Leimgruber P, Abi-Mansour P, Tate J, Gruentzig AR: Restenosis after multi-lesion and multi-vessel coronary angioplasty (PTCA). J Am Coll Cardiol 7:22A, 1986 (abstr).

Rupprecht HJ, Brennecke R, Bernhard G, et al.: Analysis of risk factors for restenosis after PTCA. Cathet Cardiovasc Diagn 19:151–159, 1990.

San Francisco Heart Institute, San Francisco-Peninsula Cardiovascular Medical Corporation, inc., and then-associated member doctors; slides, charts, data, statistics, computer databases, files and tapes, illustrations and other materials, 1984–1988.

Schmitz HJ, Essen RV, Meyer J, Effert S: The role of balloon size for acute and late angiographic results in coronary angioplasty. Circulation 70[Suppl II]:II-295, 1984 (abstr).

Shaw RE, Myler RK, Fishman-Rosen J, Murphy MC, Stertzer SH, Topol EJ: Clinical and morphologic factors in prediction of restenosis after multiple vessel angioplasty. J Am Coll Cardiol 7:63A, 1986 (abstr).

Shaw RE, Myler RK, Stertzer SH, et al.: Recurrence after coronary angioplasty: prediction and prevention. Cardiology 4:42–45, 1987.

Stertzer SH, Myler RK, Bruno MS, Wallsh E: Transluminal coronary artery dilation. Pract Cardiol 5:25–31, 1979.

Stone GW, Rutherford BD, McConahay DR, et al.: A randomized trial of corticosteroids for the prevention of restenosis in 102 patients undergoing repeat coronary angioplasty. Cathet Cardiovasc Diagn 18:227–231, 1989.

Uebis R, von Essen R, vom Dahl J, Schmitz HJ, Seiger K, Effert S: Recurrence rate after PTCA in relationship to the initial length of coronary artery narrowing. J Am Coll Cardiol 7:62A, 1986 (abstr).

VanDormael MG, Chaitman BR, Ischinger T, et al.: Immediate and short-term benefit of multilesion coronary angioplasty: Influence of degree of revascularization. J Am Coll Cardiol 6:983–991, 1985.

Waller BF, Pinkerton CA, Foster LN: Morphologic evidence of accelerated left main coronary artery stenosis: A late complication of percutaneous transluminal balloon angioplasty of the proximal left anterior descending coronary artery. J Am Coll Cardiol 9:1019–1023, 1987.

White CW, Wright CB, Doty DB, et al.: Does visual interpretation of coronary arteriogram predict the physiologic importance of a coronary stenosis? N Engl J Med 310:819–824, 1984.

Whitworth HB, Pilcher GS, Roubin GS, Gruentzig AR: Do proximal lesions involving the origin of the left anterior descending artery (LAD) have a higher resenosis rate after coronary angioplasty (PTCA)? Circulation 72[Suppl III]:III-398, 1985 (abstr).

CHAPTER 11. COMPLICATIONS OF CORONARY ANGIOPLASTY

Arora RR, Raymond RE, Dimas AP, et al.: Side branch occlusion during coronary angioplasty: Incidence, angiographic characteristics, and outcome. Cathet Cardiovasc Diagn 18:210–212, 1989.

Chesler E, Gornick CE, Pierpont G, Weir EK: High incidence of acute coronary occlusions complicating percutaneous transluminal coronary angioplasty for angina pectoris. Am J Cardiol 64:665–667, 1989.

Ciampricotti R, Dekkers PJWM, El Camal MIH, et al.: Catheter reperfusion for failed emergency coronary angioplasty without subsequent bypass surgery. Cathet Cardiovasc Diagn 18:159–64, 1989.

Clark DA: "Coronary Angioplasty." New York: Alan R. Liss, Inc., 1987.

Colombo A, Skinner JM: Balloon entrapment in a coronary artery: Potential serious complications of balloon rupture. Cathet Cardiovasc Diagn 19:23–25, 1990.

Ellis SG, Roubin GS, King SB III, et al.: In-hospital cardiac mortality after acute closure after coronary angioplasty: Analysis of risk factors from 8,207 procedures. J Am Coll Cardiol 11:211–216, 1988.

Esplugas E, Cequier AR, Sabate X, Jara F: False coronary dissection with the new monorail angioplasty balloon catheter. Cathet Cardiovasc Diagn 19:30–33, 1990.

Finci L, Meier B, Roy P, Steffenino G, Rutishanser W: Clinical experience with the Monorail balloon catheter for coronary angioplasty. Cathet Cardiovasc Diagn 14: 206–212, 1988.

Hadjimiltiades H, Goldbaum TS, Mostel E, et al.: Coronary air embolism during coronary angioplasty. Cathet Cardiovasc Diagn 16:164–167, 1989.

Hartzler GO, Rutherford BD, McConahay DR: Removal of angioplasty debris from the coronary and systemic arterial circulation—Is it necessary? J Am Coll Cardiol 9(2):107A, 1987 (abstr).

King SB III: Prediction of acute closure in percutaneous transluminal coronary angioplasty. Circulation 81:IV-2–IV-4, 1990.

Matthews BJ, Ewels CJ, Kent KM: Coronary dissection: A predictor of restenosis? Am Heart J 115:547–554, 1988.

Redd DCB, Roubin GS, Leimgruber PP, et al.: The transstenotic pressure gradient trend as a predictor of acute complications after percutaneous transluminal coronary angioplasty. Circulation 4:792–801, 1987.

Rizzo TF, Werres R, Ciccone J, et al.: Entrapment of an angioplasty balloon catheter: A case report. Cathet Cardiovasc Diagn 14:255–257, 1988.

San Francisco Heart Institute, San Francisco-Peninsula Cardiovascular Medical Corporation, Inc., and then-associated member doctors; slides, charts, data, statistics, computer databases, files and tapes, illustrations and other materials, 1984–1988.

Rothschild R, Voda J: Coronary artery dissection caused by angioplasty balloon rupture. Cathet Cardiovasc Diagn 19:26–29, 1990.

Takatsu F, Kinoshita A: Case of spontaneous healing of occlusive dissection on percutaneous transluminal coronary angioplasty. Cathet Cardiovasc Diagn 18:249–254, 1989.

Vrolix M, Vanhaecke J, Pliessens J, DeGeest H: An unusual case of guide wire fracture during percutaneous transluminal coronary angioplasty. Cathet Cardiovasc Diagn 15:99–102, 1988.

Watson LE: Snare loop technique for removal of broken steerable PTCA wire. Cathet Cardiovasc Diagn 13:44–49, 1987.

CHAPTER 12. PATIENT CARE ASPECTS OF PTCA

Bouman C: Intracoronary thrombolysis and percutaneous transluminal coronary angioplasty. Am J Cardiol 19: 397–409, 1984.

Cimini DM, Goldfarb J: Standard of care for the patient with percutaneous transluminal coronary angioplasty. Crit Care Nurse 3(6):76–78, 1983.

Clark DA: "Coronary Angioplasty." New York: Alan R. Liss, Inc., 1987.

Doran KA, Hansen C: PTCA: Patient education. Dimen Crit Care Nurs 2:56–64, 1983.

Ellis SG, Roubin GS, Wilentz J, Douglas JS. King SB: Effect of 18- to 24-hour heparin administration for prevention of restensois after uncomplicated coronary angioplasty. Am Heart 117:777–781, 1989.

Faxon DP: Current status of coronary angioplasty. Hosp Pract:59–71, 1987.

Finesilver C: Preparation of adult patients for cardiac catheterization and coronary aneoangiography. Int J Nurs Stud 15:214–221, 1978.

Gabliani G, Deligonul M, Kern MJ, Vandormael M: Acute coronary occlusion occurring after successful percutaneous transluminal coronary angioplasty: Temporal relationship to discontinuation of anticoagulation. Am Heart J 116:696–700, 1988.

Galan K, Gruentzig A, Hollman J: Significance of early chest pain after coronary angioplasty. Heart Lung 14: 109–111, 1985.

Lanoue AS, Snyder BA, Galan KM: Percutaneous transluminal coronary angioplasty: Nonoperative treatment of coronary artery disease. J Cardio/Nurs 1(1):30–44, 1986.

Lynn-McHale DJ: Interventions for acute myocardial infarction: PTCA and CABGS. Crit Care Nurse 12(2):28–38, 1989.

McCarthy C: Percutaneous transluminal coronary angioplasty: Therapeutic intervention in the cardiac catheterization laboratory. Heart Lung 11:294–298, 1982.

Mullin SM: Percutaneous transluminal coronary angioplasty (PTCA). Occup Health Nurs 32(2):75–77, 1984.

Newton K: Cardiac catheterization. In Underhill S, Woods S, Sivarajan E, Halfpenny C (eds): "Cardiac Nursing." Philadelphia: J.B. Lippincott, 1982.

Ott B: Percutaneous transluminal coronary angioplasty and nursing implications. Heart Lung 11;294–298, 1982.

Partridge S: The nurse's role in percutaneous transluminal coronary angioplasty. Heart Lung 11:505–511, 1982.

Popma JJ, Dehmer GJ: Care of the patient after coronary angioplasty. Ann Int Med 110(7):547–559, 1989.

Rudisill PT, Moore LA: Relationship between arterial and venous activated partial thromboplastin time values in patients after percutaneous transluminal coronary angioplasty. Heart Lung 18(5):514–519, 1989.

Shaw R, Cohen F, Fishman-Rosen J, et al.: The impact of coping, anxiety and cardiac information level on late complications, restenosis and psychosocial adjustment in patients following coronary angioplasty. Psychosomatic Med 48(8): 582–597, 1986.

Sipperly ME: Expanding role of coronary angioplasty: Current implications, limitations, and nursing considerations. Heart Lung 18(5):507–513, 1989.

CHAPTER 13. NEW TECHNOLOGIES FOR THE TREATMENT OF OBSTRUCTIVE ARTERIAL DISEASE

1. Chesler E, Gornick C, Pierpont G, Weir EK: High incidence of acute coronary occlusions complicating percutaneous transluminal coronary angioplasty for angina pectoris. Am J Cardiol 64:665–667, 1989.

2. Taley JD, Jones EL, Weintraub WS, King SB III: Coronary artery bypass surgery after failed elective percutaneous transluminal coronary angioplasty. Circulation 79[Suppl I]:I-126–I-131, 1989.

3. Liu MW, Roubin GS, King SB III: Restenosis after coronary angioplasty: Potential biologic determinants and role of intimal hyperplasia. Circulation 79:1369–1373, 1989.

4. Fanelli C, Aronoff R: Restenosis following coronary angioplasty. Am Heart J 119:357–368, 1990.

5. Detre K, Holubkov R, Kelsey S, et al.: Percutaneous transluminal coronary angioplasty in 1985–1986 and 1977–1981. N Engl J Med 318:265–270, 1988.

6. Gardiner GA Jr, Meyerovitz MF, Harrington DP, et al.: Dissection complicating angioplasty. AJR 145:627–631, 1985.

7. Cowley MJ, Dorros G, Kelsey SF, et al.: Acute coronary events associated with percutaneous transluminal coronary angioplasty. Am J Cardiol 53:12C–16C, 1984.

8. Fischell TA, Derby G, Tse TM, Stadius ML: Coronary artery vasoconstriction routinely occurs after percutaneous transluminal coronary angioplasty: A quantitative arteriographic analysis. Circulation 78:1323–1334, 1988.

9. Mabin TA, Holmes DR Jr, Smith HC, et al.: Intracoronary thrombus: Role in coronary occlusion complicating percutaneous transluminal coronary angioplasty. J Am Coll Cardiol 5:198–202, 1985.

10. Buccino KR, Brenner AS, Browne KF: Acute reocclusion during percutaneous transluminal coronary angioplasty: Immediate and long-term outcome. Cathet Cardiovasc Diagn 17:75–79, 1989.

11. Ischinger T, Gruentzig AR, Meier B, Galan K: Coronary dissection and total coronary occlusion associated with percutaneous transluminal coronary angioplasty:

286   Bibliography and Suggested Readings

Significance of initial angiographic morphology of coronary stenoses. Circulation 74:1371–1378, 1986.

12. Ellis SG, Roubin GS, King SB III: Angiographic and clinical predictors of acute closure after native vessel coronary angioplasty. Circulation 77:372–379, 1988.

13. Holmes DR Jr, Vliedyts RE, Smith HC, et al.: Restenosis after percutaneous transluminal coronary angioplasty (PTCA): A report from the PTCA Registry of the National Heart, Lung and Blood Institute. Am J Cardiol 53:77C–81C, 1984.

14. Leimgruber PP, Roubin GS, Hollman J: Restenosis after successful coronary angioplasty in patients with single-vessel disease. Circulation 73:710–717, 1986.

15. Meier B, King SB III, Gruentzig AR, et al.: Repeat coronary angioplasty. J Am Cardiol 4:463–466, 1984.

16. Nobuyoshi M, Kimura T, Nosaka H, et al.: Restenosis after successful percutaneous transluminal coronary angioplasty: Serial angiographic follow-up of 229 patients. J Am Coll Cardiol 12:616–623, 1988.

17. Quigley P, Kereiakes D, Hinohara J, et al.: Efficacy of gradual prolonged balloon inflation during coronary angioplasty in humans using an autoperfusion catheter. Circulation [Suppl II]:II-449, 1988.

18. Roubin G, Douglas J, Ming S, et al.: Influence of balloon size on initial success, acute complications, and restenosis after percutaneous transluminal coronary angioplasty. Circulation 78:557–565, 1988.

19. Blackshear JL, O'Callaghan WG, Califf RM: Medical approaches to prevention of restenosis after coronary angioplasty. J Am Coll Cardiol 9:834–848, 1987.

20. Schwartz L, Bourassa MG, Lesperance J, et al.: Aspirin and dipyridamole in the prevention of restenosis after percutaneous transluminal coronary angioplasty. N Engl J Med 318:1714–1718, 1988.

21. Faxon DP, Sanborn TA, Haudenschild CC, Ryan TJ: Effect of antiplatelet therapy on restenosis after experimental angioplasty. Am J Cardiol 53:72C–76C, 1984.

22. Thornton MA, Gruentzig AR, Hollman J, King SB III, Douglas JS: Coumadin and aspirin in prevention of recurrence after transluminal coronary angioplasty: A randomized study. Circulation 69:721–727, 1984.

23. Corcos T, David PR, Val PG: Failure of diltiazem to prevent restenosis after percutaneous transluminal coronary angioplasty. Am Heart J 109:926–931, 1985.

24. Whitworth HB, Roubin GS, Hollman J, et al.: Effect of nifedipine on recurrent stenosis after percutaneous transluminal coronary angioplasty. J Am Coll Cardiol 8:1271–1276, 1986.

25. Dehmer GJ, Popma JJ, van den Berg EK, et al.: Reduction in the rate of early stenosis after coronary angioplasty by a diet supplemented with n-3 fatty acids. N Engl J Med 319:733–740, 1988.

26. Clowes AW, Reidy MA, Clowes MM: Mechanisms of stenosis after arterial injury. Lab Invest 49:208–215, 1983.

27. Gerrity RG, Loop FD, Golding LAR, Ehrhart LA, Argenyi ZB: Arterial response to laser operation for removal of atherosclerotic plaques. J Thorac Cardiovasc Surg 85:409–421, 1983.

28. Abela GS, Crea F, Seeger JM, et al.: The healing process in normal canine arteries and in artherosclerotic monkey arteries after transluminal laser irradiation. Am J Cardiol 56:983–988, 1985.

29. Higginson LA, Farell EM, Walley VM, Taylor RS, Keon WJ: Arterial response to excimer and argon laser irradiation in atherosclerotic swine. Lasers Med Sci 4:85–92, 1989.

30. Demopulos PA, Olin EV, Yee W, Kernoff RS, Fischell TA, Ginsburg R: Balloon angioplasty and rotational tip (Kensey) catheter in the rabbit model of atherosclerosis: Acute and chronic results. J Am Coll Cardiol 9(2):202A, 1988 (abstr).

31. Ellis SG, Shaw RE, Gershony G, et al.: Risk factors, time course and treatment effect for restenosis after successful percutaneous transluminal coronary angioplasty of chronic total occlusion. Am J Cardiol 63:897–901, 1989.

32. Kereiakes DJ, Selmon MR, McAuley BJ, McAuley DB, Sheehan DJ, Simpson JB: Angioplasty in total coronary artery occlusion: Experience in 76 consecutive patients. J Am Coll Cardiol 6:526–533, 1985.

33. DiSciascio G, Vetrovec GW, Cowley MJ, Wolfgang TC: Early and late outcome of percutaneous transluminal coronary angioplasty for subacute and chronic total coronary occlusion. Am Heart J 111:833–839, 1986.

34. McGuff PE, Bushnell D, Saroff HS, Deterling RA: Studies of surgical applications of laser light. Surg Forum 14:143–145, 1963.

35. Abela GS, Normann S, Cohen D, Feldman RL, Geiser EA, Conti CR: Effects of carbon dioxide, Nd:YAG, and argon laser radiation on coronary atheromatous plaques. Am J Cardiol 50:1199–1205, 1982.

36. Fenech A, Abela GS, Crea F, Smith W, Feldman RL, Conti CR: A comparative study of laser beam characteristics in blood and saline media. Am J Cardiol 55:1389–1392, 1985.

37. Abela GS, Normann SJ, Cohen DM, et al.: Laser recanalization of occluded atherosclerotic arteries in vivo and in vitro. Circulation 71:403–411, 1985.

38. Lee G, Ikeda R, Herman I, et al.: The qualitative effects of laser irradiation on human arteriosclerotic disease. Am Heart J 105:885–889, 1983.

39. Geschwind H, Fabre M, Chaitman BR, et al.: Histopathology after Nd:YAG laser percutaneous transluminal coronary angioplasty of peripheral arteries. J Am Coll Cardiol 8:1089–1095, 1986.

40. Isner JM, Donaldson RF, Deckelbaum LI: The excimer laser: Gross, light microscopic and ultrastructural analysis of potential advantages for use in laser therapy of cardiovascular disease. J Am Coll Cardiol 6:1102–1109, 1985.

41. Deckelbaum LI, Isner JM, Donaldson RF, et al.: Reduction of laser-induced pathologic tissue injury using pulsed energy delivery. Am J Cardiol 56:662–667, 1985.

42. Grundfest W, Litvack F, Forrester JS, et al.: Laser ablation of human atherosclerotic plaque without adjacent tissue injury. J Am Coll Cardiol 5:929–933, 1985.

43. Crea F, Fenech A, Smith W, Conti CR, Abela GS: Laser recanalization of acutely thrombosed coronary arteries in live dogs: Early results. J Am Coll Cardiol 6:1052–1056, 1985.

44. Choy DSJ, Stertzer SH, Myler RK, Marco J, Fournial G: Human coronary laser recanalization. Clin Cardiol 7:377–381, 1984.

45. Ginsburg R, Wexler L, Mitchell RS, Profitt D: Percutaneous transluminal laser angioplasty for treatment of peripheral vascular disease. Clinical response with 16 patients. Radiology 156:619–624, 1985.

46. Abela GS, Seeger JM, Barbieri E, et al.: Laser angioplasty with angioscopic guidance in humans. J Am Coll Cardiol 8:184–192, 1986.

47. Prevosti LG, Lawrence JB, Leon MB, et al.: Surface thrombogenicity after excimer laser and hot-tip thermal ablation of plaque: Morphometric studies using an annular perfusion chamber. Surg Forum 38:330–340, 1986.

48. Ginsburg R, Wexler L, Mitchell RS, Profitt D: Percutaneous transluminal laser angioplasty for treatment of peripheral vascular disease. Clinical response with 16 patients. Radiology 156:619–624, 1985.

49. Abela GS, Seeger JM, Pry RS, et al.: Percutaneous laser recanalization of totally occluded human peripheral arteries: A technical approach. Dynamic Cardiovasc Imag 1:302–308, 1988.

50. Linnemeier TJ, Cumberland DC, Rothbaum DA, Landin RJ, Ball MW: Human percutaneous laser-assisted coronary angioplasty: Efforts to reduce spasm and thrombosis. J Am Coll Cardiol 13:16A, 1989 (abstrt).

51. Gal D, Gabriel S, Rongione AJ, et al.: Vascular spasm complicates continuous wave but not pulsed laser irradiation. Circulation 76[Suppl IV]:IV-525, 1987 (abstr).

52. Abela GS, Seeger JM, Barbieri E, et al.: Laser angioplasty with angioscopic guidance in humans. J Am Coll Cardiol 8:184–192, 1986.

53. Abela GS, Crea F, Smith W, Pepine CJ, Conti CR: In vitro effects of argon laser radiation on blood: Quantitation and morphologic analysis. J Am Coll Cardiol 5:231–237, 1985.

54. Nordstrom LA, Castaneda-Zuniga WR, Grewe DD, Schoster DVM: Laser enhanced transluminal angioplasty: The role of coaxial fiber placement. Semin Intervent Radiol 3:47–52, 1986.

55. Nordstrom LA, Castaneda-Zuniga WR, Young EG, Von Seggern KB: Direct argon laser exposure for recanalization of peripheral arteries: Early results. Radiology 168:359–364, 1988.

56. Nordstrom LA, Dorros G: Laser enhanced angioplasty: An alternative to thermal contact plaque ablation. Circulation 76[Suppl IV]:IV-47, 1987 (abstrt).

57. Foschi AE, Myers GE, Flamm MD, Jacobs WC: Laser-enhanced coronary angioplasty: Combined early results of direct argon laser exposures in atherosclerotic native arteries and bypass grafts. J Am Coll Cardiol 15:56A, 1990 (abstrt).

58. Grundfest WS, Litvack F, Doyle L, et al.: Comparison of in vitro and in vivo thermal effects of argon and excimer lasers for laser angioplasty. Circulation 74[Suppl II]:II-204, 1986 (abstrt).

59. Grundfest WS, Litvack F, Goldenberg T, et al.: Pulsed ultraviolet lasers and the potential for safe laser angioplasty. Am J Surg 150:220–226, 1985.

60. Garrison BJ, Srinivasan R: Microscopic model for the ablative photodecomposition of polymers by far ultraviolet radiation. Appl Phys Lett 44:849–851, 1984.

61. Brannon JH, Lankard Baise Al, Burns F, Kaufman J: Excimer laser etching of polyimide. J Appl Phys 58:2036–2043, 1985.

62. Higginson LAJ, Farrell EM, Walley VM, Taylor RS, Keon WJ: Arterial response to excimer and argon laser irradiation in the atherosclerotic swine. Lasers Med Sci (in press).

63. Litvack F, Grundfest WS, Adler L, et al.: Percutaneous excimer laser angioplasty of the lower extremities: Results of an initial clinical trial. Radiology 172:331–335, 1989.

64. Litvack F, Grundfest WS, Eigler N, et al.: Percutaneous excimer laser coronary angioplasty. Lancet 2:102–103, 1989.

65. Litvack F, Margolis J, Eigler N, et al.: Percutaneous excimer laser coronary angioplasty: Results of the first 110 procedures. J Am Coll Cardiol 15:25A, 1990 (abstr).

66. Werner GS, Buchwald A, Unterberg C, Voth E, Kreuzer H, Wiegand V: Recanalization of chronic coronary occlusion by excimer-laser angioplasty. J Am Coll Cardiol 15:245A, 1990 (abstr).

67. Banga I, Bihari-Varga M: Investigations of free and elastin-bound fluorescent substances present in the atherosclerotic lipid and calcium plaques. Connect Tissue Res 2:237–241, 1974.

68. Blankenhorn DH, Braunstein H: Carotenoids in man. III. The microscopic pattern of fluorescence in atheromas and its relation to their growth. J Clin Invest 37:160–165, 1958.

69. Decklebaum LI, Lam JK, Cabin HS, Clubb KS, Long MB: Discrimination of normal and atherosclerotic aorta by laser-induced fluorescence. Lasers Surg Med 7:330–335, 1987.

70. Anderson PS, Gustafson A, Sternram U, Svanberg K, Svanberg S: Diagnosis of arterial atherosclerosis using laser-induced fluorescence. Lasers Med Surg 2:261–266, 1987.

288   Bibliography and Suggested Readings

71. Leon MB, Lu DY, Prevosti LG, et al.: Human arterial surface fluorescence: Atherosclerotic plaque identification and effects of laser atheroma ablation. J Am Coll Cardiol 12:94–102, 1988.

72. Leon MB, Prevosti LG, Smith PD, et al.: Probe and fire laser angioplasty: Fluorescence atheroma detection and selective laser atheroma ablation. Circulation 76 [Suppl IV]:IV-409, 1987 (abstr).

73. Leon MB, Prevosti LG, Smith PD, et al.: In vivo laser-induced fluorescence plaque detection: Preliminary results in patients. Circulation 76 [Suppl IV]:IV-408, 1987 (abstr).

74. Bartorelli AL, Bonner RF, Almagor Y, et al.: Enhanced recognition of plaque composition in vivo using laser-excited fluorescence spectroscopy. J Am Coll Cardiol 13:55A, 1989 (abstr).

75. Leon MB, Lu DY, Prevosti LG, et al.: Human arterial surface fluorescence: Atherosclerotic ablation. J Am Coll Cardiol 12:94–102, 1988.

76. Leon MB, Bartorelli AL, Almagor Y, et al.: Flourescence-guided laser angioplasty: Updated clinical results and future directions. J Am Coll Cardiol 15:26A, 1990 (abstr).

77. Sanborn TA, Faxon DP, Haudenschild CC, Ryan TJ: Experimental angioplasty: Circumferential distribution of laser thermal energy with a laser probe. J Am Coll Cardiol 5:934, 1985.

78. Sanborn TA, Cumberland DC: Laser Probe. In Isner JM, Clarke RH (eds.): "Cardiovascular Laser Therapy." New York: Raven Press, 1989, p 149.

79. Sanborn TA, Haudenschild CC, Gottsman SB, Ryan TJ: The mechanism of transluminal angioplasty; evidence for formation of aneurysms in experimental atherosclerosis. Circulation 68:1136, 1983.

80. Sanborn TA, Cumberland DC, Tayler DI, Ryan TJ: Human percutaneous laser thermal angioplasty. Circulation 72 [Suppl III]:III-303, 1985 (abstr).

81. Sanborn TA, Cumberland DC, Greenfield AJ, Tayler DI, Welch CL, Guben JK, Ryan TJ: Six-month follow-up of laser probe assisted balloon angioplasty. Circulation 74[Suppl II]:II-457, 1986 (asbtr).

82. Sanborn TA, Cumberland DC, Greenfield AJ, et al.: Peripheral laser-assisted balloon angioplasty: Initial multicenter experience in 219 peripheral arteries. Arch Surg 124:1099, 1989.

83. Sanborn TA, Faxon DP, Kellett MA, Ryan TJ: Percutaneous coronary laser thermal angioplasty. J Am Coll Cardiol 8:1437, 1986.

84. Linnemeier TJ, Cumberland DC, Rothbaum DA, Landin RJ, Ball MW: Human percutaneous laser-assisted coronary angioplasty: Efforts to reduce spasm and thrombosis. J Am Coll Cardiol 13:61A, 1989.

85. Linnemeier TJ, Cumberland DC: Percutaneous laser coronary angioplasty without balloon angioplasty. Lancet 1:154–155, 1989.

86. Spears JR: Sealing. In Isner J, Clarke R (eds): "Cardiovascular Laser Therapy." New York: Raven Press, 1989, p 177.

87. Hiehle JF Jr, Bourgelais D, Shapshy S, Schoen FJ, Spears JR: Nd:YAG laser fusion of human atheromatous placque material wall separations in vitro. Am J Cardiol 56:953, 1985.

88. Sanborn TA, Faxon DP, Haudenschild C, Gottsman SB, Ryan TJ: The mechanism of transluminal angioplasty: Evidence for formation of aneurysms in experimental atherosclerosis. Circulation 63:1136–1140, 1983.

89. Block PC, Myler RK, Stertzer S, Fallon JT: Morphology after transluminal angioplasty in human beings. N Engl J Med 305:382–385, 1981.

90. Spears JR: Percutaneous transluminal coronary angioplasty restenosis: Potential prevention with laser balloon angioplasty. Am J Cardiol 60:61B–64B, 1987.

91. Jenkins RD, Sinclair IN, Anand R, Kalil AG, Schoen FJ, Spears JR: Laser balloon angioplasty: Effect of tissue temperature on weld strength of human postmortem intima-media separations. Laser Surg Med 8:30–39, 1988.

92. Spears JR, Dear WE, Safian RD, et al.: Laser balloon angioplasty: Angiographic results of a multicenter trial. Circulation 80[Suppl II]:II-476, 1989 (abstr).

93. Spears JR, Reyes VP, Plokker HWT, Ferguson JJ, Dear WE, Sinclair IN, King SB, Jenkins RD, Safian RD, Rickards A, Schwartz L, LBA Study Group: Laser balloon angioplasty: Coronary angiographic follow-up of a multicenter trial. J Am Coll Cardiol 15(2):26A, 1990 (abstr).

94. Marchesini R, Andreola S, Emanuelli H, Mellone E, Schiroli A, Spinelli P, Fava G: Temperature rise in biologic tissue during Nd:YAG laser irradiation. Laser Surg Med 5:75, 1985.

95. Spears JR, James LM, Leonard BM, Sinclair IN, Jenkins RD, Motamedi M, Sinofsky EL: Plaque-media rewelding with reversible tissue optical property changes during receptive cw Nd:YAG laser exposure. Laser Surg Med 8:477–485, 1988.

96. Jenkins RD, Sinclair IN, Anand RK, James LM, Spears JR: Laser balloon angioplasty: Effect of exposure duration on shear strength of welded layers of postmortem human aorta. Laser Surg Med 8:392–396, 1988.

97. Jenkins RD, Sinclair IN, Leonard BM, Sandor T, Schoen FJ, Spears JR: Laser balloon angioplasty versus balloon angioplasty in normal rabbit iliac arteries. Laser Surg Med 9:237–247, 1988.

98. Alexopoulos D, Sanborn TA, Marmur JD, Badimon JJ, Badimon L: Biological response to laser balloon angioplasty in the atherosclerotic rabbit. Circulation 80(4)[Suppl II]:II-476, 1989 (abstr).

99. Sinclair IN, Dear WE, Safian RD, Plokker TM, Spears JR, LBA Study Group: Acute closure post PTCA successfully treated with laser balloon angioplasty. Circulation 80(4)[Suppl II]:II-476, 1989 (abstr).

100. Knudtson ML, Spindler BM, Traboulsi, Spears JR: Coronary laser balloon angioplasty in chronic total occlusion provides excellent short-term results. Circulation 80[Suppl II]:II-476, 1989.

101. Ferguson JJ, Dear WE, Leatherman LL, Safian RD, King SB, Douglas JS, Spears JR, LBA Study Group: A multi-center trial of laser balloon angioplasty for abrupt closure following PTCA. J Am Coll Cardiol 15(2):26A, 1990 (abstr).

102. Kirn T: Atheroma curettage: An idea whose time may come as several devices begin trials. JAMA 261:498–499, 1989.

103. Lam JY, Chesebro JH, Steele PM, et al.: Deep arterial injury during experimental angioplasty: Relation to a positive indium-111-labeled platelet scintigram, quantitative platelet deposition and mural thrombosis. J Am Coll Cardiol 8:1380–1386, 1986.

104. Sarembock IJ, LaVeau PJ, Sigal SL, et al.: Influence of inflation pressure and balloon size on the development of intimal hyperplasia after balloon angioplasty: A study in the atherosclerotic rabbit. Circulation 80:1029–1040, 1989.

105. Badimon L, Badimon JJ, Galvez A, et al.: Influence of arterial damage and wall shear rate on platelet deposition. Ex vivo study in a swine model. Arteriosclerosis 6:312–320, 1986.

106. Simpson JB, Johnson DE, Thapliyal HV, et al.: Transluminal atherectomy: A new approach to the treatment of atherosclerotic vascular disease. Circulation 72 [Suppl III]:III-146, 1985 (abstr).

107. Vlietstra RE, Abbotsmith CW, Douglas JS, et al.: Complications with directional coronary atherectomy. Experience at eight centers. Circulation 80[Suppl II]:II-582, 1989 (abstr).

108. Topol EJ, Robertson G, Pinkerton CA, et al.: Reduction in abrupt closure after excisional, directed coronary atherectomy: Report of multicenter SHAVE study group. Circulation (in press).

109. Garratt KN, Kaufman UP, Edwards WD, Vlietstra RE, Holmes DR Jr: Safety of percutaneous coronary atherectomy with deep arterial resection. Am J Cardiol 64:538–540, 1989.

110. Topol EJ: Emerging strategies for failed percutaneous transluminal coronary angioplasty. Am J Cardiol 63:249–250, 1989.

111. Kaufman UP, Garratt KN, Vlietstra RE, Menke KK, Holmes DR Jr: Coronary atherectomy: First 50 patients at the Mayo Clinic. Mayo Clinic Proc 64:747–752, 1989.

112. Simpson J, Rowe M, Robertson G, et al.: Directional coronary atherectomy: Success and complication rates and outcome predictors. J Am Coll Cardiol 15:196A, 1990 (abstr).

113. Selmon M, Rowe M, Simpson J, et al.: Directional coronary atherectomy for angiographically unfavorable lesions. J Am Coll Cardiol 15:58A, 1990 (abstr).

114. Simpson JB, Robertson GC, Selmon MR, Sipperly ME, Braden LJ, Hinohara T: Restenosis following successful directional coronary atherectomy. Circulation 80[Suppl II]:II-582, 1989 (abstr).

115. Hinohara T, Rowe M, Sipperly ME, et al.: Restenosis following directional coronary atherectomy of native coronary arteries. J Am Coll Cardiol 15:196A, 1990 (abstr).

116. Ghazzal Z, Ba'albaki HA, Sewell CW, et al.: Restenosis following coronary atherectomy: Angiographic follow-up and pathologic correlates. J Am Coll Cardiol 15:57A, 1990 (abstr).

117. Rogers PJ, Garratt KN, Kaufman UP, et al.: Restenosis after atherectomy versus PTCA: Initial experience. J Am Coll Cardiol 15:197A, 1990 (abstr).

118. Emy RE, Gelbfish JS, Safian RD, Diver DJ, Baim DS: Does tissue removal explain all atherectomy improvement? Circulation 80[Suppl II]:II-582, 1989 (abstr).

119. Chesebro JH, Lam JYT, Bedimon L, Fuster V: Restenosis after arterial angioplasty. Am J Cardiol 60:10B–16B, 1987.

120. Yock PG, Fitzgerald PJ, Jang YT, et al.: Initial trials of a combined ultrasound imaging/mechanical atherectomy catheter. J Am Coll Cardiol 15:105A, 1990 (abstr).

121. Hansen DD, Auth DC, Vrocko R, Ritchie JL: Rotational atherectomy in atherosclerotic rabbit iliac arteries. Am Heart J 115:160–165, 1988.

122. Fourrier JL, Auth DC, LaBlanche JM, Brunetaud JM, Gommeaux A, Bertrand ME: Human percutaneous coronary rotational atherectomy: Preliminary results. Circulation 78[Suppl II]:II-82, 1988 (abstr).

123. Ahn SS, Auth DC, Marcus DR, Moore WS: Removal of focal atheromatous lesions by angioscopically guided high speed rotary atherectomy. J Vasc Surg: 292–299, 1988.

124. Fourrier JL, Bertrand ME, Auth DC, Gommeaux A, LaBlanche JM: Percutaneous coronary rotational angioplasty. Symposium on Transcatheter Coronary Therapeutics—1989. Presented by the Georgetown University School of Medicine and Hospital, Washington, DC, 1989.

125. Zacca NM, Raizner AE, Noon GP, et al.: Short-term follow-up of patients treated with a recently developed rotational atherectomy device and in vivo assessment of the particles generated. J Am Coll Cardiol 11:109A, 1988 (abstr).

290   Bibliography and Suggested Readings

126. Fourrier JL, Stankowiak C, Lablanche JM, Prat A, Brunetaud JM, Bertrand ME: Histopathology after rotational angioplasty of peripheral arteries in human beings. J Am Coll Cardiol 11:109A, 1988 (abstr).

127. Hansen DD, Auth DC, Hall M, Ritchie JL: Rotational endarterectomy in normal canine coronary arteries. Preliminary report. J Am Coll Cardiol 11:1073–1077, 1988.

128. Zacca N, Heibig J, Harris S, et al.: Percutaneous coronary high speed rotational atherectomy: New, but how safe? J Am Coll Cardiol 15:58A, 1990 (abstr).

129. Teirstein PS, Ginsburg R, Warth DC, Hoq N, Jenkins NS, McCowan L: Complications of human coronary rotoblation. J Am Coll Cardiol 15:47A, 1990 (abstr).

130. Niazi KA, Brodsky M, Friedman HZ, et al.: Restenosis after successful mechanical rotary atherectomy with the Auth Rotoblator. J Am Coll Cardiol 15:57A, 1990 (abstr).

131. Stack RS: New interventional technologies in cardiology. Mayo Clin Proc 64:867–870, 1989.

132. Siegel RJ, Fishbein MC, Forrester J, et al.: Ultrasonic plaque ablation. A new method for recanalization of partially or totally occluded arteries. Circulation 78:1443–1448, 1988.

133. Siegel RJ, Cumberland DC, Myler RK: Ultrasonic angioplasty: Initial clinical experience. Circulation 80[Suppl II]:II-304, 1989 (abstr).

134. Wholey MH: The "TEC" atherectomy catheter: Results in the first 100 patients. Program of the International Symposium on Peripheral Vascular Intervention, presented by the Miami Vascular Institute, Miami, Florida, 1989, p 168.

135. Stack RS, Phillips HR, Quigley PJ, et al.: Multicenter registry of coronary atherectomy using the transluminal extraction-endarterectomy catheter. J Am Coll Cardiol 15:196A, 1990 (abstr).

136. Wholey MH, Smith JAM, Godlewski P, Nagurka M: Recanalization of total arterial occlusions with the Kensey dynamic angioplasty catheter. Radiology 172:95–98, 1989.

137. Vallbracht C, Liermann DD, Prignitz I, et al.: Low-speed rotational angioplasty in chronic peripheral artery occlusions: Experience in 83 patients. Radiology 172:327–330, 1989.

138. Dotter CT: Transluminally placed coilspring endoarterial tube grafts. Long-term patency in canine popliteal artery. Invest Radiol 4:327–332, 1969.

139. Schetky LM: Shape-memory alloys. Sci Am 241:74–83, 1979.

140. Dotter CT, Buschmann RW, McKinney MK, Rosch J: Transluminal expandable nitinol coil stent grafting: Preliminary report. Radiology 147:259–260, 1983.

141. Cragg A, Lund G, Rysavy J, Castaneda F, Castaneda-Zuniga W, Amplatz K: Nonsurgical placement of arterial endoprostheses: A new technique using nitinol wire. Radiology 147:261–263, 1983.

142. Masss D, Zollikofer L, Largiader F, Senning A: Radiological follow-up of transluminally inserted vascular endoprostheses: An experimental study using expanding spirals. Radiology 152:659–663, 1984.

143. Wright KC, Wallace S, Charnsangavej C, Carrasco CH, Gianturco C: Percutaneous endovascular stents: An experimental evaluation. Radiology 156:69–72, 1985.

144. Palmaz JC, Sibbitt RR, Reuter SR, Tio FO, Rice WJ: Expandable intraluminal graft: A preliminary study. Radiology 156:73–77, 1985.

145. Palmaz JC: Balloon-expandable intravascular stent. Am J Radiol 150:1263–1269, 1988.

146. Schatz RA: A view of vascular stents. Circulation 79:445–457, 1989.

147. Sigwart U: The self-expanding mesh stent. In Topol EJ (ed): "Textbook of Interventional Cardiology." Philadelphia: W.B. Saunders, 1990, p 622.

148. Ellis SG: The Palmaz-Schatz stent: Potential coronary applications. In Topol EJ (ed): "Textbook of Interventional Cardiology." Philadelphia: W.B. Saunders, 1990, p 625.

149. Sigwart U, Puel J, Mirkovitch V, Joffre F, Kappenberger L: Intravascular stents to prevent occlusion and restenosis after transluminal angioplasty. N Engl J Med 316:701–706, 1987.

150. Sigwart U, Vogt P, Goy JJ, Urban P, Stauffer JC, Kappenberger L, Fischer A: Creatinin kinase levels after bail-out stenting for post angioplasty coronary occlusion. Circulation 80[Suppl II]:II-258, 1989 (abstr).

151. Serruys PW, Beatt KJ, Bertrand M, Meier B, Puel J, Rickard T, Sigwart U: Restenosis rate after coronary stent implantation. Angiographic assessment of the initial series. Circulation 80[Suppl II]:II-173, 1989 (abstr).

152. Palmaz JC, Garcia OJ, Copp DT, et al.: Balloon expandable intra-arterial stents: Effect of anticoagulation on thrombus formation. Circulation 76[Suppl IV]:IV-45, 1987 (abstr).

153. Palmaz JC, Schatz RA, Richter G, Gardiner A, Becker G, Garcia O: Transluminal stenting of iliac artery stenosis: Preliminary report of a multicenter trial. Circulation [Suppl II]:II-415, 1988 (abstr).

154. King SB III: Vascular stents and atherosclerosis. Circulation 79:458–459, 1989.

155. Schatz RA, Leon M, Baim D, et al.: Short-term clinical results and complications with the Palmaz-Schatz coronary stent. J Am Coll Cardiol 1990;15[Suppl A]:117A, 1990 (abstr).

156. Ellis SG, Savage M, Baim D, et al.: Intracoronary stenting to prevent restenosis: Preliminary results of a

multicenter study using the Palmaz-Schatz stent suggest benefit in selected high risk patients. J Am Coll Cardiol 15[Suppl A]:118A, 1990 (abstr).

157. Duprat G Jr, Wright KC, Charnsangavej C, Wallace S, Gianturco C: Flexible balloon expandable stent for small vessels. Radiology 162:276–278, 1987.

158. Roubin GS, Robinson KA: The Gianturco-Roubin stent. In Topol EJ (ed): "Textbook of Interventional Cardiology." Philadelphia: W.B. Saunders, 1990, p 633.

159. Roubin GS, Robinson KA, King S, Gianturco C, Black AJ, Brown JE, Siegel RJ, Douglas JS: Early and late results of intracoronary arterial stenting after coronary angioplasty in dogs. Circulation 76:891–897, 1987.

160. Robinson KA, Roubin GS, Siegel RJ, Black AJ, Apkarian RP, King SB III: Intra-arterial stenting in the atherosclerotic rabbit. Circulation 78:646–653, 1988.

161. Roubin GS, Douglas JS Jr, Lenbo NJ, Black AJ, King SB III: Intracoronary stenting for acute closure following percutaneous transluminal coronary angioplasty. Circulation 78[Suppl II]:II-407, 1988 (abstr).

162. Slepian MJ: Polymeric endoluminal paving and sealing: Therapeutics at the crossroad of biomechanics and pharmacology. In Topol EJ (ed): "Textbook of Interventional Cardiology." Philadelphia: W.B. Saunders, 1990, p 647.

163. Murphy JG, Schwartz RS, Kennedy K, et al.: A new, biocompatible polymeric coronary stent: Design and early results in a pig model. J Am Coll Cardiol 15[Suppl A]:105A, 1990 (abstr).

164. Wilson JM, Birinyi LK, Salomon RN, Libby P, Callow AD, Mulligan RC: Implantation of vascular grafts lined with genetically modified endothelial cells. Science 244:1344–1346, 1989.

165. Dichek DA, Neville RF, Zweibel JA, Freeman SM, Leon MB, Anderson WF: Seeding of intravascular stents with genetically engineered endothelial cells. Circulation 80:1347–1353, 1989.